MANAGING
METABOLIC ABNORMALITIES
IN THE PSYCHIATRICALLY ILL

A Clinical Guide for Psychiatrists

Edited by

Richard A. Bermudes, M.D.
Paul E. Keck Jr., M.D.
Susan L. McElroy, M.D.

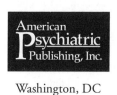

American Psychiatric Publishing, Inc.

Washington, DC
London, England

Copyright © 2007 American Psychiatric Publishing, Inc.
ALL RIGHTS RESERVED

Manufactured in the United States of America on acid-free paper
10   09   08   07   5   4   3   2
First Edition

Typeset in Adobe's AGaramond and Frutiger.

American Psychiatric Publishing, Inc.
1000 Wilson Boulevard
Arlington, VA 22209-3901
www.appi.org

Library of Congress Cataloging-in-Publication Data
Managing metabolic abnormalities in the psychiatrically ill : a clinical guide for psychiatrists
/ edited by Richard A. Bermudes, Paul E. Keck Jr., Susan L. McElroy.
        p. ; cm.
    Includes bibliographical references and index.
    ISBN 1-58562-241-9 (pbk. : alk. paper)
    1. Metabolism–Disorders. 2. Cardiovascular system–Diseases. 3. Mentally ill—
Diseases. 4. Mentally ill—Health and hygiene. 5. Psychotropic drugs—Side effects.
    I. Bermudes, Richard A., 1967– II. Keck, Paul E. III. McElroy, Susan L. [DNLM:
    1. Mental Disorders—complications. 2. Antipsychotic Agents—adverse effects.
    3. Cardiovascular Diseases—complications. 4. Diabetes Complications. 5. Metabolic
Syndrome X—complications. 6. Obesity—complications. WM 140 M266 2007]
    RC627.6.M36 2007
    616.3′9—dc22
                                                                    2006031098

British Library Cataloguing in Publication Data
A CIP record is available from the British Library.

CONTENTS

CONTRIBUTORS

Richard A. Bermudes, M.D.
Assistant Clinical Professor, Department of Psychiatry and Behavioral Sciences, University of California, Davis Medical Center, Sacramento, California

Kamran Bordbar, M.D.
Resident in Psychiatry, Centre of Addiction & Mental Health, Toronto, Ontario, Canada

David D'Alessio, M.D.
Professor, Department of Medicine, Vontz Chair for Diabetes Research, University of Cincinnati, Cincinnati, Ohio

Anna Guerdjikova, Ph.D.
Postdoctoral Fellow, Psychopharmacology Research Program, Department of Psychiatry, University of Cincinnati College of Medicine, Cincinnati, Ohio

Rakesh Kaneria, M.D.
Assistant Professor of Clinical Psychiatry, Psychopharmacology Research Program, Department of Psychiatry, University of Cincinnati College of Medicine, Cincinnati, Ohio

Paul E. Keck Jr., M.D.
President and CEO of the Craig and Frances Lindner Center of HOPE and Lindner Professor of Psychiatry and Neuroscience and Executive Vice Chairman of the Department of Psychiatry at the University of Cincinnati College of Medicine in Cincinnati, Ohio

Craig R. Keenan, M.D.
Assistant Clinical Professor, Department of Internal Medicine, University of California, Davis, Sacramento, California

Jakub Z. Konarski, M.Sc.
Doctoral candidate, Institute of Medical Science, University of Toronto, Toronto, Ontario, Canada

Renu Kotwal, M.D.
Assistant Professor of Clinical Psychiatry, Psychopharmacology Research Program, Department of Psychiatry, University of Cincinnati College of Medicine, Cincinnati, Ohio

Robert M. McCarron, D.O.
Assistant Clinical Professor, Department of Psychiatry and Behavioral Sciences, Department of Internal Medicine, University of California, Davis, Sacramento, California

Susan L. McElroy, M.D.
Professor of Psychiatry and Neuroscience, Psychopharmacology Research Program, Department of Psychiatry, University of Cincinnati College of Medicine, Cincinnati, Ohio

Roger S. McIntyre, M.D., F.R.C.P.C.
Associate Professor, Department of Psychiatry and Pharmacology, University of Toronto; Head, Mood Disorders Psychopharmacology Unit, University Health Network, Toronto, Ontario, Canada

Jonathan M. Meyer, M.D.
Assistant Professor of Psychiatry in Residence, University of California, San Diego; Staff Psychiatrist, Veterans Affairs San Diego Healthcare System, San Diego, California

John W. Newcomer, M.D.
Professor of Psychiatry, Psychology, and Medicine; Medical Director, Clinical Studies, Washington University School of Medicine, St. Louis, Missouri

Joanna K. Soczynska, B.Sc.
Masters of Science Candidate, Institute of Medicine, University of Toronto, Toronto, Ontario, Canada

Disclosure of Competing Interests

Richard A. Bermudes, M.D.—*Research:* Abbott Laboratories; Eli Lilly and Company; *Speaker bureau:* Abbott Laboratories; Bristol-Myers Squibb, Eli Lilly and Company, Pfizer

Kamran Bordbar, M.D.—None to report

David D'Alessio, M.D.—*Grant support:* Amylin, Eli Lilly and Company, Novartis; *Consultant:* Amylin, Merck, Novartis

Anna Guerdjikova, Ph.D.—None to report

Rakesh Kaneria, M.D.—None to report

Paul E. Keck Jr., M.D.—*Consultant or Scientific Advisory Board Member:* Abbott Laboratories, AstraZeneca Pharmaceuticals, Bristol-Myers Squibb, Eli Lilly and Company, GlaxoSmithKline, Memory Pharmaceuticals, Neurocrine Biosciences, Pfizer, Shire; *Principal Investigator or Co-investigator on Research Studies Sponsored by:* Abbott Laboratories, American Diabetes Association, AstraZeneca Pharmaceuticals, Bristol-Myers Squibb, Eli Lilly and Company, GlaxoSmithKline, Janssen Pharmaceutica, Memory Pharmaceuticals, Merck, National Institute of Mental Health, National Institute on Drug Abuse, Pfizer, Stanley Medical Research Institute, UCB Pharma

Craig R. Keenan, M.D.—None to report

Jakub Z. Konarski, M.Sc.—*Grant support:* Eli Lilly and Company, Ontario Graduate Scholarship; *Paid consultant:* Astra-Zeneca, Janssen-Ortho, Wyeth; *Travel honoraria:* Astra-Zeneca, Wyeth

Renu Kotwal, M.D.—*Speaker's bureau:* Bristol-Myers Squibb, Cyberonics; *Grant support:* Eisai Pharmaceuticals.

Robert M. McCarron, D.O.—*Speaker and Advisor:* Eli Lilly and Company

Susan L. McElroy, M.D.—*Consultant or Scientific Advisory Board Member:* Abbott Laboratories, Eli Lilly and Company, GlaxoSmithKline, Janssen Pharmaceutica, Ortho-McNeil, Wyeth-Ayerst; *Principal Investigator or Co-investigator on Research Studies Sponsored by:* Abbott Laboratories, Bristol-Myers Squibb, Eisai Pharmaceuticals, Eli Lilly and Company, Forest Labs, National Institutes of Health, Ortho-McNeil, Pfizer, Sanofi-Synthelabo, Somaxon Pharmaceuticals; *Patents:* Inventor on U.S. Patent No. 6,323,236B2, Use of Sulfamate Derivatives for Treating Impulse Control Disorders, and, along with the patent's assignee, University of Cincinnati, Cincinnati, OH, receives payments from Johnson & Johnson Pharmaceutical Research & Development, L.L.C., which has exclusive rights under the patent.

Roger S. McIntyre, M.D., F.R.C.P.C.—*Consultant and speaker:* Astra-Zeneca, Biovail, Eli Lilly and Company, GlaxoSmithKline, Janssen-Ortho, Lundbeck, Organon, Oryx, Pfizer, Prestwick, Wyeth; *Research funding:* Astra-Zeneca, GlaxoSmithKline, Merck, Servier, Wyeth

Jonathan M. Meyer, M.D.—*Consultant and speaker:* Bristol-Myers Squibb, Janssen Pharmaceutica, Pfizer; *Research grant support:* Bristol-Myers Squibb

John W. Newcomer, M.D.—*Consultant:* Astra-Zeneca, Bristol-Myers Squibb, GlaxoSmithKline, Janssen Pharmaceutica, Organon, Pfizer, Solvay, Wyeth; *Grant support:* Bristol-Myers Squibb, Janssen Pharmaceutica, National Alliance for Research on Schizophrenia and Depression, National Institute of Mental Health, Pfizer, Sidney R. Baer Foundation; *Data Safety Monitoring Committee member:* Organon; *Product development royalties (for metabolic screening form):* Compact Clinicals

Joanna K. Soczynska, B.Sc.—*Travel funds:* Janssen Pharmaceutica, Organon, Wyeth

PREFACE

Dramatic shifts in the delivery of mental healthcare are anticipated in the next few years. A number of important recommendations emanating from the Institute of Medicine's (2006) *Quality Chasm Series: Improving the Quality of Health Care for Mental and Substance-Use Conditions* (Washington, DC, National Academies Press, 2006) are likely to inform and influence the treatment of patients with psychiatric disorders. One of the most important unmet needs of patients with psychiatric disorders identified by the report is the lack of integration of general medical care with psychiatric care and the related problem of barriers to collaboration and communication among healthcare providers. The recognition of this gap in comprehensive healthcare for patients with psychiatric disorders coincides with an evolving body of research evidence that indicates that patients with psychotic, mood, and alcohol and substance use disorders, compared with the general population of the United States, have elevated rates of morbidity and mortality from a number of medical illnesses. These heightened morbidity and mortality rates are all the more striking because morbidity and mortality rates from cardiovascular disease, obesity, type II diabetes, and the metabolic syndrome are already high and are continuing to rise in the general population. Moreover, there is an increasing appreciation of the potential adverse effects on metabolic and cardiovascular health of specific medications with demonstrated efficacy in a number of psychiatric disorders. These risks need to be considered in the overall context of potential risks and benefits of treatment, background risks of medical illnesses associated with specific psychiatric disorders themselves, and means of applying these data to treatment recommendations, monitoring, and clinical practice.

This book represents an attempt to distill the available research regarding the relationships among major psychiatric illnesses, obesity, diabetes, the metabolic syndrome, and cardiovascular disease. The authors of each chapter have attempted to synthesize and critically evaluate the available literature on these topics and apply this information to clinical practice. A substantial amount of knowledge from medical and psychiatric research has been gleaned in the past decade or longer, enough to begin to improve the lives of our patients by importing this knowledge to practice.

Richard A. Bermudes, M.D.
Paul E. Keck Jr., M.D.
Susan L. McElroy, M.D.

Chapter 1

DIABETES

An Overview

David D'Alessio, M.D.

Diabetes mellitus is a disease with a history going back to ancient times, yet it is a growing scourge in the modern world. Most broadly, diabetes can be defined as disorders of nutrient metabolism that result in abnormalities in circulating glucose and, frequently, lipids. These abnormalities confer an increased risk for vascular diseases, infectious complications, and other morbidities. It is currently estimated that nearly 20 million Americans, 7%–8% of the population, have diabetes (Boyle et al. 2001). Although a number of distinct syndromes exist, diabetes is generally caused by impaired insulin secretion with or without abnormal sensitivity to insulin action. The vast majority of affected patients have either type 1 diabetes mellitus (T1DM) or type 2 diabetes mellitus (T2DM), and although these diseases share several clinical features, their pathogenesis is markedly different (Table 1–1). Of the two types of diabetes, T2DM is eight to nine times more common and is closely related to obesity, a problem that is on the rise worldwide. Although T1DM was previously called juvenile-onset diabetes and T2DM was called adult-onset diabetes, it is now clear that both diseases affect people from childhood to older age. Because the incidence of both types of diabetes has increased markedly since the 1980s—a trend that is predicted to continue (Boyle et al. 2001)—diabetes will be one of the major public health burdens for the foreseeable future.

Large intervention studies initiated in the late 1970s have firmly established the role of chronic hyperglycemia in causing microvascular complications, including renal, retinal, and neurological disease (American Diabetes Association 2003a, 2003b). It is also clear that the disordered metabolism of diabetes contributes to macrovascular disease, with increased rates of cardiac, cerebral, and periph-

1

TABLE 1–1. Important definitions related to diabetes

Type 1 diabetes	Result of autoimmune destruction of the insulin-producing β-cells of the pancreas; referred to in the literature and in clinical settings as "childhood" or "juvenile-onset" diabetes or "insulin-dependent" diabetes mellitus. Patients with Type 1 diabetes are by definition insulin dependent.
Type 2 diabetes	Most prevalent form of diabetes; also referred to as non-insulin-dependent diabetes, adult-onset diabetes, or obesity-related diabetes. Caused by the combination of impaired insulin secretion and insulin resistance.
Gestational diabetes mellitus	Diabetes developing during pregnancy. Pregnancy is associated with a reduction in the sensitivity of tissues to the actions of insulin. Gestational diabetes occurs when insulin secretion is inadequate to compensate for the insulin resistance of pregnancy. Approximately 2% of pregnant women develop gestational diabetes, and those who do have an increased risk for later development of diabetes.
Insulin resistance	Characterized by reduced sensitivity of muscle, adipose tissue, and hepatic cells to insulin. There is no single laboratory test for insulin resistance; however, individuals with the metabolic syndrome (see Chapter 2, "The Metabolic Syndrome," this volume), which has been referred to as the "insulin resistance syndrome," often have insulin resistance. Other clinical manifestations include increased waist circumference, elevated fasting glucose levels, abnormally high plasma glucose 2 hours after an oral glucose tolerance test, elevated fasting and postprandial plasma insulin concentrations, and changes in the lipid profile (elevated triglycerides, decreased high-density lipoprotein, and small low-density lipoprotein particles).

eral arterial disease in diabetic persons (American Diabetes Association 1998; Kannel and McGee 1979; Stamler et al. 1993). These long-term complications of diabetes account for the dramatically increased morbidity and mortality among diabetic patients, and thus prevention of end-organ disease is the principal goal of diabetic treatment.

Diabetes accounts for a disproportionate share of medical costs in the United States because of the prevalence of the condition and the burden of its associated morbidities. Estimated direct costs in 2002 were approximately $100 billion, with expenses due to work losses, disability, and mortality approaching another $40 billion (Hogan et al. 2003). On the basis of 2002 data, 20% of healthcare expenditures were attributable to patients with diabetes (Hogan et al. 2003). Given the increasing rates of diabetes, and especially its occurrence in younger people, the overall impact of diabetes on the American healthcare system is truly daunting.

Epidemiology

T2DM is the most common form of diabetes in the United States, and recent estimates are that more than 5% of Americans have this condition, with perhaps three times more being at risk (Bennett et al. 2002; Mokdad et al. 2003). Although trends in the industrialized world have been similar, there are now alarming increases in rates of T2DM in countries such as China and India, where the disease was previously rare (Zimmet et al. 2001). The prevalence of T2DM has been increasing since the mid-1970s, and although the cause for this trend is not entirely clear, the increase in the number of elderly and overweight people in the United States during that time certainly has had a major impact, given that aging and obesity are the two most important risk factors for developing diabetes.

There are very clear ethnic variations in diabetes prevalence in the United States. Rates among adult Native Americans (15%), Hispanics (12%) and African Americans (12%) are greater than those among persons of European ancestry (8%) (Bennett et al. 2002; Centers for Disease Control and Prevention 2003; Fujimoto 1995). Some Native American tribes have very high rates of diabetes; for example, more than 40% of Pima Indians are diabetic. The variation in diabetes rates among persons of similar heritage is consistent with prominent genetic effects on the expression of this condition. However, despite considerable effort, identification of the important diabetes genes is still under investigation (Shuldiner and McLenithan 2004).

Beyond these ethnic differences, there are some socioeconomic tendencies associated with T2DM (Table 1–2; Cowie and Eberhardt 1995). T2DM is much more common in the elderly, and there is a steady increase in the prevalence with increasing age. In addition, there is an inverse relationship between rates of diabetes and educational status and personal wealth, with relatively greater percentages

TABLE 1–2. Possible risk factors for diabetes

	Type 2 diabetes	Type 1 diabetes
Less risk	Education Personal wealth	Increasing age Ethnicity (Hispanic, African American, Asian)

Higher risk	Increasing age ($\geq$45 years)[a]
	Obesity (BMI$\geq$25 kg/m^2)[a]
	Other risk factors[b]
	  Ethnicity (Hispanic, African American, Native American, Asian American, Pacific Islander)
	  Family history of type 2 diabetes (parents or siblings)
	Other conditions
	  History of gestational diabetes or of delivering a baby weighing more than 9 lb
	  Hypertension
	  Dyslipidemia (low high-density lipoprotein, elevated triglycerides > 250 mg/dL)
	  Polycystic ovary disease
	  History of vascular disease
		Education
		Personal wealth
		Caucasian race

Note. BMI = body mass index.

[a]Testing for diabetes should be considered by healthcare providers at 3-year intervals beginning at age 45, especially in those with a BMI$\geq$25 kg/m^2.

[b]Testing should be considered at a younger age or more frequently than 3-year intervals for individuals who have a BMI$\geq$25 kg/m^2 and who have one or more other risk factors (American Diabetes Association 2004).

of diabetic individuals living in poverty. Finally, a disproportionate percentage of T2DM patients are military veterans. Although the cause for this link is not clear, there are epidemiological studies to support exposure to toxic agents, such as Agent Orange, as a risk factor for developing future diabetes (Henriksen et al. 1997).

A very disturbing trend in T2DM has been the sharply rising incidence in adolescents (Fagot-Campagna et al. 2001; Rosenbloom et al. 1999). Whereas in the early 1980s this form of diabetes was virtually never seen in young people, the prevalence in children and adolescents has increased steadily since, and T2DM now accounts for up to 25% of new-onset cases in pediatric diabetes clinics (Pinhas-Hamiel et al. 1996). It seems very likely that the earlier development of diabetes in younger cohorts is related to increased rates of obesity in children (Ogden et al. 2002).

It is currently estimated that T1DM accounts for 5%–10% of diagnosed cases of diabetes in the United States (Bennett et al. 2002). In approximately 40% of these cases, the patient is younger than 20 years of age, making this one of the more common chronic diseases of childhood (Rewers et al. 1988). However, it is not strictly a disease of young people as previously thought, and almost 1% of persons living in this country will develop T1DM over the course of their lifespan. The incidence of T1DM is increasing by 3%–5% per year (EURODIAB ACE Study Group 2000; Onkamo et al. 1999), an alarming trend for which no cause has yet been determined. T1DM is most prevalent in the Scandinavian countries, whereas persons of Asian origin are least likely to be affected (Bennett et al. 2002; Fujimoto 1995). In the United States, Caucasians are 1.5 times more likely to develop T1DM than are Hispanics or African Americans. There are socioeconomic trends that can be discerned for T1DM as well. Persons with T1DM earn, on average, slightly more money than those without diabetes and are more likely to be employed (Cowie et al. 1995).

Pathogenesis

In fundamental terms, diabetes results when there is insufficient insulin action to maintain plasma glucose levels in the normal range. In nondiabetic humans, blood glucose is tightly controlled, with fasting and postprandial values ranging over a roughly 50-mg/dL spectrum (80–130 mg/dL) in adults eating normal diets. The pancreatic β-cell is central in this homeostatic process, adjusting the amount of insulin secreted precisely in order to regulate glucose output from the liver and promote glucose uptake after meals. Both T1DM and T2DM result from deficits in insulin secretion. In patients developing T1DM there is autoimmune destruction of the β-cells and an almost complete lack of insulin secretion. Untreated, this condition is fatal because of the essential role insulin plays in fuel metabolism. The cause of T2DM is more complex and the disease is more insidious. Affected patients have impaired sensitivity of the normal important targets for insulin: the liver, skeletal muscle, and adipose tissue (see Figure 1–1; Pessin and Saltiel 2000; Shulman 2000). In addition, insulin secretion is impaired (Cavaghan et al. 2000; Porte 1999), although not absent as in T1DM. The underlying factors leading to these general pathogenetic mechanisms are listed below.

GENETICS

T1DM is a complex multigenic disease. Although the risk of T1DM is significantly higher in persons with an affected first-degree relative, only 10% of all patients with this condition have a positive family history (Lorenzen et al. 1994). The primary genetic susceptibility for T1DM is the human leukocyte antigen (*HLA*) loci and the immune functions governed by these genes. Approximately 95% of patients with T1DM have either *HLA-DR3* or *HLA-DR4* (Bennett et al. 2002). However, twin and family studies indicate that genetic factors alone cannot explain the development of T1DM (Kaprio et al. 1992).

A number of environmental risk factors have been proposed for T1DM, but none has been conclusively proved as an etiology. Viral infections—particularly mumps, rubella, and enteroviruses—have been linked to outbreaks of T1DM and may explain the seasonal patterns of new diagnoses that have been observed in several regions (Bennett et al. 2002).

Most T2DM also involves the contribution of multiple genes. There are several rare monogenic forms of diabetes, termed *maturity-onset diabetes in youth* (MODY), that have some clinical similarity to T2DM and are the result of mutations in key factors for β-cell function that cause modest insulin secretory defects (Bell and Polonsky 2001; Shuldiner and McLenithan 2004). The concordance of these purely β-cell disorders with T2DM serves to emphasize the important role that impaired insulin secretion plays in this condition. Typically, inheritance is expressed to a greater extent in T2DM than in T1DM. More than 50% of all patients with T2DM have a positive family history of diabetes (Rewers and Hamman 1995), and the concordance rates in identical twins are approximately 70%. Clearly, genetics is a major factor in the ethnic variation in rates of diabetes, but it is likely that environmental factors are equally important in the development of T2DM. Obesity is the most commonly appreciated of these factors, with physical inactivity and aging also contributing significantly (Goodpaster et al. 2003; Harris 1991).

It seems likely that the genetic makeup conferring susceptibility to diabetes (e.g., the tendency to become insulin resistant or to have subtle defects in insulin secretion) is common among modern humans, affecting 25%–30%. In the face of these inherent abnormalities, the dramatic shifts in environmental factors that have occurred in the past half century, such as more generalized sedentary behavior and caloric overconsumption, have combined to drive the rates of diabetes upward.

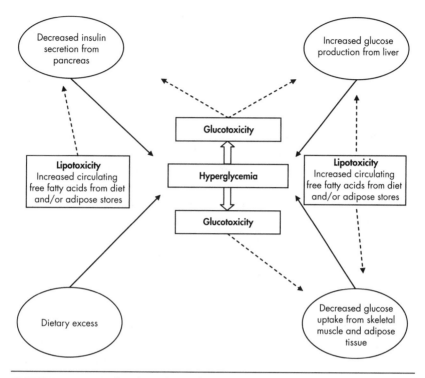

FIGURE 1–1. Pathophysiology of type 2 diabetes.

PATHOPHYSIOLOGY OF HYPERGLYCEMIA

Impaired Insulin Secretion

In healthy humans, β-cell function is primarily controlled by plasma glucose concentrations. Elevations of blood glucose are necessary for insulin release above basal levels, and other stimuli are relatively ineffective when plasma glucose is in the fasting range (80–100 mg/dL). These other stimuli, including circulating nutrients, insulinotropic hormones released from the gastrointestinal tract, and autonomic neural pathways, play important adjunctive roles, adjusting insulin output appropriately for meal size or physiological setting (D'Alessio 2002; D'Alessio et al. 2001; Kahn and Porte 2002). When blood glucose levels increase after meal consumption, stimulatory hormones and neural transmitters can amplify β-cell release to meet the needs for normal glucose disposition.

In persons with T2DM the sensitivity of the β-cell to glucose is impaired, and there is also a loss of responsiveness to other stimuli (Bell and Polonsky 2001; Porte 1999). These effects result in a delayed and insufficient amount of circulating insulin, which in turn allows the blood glucose to rise dramatically after meals and fails to restrain liver glucose release during fasting. Defective β-cell sensitivity to glucose appears to have a strong genetic component, but except in rare cases, the specific genes involved are not known. Beyond the defect in functional properties of the β-cell, such as a relative insensitivity to glucose, the absolute mass of β-cells is reduced in T2DM patients. It has been estimated that at the time of diagnosis, persons with T2DM have approximately 50% of the normal complement of β-cells (Butler et al. 2003). This initial deficit is compounded by a gradual loss of β-cell mass over time, potentially related to toxic effects of hyperglycemia. Progressive reduction of β-cell mass explains the natural history of T2DM in most patients who require steadily increasing therapy to maintain some degree of glucose control.

In T1DM the β-cells of the pancreatic islet are specifically targeted by an auto-immune inflammatory response that eliminates most endogenous insulin production. The general consensus has been that this process occurs over several years, with the onset of clinical disease frequently delayed until 90% of β-cell mass is gone. The autoimmune nature of this process is almost always marked by the presence of circulating antibodies to islet cell antigens, including insulin. These markers have become important in the determination of diabetes etiology and are available in most clinical laboratories. Once the autoimmune process has run its course, significant regeneration of β-cells does not occur.

Several drugs have been reported to impair insulin secretion, including thiazide diuretics, phenytoin, phenothiazines, and cyclosporine (Pandit et al. 1993). However, these effects are uncommon and generally occur only when very high dosages of these medications are used. The mechanisms of β-cell impairment are not clear, but direct toxicity is frequently cited, and elevation of catecholamines, a physiological inhibitor of insulin secretion, may also be involved.

Insulin Resistance

Insulin sensitivity is a quantifiable parameter that is measured as the amount of glucose cleared from the blood in response to a dose of insulin. Insulin sensitivity varies within individuals over time and across groups or populations of subjects; some healthy people are relatively more insulin sensitive and others more resistant than the population average. *Insulin resistance* is a relative designation, for example, the lowest quintile of insulin sensitivity within a population of nondiabetic subjects or the mean insulin sensitivity in a group of obese compared with lean subjects. The major insulin-responsive tissues are skeletal muscle, adipose tissue, and the liver. Insulin resistance in muscle and fat is generally marked by a decrease in transport of glucose from the circulation. *Hepatic insulin resistance* generally refers to a blunted ability of insulin to suppress glucose production.

It is known that insulin sensitivity is under genetic control, but it is unclear whether insulin-resistant individuals have mutations in specific components of the insulin signaling cascade or a complement of signaling effectors that operate at the lower range of normal (Pessin and Saltiel 2000; Withers and White 2000). Regardless, it is apparent that insulin resistance clusters in families and is a major risk factor for the development of diabetes. Cases of insulin receptor mutations causing insulin resistance are known but are exceedingly rare (Pessin and Saltiel 2000).

It is clear that environmental factors can lead to insulin resistance (Kahn et al. 2001), with obesity probably the most clinically significant risk factor (Pessin and Saltiel 2000). Individuals who gain weight become more insulin resistant, and weight loss improves insulin sensitivity. Rates of insulin resistance are doubled in obese subjects compared with lean subjects, but it is important to note that not all obese people are insulin resistant (Ferrannini et al. 1997). However, among the obese there is an increase in insulin resistance, with greater body weight demonstrating a "dose" effect of body adiposity on insulin sensitivity (Kahn and Flier 2000; Wajchenberg 2000). High levels of circulating fatty acids can cause insulin resistance and provide a potential explanation for the connection between obesity and impaired insulin sensitivity (Shulman 2000). Beyond the effect of body weight, per se, on impaired insulin sensitivity, the distribution of adipose tissue has a major impact on insulin resistance. Central or visceral adiposity (fat stored in the abdominal cavity) has more deleterious effects on insulin sensitivity than subcutaneous or gluteal-femoral fat stores (Kahn and Flier 2000; Wajchenberg 2000). Whether central adiposity causes insulin resistance directly through biochemical or endocrine effects or whether storage of visceral fat and insulin resistance are related by a common inherited or environmental factor is unknown. In addition to central storage of lipids, it is becoming clear that excessive fat accumulation in skeletal muscle, usually in the context of obesity, is associated with insulin resistance.

Another important variable in determining insulin sensitivity is activity level. Sedentary persons are more insulin resistant than active ones, and physical training can improve insulin sensitivity beyond its effects in weight loss. Physical activity can decrease the risk of developing diabetes (Knowler et al. 2002) and improve glycemic control in persons who have diabetes (Boule et al. 2001; Hu et al. 2001). Insulin resistance is more common in the elderly, and within populations, insulin sensitivity decreases linearly with age. Older individuals tend to be less physically active, which can contribute to insulin resistance. In addition, over the normal course of aging there is a decrease in muscle mass and an increase in fat mass, with an increased percentage of fat stored in the abdominal cavity (Wajchenberg 2000). In deconditioned persons, physical training can improve glucose metabolism even with small increases in body weight due to increased muscular function and hypertrophy.

Clinical Features

TYPE 1 DIABETES

T1DM (formerly termed *juvenile-onset* or *insulin-dependent* diabetes) is caused by severe insulinopenia, and the clinical consequences directly reflect a near-complete lack of insulin action. When insulin is absent, hepatic glucose production is uncontrolled, and blood glucose levels rise. Glucose uptake by muscle and other peripheral tissues is minimal without insulin stimulation. Without inhibition by insulin, adipocytes release fatty acids at a brisk rate, and these fatty acids are metabolized in the liver to ketone bodies. The high levels of solutes in the blood overwhelm the renal threshold to retain them, and osmotic diuresis ensues. Persons with T1DM typically present with symptoms of hyperglycemia such as polyuria and polydipsia resulting from glucosuria and osmotic diuresis. Weight loss is almost invariable and results from wasting of glucose calories lost with glucosuria as well as impaired nutrient storage in the absence of insulin. Unintentional weight loss is a reliable sign of insulin deficiency, and patients with new-onset hyperglycemia and significant weight loss should be suspected of having T1DM. This is an important clinical distinction, because only insulin therapy will ultimately be effective in T1DM patients, and delay in its provision can lead to serious consequences. The occurrence of diabetic ketoacidosis (DKA) is a definitive sign of severe lack of insulin, and in this setting the diagnosis of T1DM is almost certain.

TYPE 2 DIABETES

T2DM (formerly termed *adult-onset* or *non-insulin-dependent* diabetes) is the most common form of diabetes, accounting for approximately 90% of cases in the United States (Bennett et al. 2002). It is usual for patients to have a preclinical phase of glucose intolerance or subtle elevations of fasting glucose for several years before the diagnosis of diabetes is made. Indeed, it is currently estimated that the number of patients with undiagnosed T2DM is one-third again the number of known cases (Mokdad et al. 2003). If this estimate is accurate, the number of Americans with diabetes is closer to 30 million than 20 million.

Most patients with T2DM are overweight, and the increase in this form of diabetes in the United States and many other parts of the world is strongly linked to the overall increase in obesity. This connection is most commonly explained by the effects of obesity in decreasing tissue sensitivity, thus causing insulin resistance. Insulin resistance is an invariable component of T2DM, even among patients with relatively normal body weight. However most insulin-resistant people are not diabetic, because individuals with normal β-cell function increase their insulin output manyfold to compensate for decreased insulin sensitivity (Kahn et al. 2001). In fact, T2DM can be simply conceptualized as a condition in which insulin secretion cannot compensate for insulin resistance (Bell and Polonsky 2001; Kahn and Porte 2002). Therefore, even minor defects in insulin secretion can result in hyperglycemia if insulin resistance is severe, and persons with only mildly diminished insulin sensitivity will not become diabetic unless they have more severe β-cell defects.

Patients with T2DM often do not have the dramatic symptoms of hyperglycemia and insulinopenia that typify the presentation of T1DM (Table 1–3). Typically, persons with T2DM present asymptomatically and have hyperglycemia

---

TABLE 1–3. Symptoms of type 1 and type 2 diabetes

Polydipsia or excessive thirst
Increased appetite
Polyuria
Fatigue
Unexplained weight gain or loss
Slow-healing sores or cuts
Poor sensation or tingling in feet
Blurry vision

Note. Most patients are asymptomatic when diagnosed with diabetes.

---

detected on fasting or random blood samples. In patients who do have symptoms, the symptoms tend to be related to the spilling of glucose into the urine, and complaints of polyuria and polydipsia are not uncommon. Because T2DM is not associated with severe insulinopenia, weight loss is not common on presentation. In fact, because insulin sensitivity decreases with increased levels of obesity, many patients come to diagnosis at a time of maximum body weight.

OTHER FORMS OF DIABETES

Gestational diabetes is defined as abnormal blood glucose regulation arising during pregnancy (Buchanan and Xiang 2005). Insulin resistance is a normal part of pregnancy and progresses over the course of gestation, peaking in the third trimester. The current viewpoint is that persons with inherent β-cell defects who cannot overcome this physiological insulin resistance become glucose intolerant or diabetic (Buchanan and Xiang 2005). Most revert to normal glucose tolerance in the immediate postpartum period, but up to 50% go on to develop T2DM in later years (Buchanan and Kjos 1999; O'Sullivan 1991).

Recently, an interesting variant of diabetes has been described, primarily in African American patients. This group of patients often presents with severe metabolic decompensation or even DKA, which is typical for patients with T1DM (Banerji et al. 1996; Mauvais-Jarvis et al. 2004; Umpierrez et al. 1995). However, these patients often develop a remission or significant improvement in their diabetes within several months of treatment. They are typically weaned from insulin, and their diabetes is often managed satisfactorily with oral glucose-lowering agents or diet alone. Typically these subject have other features of T2DM, including obesity and a strong family history of diabetes. The epidemiology of this atypical form of diabetes (termed variably "ketosis-prone" or "Flatbush" diabetes) has not been well worked out but probably comprises only a minority of the persons of African descent who develop diabetes.

Diabetes can arise from generalized pancreatic diseases such as chronic pancreatitis, hemochromatosis, and cystic fibrosis, which damage islets as well as acinar tissue. Endocrinopathies such as Cushing's syndrome, acromegaly, and pheochromocytoma are also frequently associated with diabetes. Importantly, a number of medications can interfere with glucose metabolism and cause or exacerbate diabetes. Niacin and glucocorticoids cause insulin resistance (Pandit et al. 1993). Pentamidine, thiazides and high dosages of aspirin can impair insulin secretion (Pandit et al. 1993).

Diagnosis

The diagnostic criteria for diabetes have been refined over the past two decades in an attempt to improve detection. The current standards are given in Table 1–4. As it has become clear that complications of hyperglycemia can occur at lower average glucose levels, the values used in diagnosis have gradually decreased. In addition, because the regulation of blood glucose across the population is a continuous measure, the risk for the development of diabetes can be predicted. The glucose criteria for diabetes and prediabetes are given in Table 1–5. The most commonly used of these is two fasting blood glucose values of 126 mg/dL or greater (American Diabetes Association 2005a). In addition, random blood glucose values greater than 200 mg/dL are diagnostic for diabetes. Oral glucose tolerance testing is probably a more sensitive measure, but because of the added time and expense, such testing is not recommended for universal screening. This is reasonable, because approximately 95% of persons with diabetes based on a 2-hour postingestion glucose level will have a fasting glucose of 126 mg/dL or greater. *Prediabetes* is a term that encompasses what was formerly called *impaired glucose tolerance* as well as other abnormalities in glucose regulation. Oral glucose tolerance testing is now used routinely only in the evaluation of pregnant women for gestational diabetes. The hemoglobin A_{1c} (HbA_{1c}) level, a measure of average glycemia over the past 3 months, is not sufficiently sensitive to use in the early detection of diabetes.

Complications

The major complications of diabetes are nephropathy (renal failure), retinopathy, neuropathy, and cardiovascular disease. These complications are common to both T1DM and T2DM. Diabetes is the leading cause of renal failure in the United States, and persons with diabetes constitute a large percentage of kidney transplant recipients. Approximately 30% of patients with T1DM will develop clinically significant renal disease (Nelson et al. 1995); a lesser percentage of T2DM patients develop renal failure due to diabetes. The incidence increases with the number of years of diabetes up to 15 or 20 years, after which it plateaus. This suggests that only a subset of persons with diabetes is susceptible to renal complications.

TABLE 1–4. Criteria for the diagnosis of diabetes mellitus

1. Symptoms of diabetes plus casual plasma glucose concentration ≥200 mg/dL (11.1 mmol/L).

   Casual is defined as any time of day without regard to time since last meal.

   Classic symptoms of diabetes include polyuria, polydipsia, and unexplained weight loss.

or

2. Fasting plasma glucose ≥126 mg/dL (7.0 mmol/L).

   Fasting is defined as no caloric intake for at least 8 hours.

or

3. 2-Hour postprandial glucose ≥200 mg/dL (11.1 mmol/L) during an oral glucose tolerance test.

   The test should be performed using a glucose load containing the equivalent of 75 g anhydrous glucose dissolved in water.

Note. In the absence of unequivocal hyperglycemia with acute metabolic decompensation, these criteria should be confirmed by repeat testing on a different day. The third measure (oral glucose tolerance test) is not recommended for routine clinical use.

Source. Adapted from the recommendations of the American Diabetes Association (2005b).

TABLE 1–5. Glucose thresholds for the diagnosis of diabetes and prediabetes

Diagnosis	Fasting glucose, mg/dL	OGTT 2-hour glucose, mg/dL
Nondiabetic	<100	<140
Prediabetes	100–125	140–199
Diabetes	≥126	>200

Note. OGTT=oral glucose tolerance test.
Source. Adapted from the recommendations of the American Diabetes Association (2005b).

Approximately two-thirds of persons with diabetes will develop some degree of retinopathy (Klein 2002). Of these, approximately 25%–30% of diabetic patients will have eye disease of a severity sufficient to cause visual impairment; diabetes is the leading cause of blindness in the United States.

Diabetic neuropathy occurs in 40%–50% of adult patients who have had diabetes for more than 10 years (Partanen et al. 1995). Symptoms typically involve decreased sensation and pain in the lower extremities, but diabetic neuropathy is implicated in a wide range of neuropathic syndromes, from cranial neuropathies to radiculopathies and amyotrophy (Harati 1987). Importantly, loss of peripheral sensation puts patients at significant risk for injuries and ulceration of the feet, and complications of these local problems are the reason why diabetes is the major cause of lower-limb amputation.

Cardiovascular disease is the leading cause of death among patients with diabetes (Haffner et al. 1998; Laakso 1999). Myocardial infarction is the primary entity, but diabetic patients also have an excess burden of congestive heart failure and stroke. There is ample evidence that hyperglycemia contributes to vascular disease, but this process is probably multifactorial in diabetic patients, with contributions from other abnormalities such as dyslipidemia and vessel inflammation.

Screening for retinopathy, nephropathy, neuropathy, and cardiovascular disease has become a standard part of diabetes care and has the potential for greatly reducing the morbidity and mortality associated with these diseases (Table 1–6). All patients with T1DM and T2DM should be seen annually by an ophthalmologist for retinal screening. Detection of advancing retinopathy and treatment with laser photocoagulation can greatly reduce vision loss and blindness. Screening of urine for microalbuminuria has the potential to detect incipient diabetic nephropathy well before it becomes symptomatic and at a stage where progression can be slowed. Neuropathy is best detected by physical examination, primarily by evaluating the feet for abnormal callous and skin breakdown and assessing the sensation to pinprick and vibration. Other cardiovascular risk factors should be sought diligently in diabetic patients, with special attention to plasma lipids, blood pressure, and smoking. Diabetic patients complaining of any symptoms that could be construed as being cardiac in origin (chest pain, dyspnea, exercise intolerance) should be worked up aggressively.

Treatment

It has now been established that treatment of hyperglycemia with insulin or oral medications will decrease the incidence of diabetic complications (American Diabetes Association 2005b). T1DM patients absolutely require insulin as therapy. The results of the Diabetes Control and Complications Trial (DCCT; American Diabetes Association 2003a) demonstrated that in T1DM, intensive insulin treatment with a goal of lowering blood glucose to average levels approaching those of nondiabetic persons significantly decreased the incidence of nephropathy, retinopathy, and neuropathy. The United Kingdom Prospective Diabetes Study (UKPDS; American Diabetes Association 2003b) showed similar results for glucose lowering with oral agents, insulin,

TABLE 1–6.　Standard screening procedures for diabetic complications

Complication	Recommended evaluation
Retinopathy	Dilated funduscopic examination by experienced ophthalmologist
Nephropathy	Urinary determination of albumin excretion
Neuropathy	Physical examination
Cardiovascular disease	Measurement of blood lipids, blood pressure; smoking cessation

Note.　Screening should be performed at least annually.

and their combination in patients with T2DM. To date, no trial has demonstrated an effect for treatment of blood glucose in lowering the incidence of cardiovascular disease, although there is suggestive evidence that this occurs. Advances in laser photocoagulation therapy and emphasis on early and regular retinal examinations have had a major impact on decreasing the morbidity of diabetic retinopathy and preserving vision. Likewise, the course of diabetic nephropathy has been significantly improved with the use of angiotensin-converting enzyme inhibitors and angiotensin receptor blockers to treat hypertension and early renal disease in diabetic patients.

FORMS OF DIABETES

Type 1 Diabetes

Patients with severe insulin deficiency are dependent on insulin for health and functioning. In the absence of insulin, blood glucose levels remain elevated and storage of nutrients is so impaired that rapid weight loss ensues. Any concurrent stress can precipitate DKA, a life-threatening condition that results from severe insulin deficiency in the presence of increased circulating stress hormones such as catecholamines, glucagon, and cortisol. In DKA, uncontrolled hyperglycemia leads to glucose loss in the urine and dehydration from osmotic diuresis. In the absence of insulin, fatty acid release from adipose stores is unregulated, and rampant fat oxidation leads to the production of large amounts of ketone bodies, which are weak organic acids. This can cause severe metabolic acidosis. Treatment of DKA requires vigorous fluid resuscitation, electrolyte replacement, and insulin, usually in the intensive care unit setting.

Patients with T1DM usually require multiple injections of insulin daily; there is no role for oral diabetic treatments in this condition. Because intensive treatment with the goal of maintaining plasma glucose as near normal as possible is now the standard of care, insulin regimens have become more complex and generally more effective. There are now a host of insulins and insulin analogues that differ in kinetic profile, which allows a pattern of insulinization that mimics normal human physiology (Hirsch 2005). Proper insulin treatment requires careful monitoring of blood glucose, dietary consideration for appropriate dosing, and adjustments of therapy for metabolic stressors such as infectious illness or physical exercise (American Diabetes Association 2005b). Although the indications for insulin use have increased with the advent of more intensive diabetes management, there are still substantial barriers to this treatment (Davidson et al. 1997), including the technical demands of injection and self-glucose monitoring, reluctance of physicians to prescribe a medication that can be both under- and overdosed, and the limited time and expertise for patient education required for insulin use in many primary care clinics. For this reason, initiation of insulin and management of complex or difficult cases are often left to endocrinologists and other diabetes experts.

Type 2 Diabetes

Patients with T2DM represent a wide spectrum of disease severity with a wider range of therapeutic choices. Persons with mild or early diabetes may be adequately managed with diet and exercise (Knowler et al. 2002). In this case, diet usually involves some degree of caloric restriction and reduction of saturated fat intake; the latter recommendation is part of a strategy to reduce risk for cardiovascular disease, because no studies have shown any definite benefit of dietary fat reduction for either weight loss or glucose controls. Many patients with mild or early diabetes, as well as individuals presenting with more advanced diabetes, will eventually require treatment with oral medications. Because T2DM is a progressive disease, most patients progress from the mild stage to worse levels of glycemia over time (Chan and Abrahamson 2003). The typical course involves the addition of an oral antidiabetic agent, dose titration, and stabilization for a period of months or years followed by a worsening and need for additional therapy. Most patients treated with oral agents need more than one drug, and three- and four-drug regimens are becoming more common. Eventually, most patients with T2DM require insulin to maintain adequate glycemic control, although these individuals rarely reach a state of insulin deficiency that puts them at risk for DKA.

TREATMENT GOALS

HbA_{1c} is a measure of the glycosylation of hemoglobin and generally reflects the average blood glucose level over the previous 3 months. Nondiabetic subjects generally have HbA_{1c} levels of 4%–6%; a level of 6% corresponds to an average blood glucose of 120 mg/dL (American Diabetes Association 2005b). On the basis of intervention trials, the target value for good control of both T1DM and T2DM has been determined to be an HbA_{1c} level of 7% or less. A level of 8% or more is considered an indication for increasing antidiabetes therapy. Goals of treatment are shown in Table 1–7.

TABLE 1–7. Glucose treatment goals for patients with type 1 and type 2 diabetes

Test	Target value
Hemoglobin A_{1c}	<7.0%
Fasting or premeal glucose	90–130 mg/dL
2-Hour postmeal glucose	<180 mg/dL

Source. Adapted from the recommendations of the American Diabetes Association (2005b).

SPECIFIC DRUGS USED TO TREAT DIABETES

The drugs used to treat diabetes are listed in Table 1–8 (Chan and Abramson 2003; Inzucchi 2002).

Insulin

Currently available insulins include rapid-acting insulin analogues (lispro and aspart) that are active within minutes after injection, peak in 1 hour, and have a duration of action less than 3 hours; short-acting regular insulin, which has an onset of action within 30 minutes, peaks in 2–3 hours, and lasts 4–6 hours; intermediate-acting neutral protamine hagedorn (NPH) insulin, which peaks in 6–8 hours and has activity that can extend to 12–16 hours; and glargine, a long-acting insulin analogue with a flat, nonpeaking, pharmacodynamic profile and a 20–24 hour duration of action (Hirsch 2005). Patients are usually treated with one or two injections of intermediate- or long-acting insulin daily to regulate fasting and between-meal glycemia and some form of rapid- or short-acting insulin before meals to control postprandial glucose. Insulin dosing is empiric, and specific regimens for particular patients are arrived at by adjustment and glucose monitoring over time. In general, insulin needs are proportional to body weight. In addition, patients with T2DM, who have a more prominent component of insulin resistance than patients with T1DM, will require more insulin for good glycemic control. On average, patients with T1DM will take 0.5–1 units of insulin per kilogram of body weight daily, whereas insulin-requiring patients with T2DM will use more than 1 unit/kg daily.

The most common side effect of insulin therapy is *hypoglycemia,* and this is much more common in insulin-sensitive patients with T1DM than in insulin-resistant T2DM patients. Hypoglycemia in insulin-requiring patients is often related to an abnormal reduction of food intake or missing a meal. In addition, many patients have "insulin reactions" after a bout of increased physical activity, when increased muscle glucose utilization is added to the usual glucose lowering of a typical insulin dose.

TABLE 1–8.   Treatment approaches for diabetes

Class	Agents	Mechanism of action
α-Glucosidase inhibitors	Acarbose Miglitol	Decreases dietary carbohydrate absorption
Biguanides	Metformin	Reduce liver glucose output
Insulin	Various preparations	Replaces absent or decreased pancreatic β-cell insulin production
Nonsulfonylurea secretagogues	Nateglinide Repaglinide	Stimulate pancreatic β-cells to increase insulin production
Sulfonylureas	Chlorpropamide Glimepiride Glipizide Glyburide	Stimulate pancreatic β-cells to increase insulin production
Thiazolidinediones	Pioglitazone Rosiglitazone	Reduce liver glucose output Increase glucose uptake by muscle and adipose tissue

Insulin treatment also predictably causes weight gain. Some of this effect may be due to improved glycemic control and reduced calories in the form of glucosuria. In addition, insulin is necessary for lipogenesis and probably promotes adipose accretion directly. Finally, because hypoglycemia is a potent stimulus to eat, clinically apparent or subtle reductions of blood glucose from insulin treatment may promote food intake.

Injection-site reactions and immunological phenomena common in the era of animal insulins are very rare since the advent of human insulins as therapeutics.

Sulfonylureas

Sulfonylureas are a class of orally administered insulin secretagogues (chlorpropamide, glimepiride, glipizide, glyburide). These compounds are commonly used as first agents in T2DM and have an expected effect of reducing HbA_{1c} by 1% when initiated in untreated patients or added to other agents. Sulfonylureas stimulate insulin release from islet β-cells and thus are not effective in T1DM or advanced T2DM, in which the majority of these cells have been lost. The stimulatory effect on insulin release is independent of the blood glucose level, so these drugs cause hypoglycemia as their major side effect. Beyond this, sulfonylureas are generally well tolerated. Like any agent that improves blood glucose and increases circulating insulin levels, sulfonylureas cause weight gain, approximately 2–5 kg over the course of treatment.

Metformin

Metformin is a biguanide that inhibits hepatic glucose production and increases insulin sensitivity. Along with sulfonylureas, metformin is most commonly used as a first-line agent in T2DM. This drug provides degrees of glycemic control equivalent to those of sulfonylureas (approximately 1% decrease in HbA_{1c}) but generally without weight gain. Side effects include abdominal pain and bloating and other gastrointestinal effects. For this reason metformin should be started at a low dosage, and the dosage should be increased gradually to minimize these symptoms. Lactic acidosis has been reported in a handful of cases related to metformin use, almost exclusively in patients with renal failure or uncompensated heart failure. A creatinine level above 1.5 mg/dL is a relative contraindication for metformin use, and more advanced states of renal failure and stage III or IV heart failure are more firm contraindications.

Thiazolidinediones

Thiazolidinediones (TZDs) are a new class of insulin sensitizers that act as agonists for the nuclear receptor PPARλ (peroxisome proliferator-activated receptor λ). The currently available TZDs are pioglitazone (Actos) and rosiglitazone (Avandia). These drugs have been shown to be similarly efficacious to sulfonylureas and metformin when started in patients with T2DM who have not been previously treated. However, because of their relatively recent introduction and greater expense TZDs are usually used as adjunctive treatment with metformin, a sulfonylurea, or insulin. Rosiglitazone and pioglitazone are generally well tolerated but predictably cause weight gain. They also cause fluid retention, which limits their use in patients with heart failure. The prototype TZD, troglitazone, was removed from the market because it caused several cases of hepatic failure. This adverse effect has not been reported for pioglitazone and rosiglitazone, although these drugs can rarely cause chemical hepatitis.

α-Glucosidase Inhibitors

α-Glucosidase inhibitors (e.g., acarbose, miglitol) are another relatively new class of drugs that act by blocking the digestion of starches and other complex carbohydrates in the intestine, delaying entry of glucose into the circulation and reducing postprandial glucose. The compound available in the United States is acarbose (Precose). Acarbose is not as potent in decreasing HbA_{1c} as the other oral agents, with reductions of approximately 0.5% in previously untreated patients. Because acarbose has its effects in the gut lumen and very little is systemically absorbed, it is a very safe compound with little drug–drug interaction. However, because it acts by reducing glucose absorption in the upper intestine, with passage of increased amounts of meal carbohydrates to the lower gut, there is an increase in bacterial metabolism in the large bowel. Thus, the predictable side effects of acarbose are increased production of abdominal gas, bloating, and flatulence. Acarbose is often used in diabetic patients who have contraindications to other oral agents or as an adjunctive therapy.

Incretin Mimetics and Incretin Enhancers

Incretin mimetics and incretin enhancers are new classes of diabetes drugs based on the properties of endogenous gastrointestinal hormones that stimulate insulin secretion and promote glucose tolerance (Ahren 2004). Incretin mimetics are peptide agonists of the glucagon-like peptide 1 receptor (GLP-1). GLP-1 is a hormone released from the small intestine that is the most potent endogenous insulin secretagogue known. Currently, one incretin mimetic, exenatide (Byetta), is available for treatment with several other compounds in advanced stages of development. Exenatide is injected twice daily and in clinical trials decreases HbA_{1c} by approximately 1% when added to sulfonylureas or metformin treatment. Exenatide has the added benefit of causing weight loss, approximately 2–6 kg over 1 year, a unique feature for diabetes therapeutics. Nausea and, less commonly, vomiting are the prominent side effects of exenatide. These are probably related to the known effects of GLP-1 to slow gastric emptying, although direct activation of central nervous system illness centers by GLP-1 is also a possible cause. These side effects have not limited long-term therapy in clinical trials.

Because GLP-1 is rapidly inactivated in the circulation, the native hormone is not a practical therapeutic. However, several compounds that block the metabolism of GLP-1 by the ubiquitous enzyme dipeptidyl peptidase IV (DPP-IV) have been developed. These compounds increase circulating concentrations of active GLP-1 in the bloodstream, extending the activity of the native peptide. In clinical trials, incretin enhancers (DPP-IV inhibitors) have been effective for glucose control and remarkably well tolerated. These agents will likely reach the market in the next 1–2 years.

Conclusion

Diabetes is a complex set of diseases that share the cardinal finding of hyperglycemia. Although only part of a spectrum of metabolic abnormalities, chronically elevated blood glucose levels lead to a common set of complications, including blindness, renal failure, and nerve damage. Because diabetes increases the risk for atherosclerotic vascular disease, it is a major risk for mortality. Susceptibility to diabetes is high in the American population, with some ethnic and racial groups having a disproportionate risk. Moreover, modern lifestyles with decreased physical activity and overconsumption of calorie-rich foods confer a strong environmental risk for the development of diabetes. Treatment of diabetes has improved in terms of both management of blood glucose and approaches to complications. However, a major goal for the American healthcare system is increased prevention of diabetes.

KEY CLINICAL CONCEPTS

- The overall incidence of both T1DM and T2DM is growing worldwide and is expected to continue to increase. Thus diabetes, and in particular T2DM, will be one of the major public health problems for the foreseeable future in psychiatric patient populations.

- Adults age 45 or older should be screened for diabetes every 3 years, particularly if they are overweight. High-risk individuals should receive screening more frequently and at a younger age.

- A fasting glucose is the most practical method to screen for diabetes. Two fasting glucose levels of 126 mg/dL or greater indicate that the patient has diabetes.

- The four major complications from diabetes are retinopathy, nephropathy, neuropathy, and cardiovascular disease. Patients with diabetes should be routinely screened for these conditions by primary care physicians and/or specialty care providers.

References

Ahren B: GLP-1 receptor agonists and DPP-4 inhibitors in the treatment of type 2 diabetes. Horm Metab Res 36:867–887, 2004

American Diabetes Association: Consensus development conference on the diagnosis of coronary heart disease in people with diabetes. Diabetes Care 21:1551–1559, 1998

American Diabetes Association: Implications of the Diabetes Control and Complications Trial. Diabetes Care 26:S25–S27, 2003a

American Diabetes Association: Implications of the United Kingdom Prospective Diabetes Study. Diabetes Care 26:S28–S32, 2003b

American Diabetes Association: Screening for type 2 diabetes. Diabetes Care 27(suppl): S11–S14, 2004

American Diabetes Association: Diagnosis and classification of diabetes mellitus. Diabetes Care 28:S37–S42, 2005a

American Diabetes Association: Standards of medical care in diabetes. Diabetes Care 28(suppl):S4–S36, 2005b

Banerji MA, Chaiken RL, Lebovitz HE: Long-term normoglycemic remission in black newly diagnosed NIDDM subjects. Diabetes 45:337–341, 1996

Bell GI, Polonsky KS: Diabetes mellitus and genetically programmed defects in beta-cell function. Nature 414:788–791, 2001

Bennett PH, Rewers MJ, Knowler WC: Epidemiology of diabetes mellitus, in Ellenberg and Rifkin's Diabetes Mellitus. Edited by Porte D Jr, Sherwin RS, Baron A. New York, McGraw-Hill, 2002, pp 277–300

Boule NG, Haddad E, Kenny GP, et al: Effects of exercise on glycemic control and body mass in type 2 diabetes mellitus: a meta-analysis of controlled clinical trials. JAMA 286:1218–1227, 2001

Boyle JP, Honeycutt AA, Narayan KM, et al: Projection of diabetes burden through 2050: impact of changing demography and disease prevalence in the U.S. Diabetes Care 24:1936–1940, 2001

Buchanan TA, Kjos SL: Gestational diabetes: risk or myth? J Clin Endocrinol Metab 84: 1854–1857, 1999

Buchanan TA, Xiang AH: Gestational diabetes mellitus. J Clin Invest 115:485–491, 2005

Butler AE, Janson J, Soeller WC, et al: Increased beta-cell apoptosis prevents adaptive increase in beta-cell mass in mouse model of type 2 diabetes: evidence for role of islet amyloid formation rather than direct action of amyloid. Diabetes 52:2304–2314, 2003

Cavaghan MK, Ehrman DA, Polonsky KS: Interactions between insulin resistance and insulin secretion in the development of glucose intolerance. J Clin Invest 106:329–333, 2000

Centers for Disease Control and Prevention: National Diabetes Fact Sheet: General Information and National Estimates on Diabetes in the United States. Atlanta, GA, Centers for Disease Control and Prevention, 2003

Chan JL, Abrahamson MJ: Pharmacological management of type 2 diabetes mellitus: rationale for rational use of insulin. Mayo Clin Proc 78:459–467, 2003

Cowie CC, Eberhardt MS: Sociodemographic characteristics of persons with diabetes, in Diabetes in America. Edited by Harris MI, Cowie CC, Stern MP, et al. Bethesda, MD, National Institutes of Health, 1995, pp 85–116

D'Alessio DA: Incretins: glucose-dependent insulinotropic polypeptide and glucagon-like peptide 1, in Ellenberg and Rifkin's Diabetes Mellitus. Edited by Porte D Jr, Sherwin RS, Baron A. New York, McGraw-Hill, 2002, pp 85–96

D'Alessio DA, Kieffer TJ, Taborsky GJ, et al: Activation of the parasympathetic nervous system is necessary for normal meal-induced insulin secretion in rhesus macaques. J Clin Endocrinol Metab 86:1253–1259, 2001

Davidson JA, Garber AJ, DiMarchi RD, et al: New advances in insulin treatment of diabetes: overcoming barriers. Endocr Pract 3:371–384, 1997

EURODIAB ACE Study Group: Variation and trends in incidence of childhood diabetes in Europe. Lancet 355:873–876, 2000

Fagot-Campagna A, Narayan KM, Imperatore G: Type 2 diabetes in children. BMJ 322: 377–378, 2001

Ferrannini E, Natali A, Bell P, et al: Insulin resistance and hypersecretion in obesity. European Group for the Study of Insulin Resistance (EGIR). J Clin Invest 100:1166–1173, 1997

Fujimoto WY: Diabetes in Asian and Pacific Islander Americans, in Diabetes in America. Edited by Harris MI, Cowie CC, Stern MP, et al. Bethesda, MD, National Institutes of Health, 1995, pp 661–682

Goodpaster BH, Krishnaswami S, Resnick H, et al: Association between regional adipose tissue distribution and both type 2 diabetes and impaired glucose tolerance in elderly men and women. Diabetes Care 26:372–379, 2003

Haffner SM, Lehto S, Ronnemaa T, et al: Mortality from coronary heart disease in subjects with type 2 diabetes and in nondiabetic subjects with and without prior myocardial infarction. N Engl J Med 339:229–234, 1998

Harati Y: Diabetic peripheral neuropathies. Ann Intern Med 107:546–559, 1987

Harris MI: Epidemiological correlates of NIDDM in Hispanics, whites, and blacks in the U.S. population. Diabetes Care 14:639–648, 1991

Henriksen GL, Ketchum NS, Michalek JE, et al: Serum dioxin and diabetes mellitus in veterans of Operation Ranch Hand. Epidemiology 8:252–258, 1997

Hirsch IB: Insulin analogues. N Engl J Med 352:174–183, 2005

Hogan P, Dall T, Nikolov P: Economic costs of diabetes in the U.S. in 2002. Diabetes Care 26:917–932, 2003

Hu FB, Leitzmann MF, Stampfer MJ, et al: Physical activity and television watching in relation to risk for type 2 diabetes mellitus in men. Arch Intern Med 161:1542–1548, 2001

Inzucchi SE: Oral antihyperglycemic therapy for type 2 diabetes: a scientific review. JAMA 287:360–372, 2002

Kahn BB, Flier JS: Obesity and insulin resistance. J Clin Invest 106:473–481, 2000

Kahn SE, Porte D Jr: Pathophysiology and genetics of type 2 diabetes mellitus, in Ellenberg and Rifkin's Diabetes Mellitus. Edited by Porte D Jr, Sherwin RS, Baron A. New York, McGraw-Hill, 2002, pp 331–336

Kahn SE, Prigeon RL, Schwartz RS, et al: Obesity, body fat distribution, insulin sensitivity and islet beta-cell function as explanations for metabolic diversity. J Nutr 131:354S–360S, 2001

Kannel WB, McGee DL: Diabetes and glucose tolerance as risk factors for cardiovascular disease: the Framingham study. Diabetes Care 2:120–126, 1979

Kaprio J, Tuomilehto J, Koskenvuo M, et al: Concordance for type 1 (insulin-dependent) and type 2 (non-insulin-dependent) diabetes mellitus in a population-based cohort of twins in Finland. Diabetologia 35:1060–1067, 1992

Klein R: Retinopathy and other ocular complications in diabetes, in Ellenberg and Rifkin's Diabetes Mellitus. Edited by Porte D Jr, Sherwin RS, Baron A. New York, McGraw-Hill, 2002, pp 663–697

Knowler WC, Barrett-Connor E, Fowler SE: Reduction in the incidence of type 2 diabetes with lifestyle intervention or metformin. N Engl J Med 346:393–403, 2002

Laakso M: Hyperglycemia and cardiovascular disease in type 2 diabetes. Diabetes 48:937–942, 1999

Lorenzen T, Pociot F, Hougaard P, et al: Long-term risk of IDDM in first-degree relatives of patients with IDDM. Diabetologia 37:321–327, 1994

Mauvais-Jarvis F, Sobngwi E, Porcher R, et al: Ketosis-prone type 2 diabetes in patients of sub-Saharan African origin: clinical pathophysiology and natural history of beta-cell dysfunction and insulin resistance. Diabetes 53:645–653, 2004

Mokdad AH, Ford ES, Bowman BA, et al: Prevalence of obesity, diabetes, and obesity-related health risk factors, 2001. JAMA 289:76–79, 2003

Nelson RG, Knowler WC, Pettitt DJ, et al: Kidney diseases in diabetes, in Diabetes in America. Edited by Harris MI, Cowie CC, Stern MP, et al. Bethesda, MD, National Institutes of Health, 1995, pp 349–400

Ogden CL, Flegal KM, Carroll MD, et al: Prevalence and trends in overweight among U.S. children and adolescents, 1999–2000. JAMA 288:1728–1732, 2002

Onkamo P, Vaananen S, Karvonen M, et al: Worldwide increase in incidence of type I diabetes: the analysis of the data on published incidence trends. Diabetologia 42:1395–1403, 1999

O'Sullivan JB: Diabetes mellitus after GDM. Diabetes 40:131–135, 1991

Pandit MK, Burke J, Gustafson AB, et al: Drug-induced disorders of glucose tolerance. Ann Intern Med 118:529–539, 1993

Partanen J, Niskanen L, Lehtinen J, et al: Natural history of peripheral neuropathy in patients with non-insulin-dependent diabetes mellitus. N Engl J Med 333:89–94, 1995

Pessin JE, Saltiel AR: Signaling pathways in insulin action: molecular targets of insulin resistance. J Clin Invest 106:165–169, 2000

Pinhas-Hamiel O, Dolan LM, Daniels SR, et al: Increased incidence of non-insulin-dependent diabetes mellitus among adolescents. J Pediatr 128:608–615, 1996

Porte D Jr: Mechanisms for hyperglycemia in the metabolic syndrome: the key role of beta-cell dysfunction. Ann N Y Acad Sci 892:73–83, 1999

Rewers M, Hamman RF: Risk factors for non-insulin-dependent diabetes, in Diabetes in America. Edited by Harris MI, Cowie CC, Stern MP, et al. Bethesda, MD, National Institutes of Health, 1995, pp 179–220

Rewers M, LaPorte RE, King H, et al: Trends in the prevalence and incidence of diabetes: insulin-dependent diabetes mellitus in childhood. World Health Stat Q 41:179–189, 1988

Rosenbloom AL, Joe JR, Young RS, et al: Emerging epidemic of type 2 diabetes in youth. Diabetes Care 22:345–354, 1999

Shuldiner AR, McLenithan JC: Genes and pathophysiology of type 2 diabetes: more than just the Randle cycle all over again. J Clin Invest 114:1414–1417, 2004

Shulman GI: Cellular mechanisms of insulin resistance. J Clin Invest 106:171–176, 2000

Stamler J, Vaccaro O, Neaton JD, et al: Diabetes, other risk factors, and 12-yr cardiovascular mortality for men screened in the Multiple Risk Factor Intervention Trial. Diabetes Care 16:434–444, 1993

Umpierrez GE, Casals MM, Gebhart SP, et al: Diabetic ketoacidosis in obese African-Americans. Diabetes 44:790–795, 1995

Wajchenberg BL: Subcutaneous and visceral adipose tissue: their relation to the metabolic syndrome. Endocr Rev 21:697–738, 2000

Withers DJ, White M: Perspective: the insulin signaling system—a common link in the pathogenesis of type 2 diabetes. Endocrinology 141:1917–1921, 2000

Zimmet P, Alberti KG, Shaw J: Global and societal implications of the diabetes epidemic. Nature 414:782–787, 2001

Chapter 2

THE METABOLIC SYNDROME

Robert M. McCarron, D.O.
Craig R. Keenan, M.D.

The metabolic syndrome is a compilation of established individual risk factors for coronary artery disease (CAD) with the potential to dramatically increase the incidence of heart disease and diabetes mellitus, and all cause mortality (Grundy et al. 2004a; Lakka et al. 2002). Hypertension, dyslipidemia, glucose dysregulation, and obesity are the core components of the metabolic syndrome and are closely associated with the one in five adult deaths from heart disease in the United States (American Heart Association 2006). Patients with psychiatric disorders have a heightened risk because they often receive suboptimal preventive medical care and are more likely to be overweight and to present with metabolic abnormalities (Druss and Rosenheck 1998; Druss et al. 2002).

Defining the Metabolic Syndrome

The assemblage of metabolic disturbances as a distinct entity was described over 80 years ago by Kylin (1923) when he found that hyperglycemia, gout, and hypertension were correlated with negative cardiovascular outcomes. In 1988, Reaven proposed the term "syndrome X" to identify the CAD risk factors of dyslipidemia, hyperglycemia, and hypertension. Currently, the metabolic syndrome—sometimes referred to as the "deadly quartet," "dysmetabolic syndrome," and "insulin resistance syndrome"—has three commonly used definitions developed by the World Health Organization (WHO), the American Association of Clinical Endocrinologists (AACE) and the National Cholesterol Education Program–Adult Treatment Panel III (NCEP-ATP III), respectively (Table 2–1). Although there are several distinctions, these descriptions share many common features while stressing the importance of CAD risk assessment.

TABLE 2–1. Common definitions of the metabolic syndrome

	Component	Abnormality
NCEP-ATP III	Three or more of the following:	
	Abdominal obesity (waist circumference)	
	Men	>40 inches (>102 cm)
	Women	>35 inches (>88 cm)
	Triglycerides[a]	≥150 mg/dL (1.695 mmol/L)
	HDL cholesterol	
	Men	<40 mg/dL (1.036 mmol/L)
	Women	<50 mg/dL (1.295 mmol/L)
	Blood pressure	≥130/≥85 mm Hg
	Fasting glucose[a,b]	≥100 mg/dL (5.6 mmol/L)
World Health Organization	Insulin resistance (indicated by one of the following)	
	Type 2 diabetes	
	Impaired fasting glucose	
	Impaired glucose tolerance	
	For those with normal fasting glucose, glucose uptake below the lowest quartile for background population under investigation under hyperglycemic, euglycemic conditions	

TABLE 2–1. Common definitions of the metabolic syndrome *(continued)*

Component	Abnormality
World Health Organization *(continued)*	
Plus two of the following:	
Blood pressure	Antihypertensive medication and/or blood pressure ≥140 mm Hg/≥90 mm Hg
Plasma triglycerides	≥150 mg/dL (1.695 mmol/L)
HDL cholesterol	
Men	<35 mg/dL (0.897 mmol/L)
Women	<39 mg/dL (1.0 mmol/L)
Obesity	Body mass index > 30 kg/m^2 and/or waist-to-hip ratio > 0.9 inches in men and > 0.85 inches in women
Renal function/Kidney disease	Urinary albumin excretion rate ≥ 20 μg/min or albumin:creatinine ratio ≥ 30 mg/g
American Association of Clinical Endocrinologists	Diagnosis depends on clinical judgment based on risk factors.
Obesity	Body mass index ≥ 25 kg/m^2
Plasma triglycerides	≥150 mg/dL (1.695 mmol/L)
HDL cholesterol	
Men	<40 mg/dL (1.036 mmol/L)
Women	<50 mg/dL (1.295 mmol/L)
Blood pressure	≥130/≥85 mm Hg

TABLE 2–1. Common definitions of the metabolic syndrome *(continued)*

Component	Abnormality
American Association of Clinical Endocrinologists *(continued)*	
Glucose	
Fasting	Between 110 mg/dL (6.1 mmol/L) and 126 mg/dL (7 mmol/L)
2-Hour postglucose challenge	>140 mg/dL (7.8 mmol/L)
Other risk factors	
Family history of type 2 diabetes, hypertension, cardiovascular disease	
Polycystic ovary syndrome	
Sedentary lifestyle	
Advancing age	
Ethnic group with high risk for type 2 diabetes or cardiovascular disease	

Note. HDL=high-density lipoprotein; NCEP-ATP III=National Cholesterol Education Program–Adult Treatment Panel III.

[a]No caloric intake for 8 hours or more.

[b]Suggested change by the American Diabetes Association from ≥110 mg/dL to ≥100 mg/dL.

Source. Adapted from Grundy et al. 2004a.

In 1998, the WHO developed the first definition of the metabolic syndrome and identified CAD as the primary clinical outcome (Alberti and Zimmet 1998). Under this definition, insulin resistance (or possible manifestations of insulin resistance) is a required component for the diagnosis. When insulin resistance is present, the diagnosis of the metabolic syndrome is established if two or more of the following are present: 1) elevated blood pressure and/or use of antihypertensive medications; 2) elevated plasma triglycerides; 3) decreased high-density lipoprotein (HDL) cholesterol; 4) increased body mass index (BMI) and/or increased waist-to-hip ratio; or 5) elevated urinary albumin excretion rate or albumin:creatinine ratio. It is often challenging to apply the WHO definition in clinical practice because the reliable determination of insulin resistance has significant time and cost limitations. Additionally, the measurement of insulin concentration and a corresponding abnormal range have not been sufficiently standardized.

The AACE also has a strong focus on insulin resistance; they use the term *insulin resistance syndrome* to describe a more comprehensive group of risk factors. Under the AACE definition, diagnosis of the metabolic syndrome depends on clinical judgment, because there is no minimum number of factors that result in having the syndrome (Einhorn et al. 2003).

The NCEP-ATP III definition of the metabolic syndrome is clearly defined, clinically useful, and often utilized to help assess risk of CAD. For a person to be diagnosed on the basis of the NCEP-ATP III guidelines, three of the following five abnormalities must exist: abdominal obesity, hypertension, decreased HDL cholesterol, hyperglycemia, or hypertriglyceridemia (National Cholesterol Education Program Expert Panel on Detection, Evaluation, and Treatment of High Blood Cholesterol in Adults 2002). This classification does not specify if patients treated with antihypertensive agents or diabetic medications still meet the criteria for hypertension and hyperglycemia, respectively. A waist circumference of more than 40 inches (>102 cm) in men and more than 35 inches (>88 cm) in females is used to determine central obesity, which is a marker for more atherogenic intraabdominal or visceral obesity. Conversely, the WHO definition uses BMI to estimate intraabdominal obesity; this measure does not reliably reflect visceral adipose tissue in various populations, including most Asians, who have a lower threshold for a diagnosis of obesity (BMI>25) (World Health Organization 2004). This distinction is important because studies have demonstrated a higher concentration of adipose-related, deleterious free fatty acids (FFAs) en route to the liver by way of the splanchnic circulation in patients with demonstrated increased visceral fat relative to those with higher subcutaneous fat (Aubert et al. 2003; Jensen et al. 1989).

PREVALENCE

The prevalence of adult obesity in the United States has increased since the early 1990s from 22.9% in 1991 to 30.5% in 2004, with more than 60% of the population currently classified as overweight or obese (Flegal et al. 2002). Given the lack of a universally accepted definition for the metabolic syndrome, it is challenging to establish an accurate rate of occurrence. With that in mind, there has been a corresponding increase in the prevalence of the NCEP-defined metabolic syndrome over the past several years. Ford et al. (2002) analyzed data from 8,814 adults in the third National Health and Nutrition Examination Survey (NHANES III; 1988–1994) and determined the overall unadjusted prevalence of the metabolic syndrome during the period 1988 to 1994 was 23.1%. Of note, the number of participants with the metabolic syndrome consistently increased with age and BMI. For example, the prevalence was 6.7% for people ages 20–29 years and greater than 40% for people over age 60. This study also demonstrated a substantial risk for Mexican Americans, for whom the prevalence was over 30%.

The NHANES IV (1999–2000) data showed an increased prevalence of 31.0% for the metabolic syndrome (Ford et al. 2004). The more conservative definition of glucose intolerance (≥100 mg/dL) used in the NHANES 1999–2000 study was responsible for about five percentage points of the increase—that is, the age-adjusted prevalence was 27% when the original NCEP-ATP III definition of glucose intolerance (≥110 mg/dL) was used. The age-adjusted prevalence increased by 23.5% (P=0.021) in women and 2.2% (P=0.831) in men. This dramatic change in women participants was due to increases in abdominal obesity, hypertension, and hypertriglyceridemia. Figure 2–1 depicts the changes in the individual components of the metabolic syndrome between the total groups as well as between men and women specifically in the two NHANES studies, NHANES III and NHANES IV. The data from these two studies indicate that the groups who are most vulnerable to the metabolic syndrome include the elderly, persons with BMIs of 25 or greater, Mexican Americans, and women (Table 2–2).

Psychiatric patients, including individuals diagnosed with schizophrenia, bipolar disorder, or major depression, may have a much higher chance of developing the metabolic syndrome (Figure 2–2). A recent report by McEvoy et al. (2005) used data from the Clinical Antipsychotic Trials of Intervention Effectiveness (CATIE) Schizophrenia Trial to assess the prevalence of the metabolic syndrome, as defined by the NCEP, in schizophrenic patients. The overall rate of occurrence was 40.9% (51.6% for women; 36.0% for men). Males in the CATIE study were 138% more likely to have the metabolic syndrome when compared with matched NHANES participants. Women in the CATIE group were 251% more likely to develop the syndrome when compared with matched NHANES participants. A recent study evaluated the presence of the metabolic syndrome in a group of patients with bipolar disorder (Fagiolini et al. 2005). Data were collected from 171 participants consecutively entering the Bipolar Disorder Center for Pennsylvanians protocol between 2003 and 2004. The study focused on the presence of the metabolic syndrome as defined by the NCEP-ATP III. Thirty

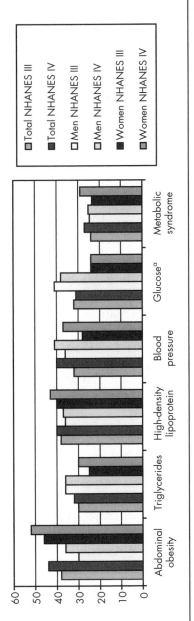

FIGURE 2–1. Age-adjusted prevalence of individual metabolic components of the metabolic syndrome among adults in the United States: National Health and Nutrition Examination Survey (NHANES) III (1988–1994) and NHANES IV (1999–2000).

[a]High fasting glucose ≥ 100 mg/dL or medication use.

Source. Adapted from Ford et al. 2004.

TABLE 2–2.   Risk groups associated with increased odds of
the metabolic syndrome

Age

Higher body mass index (≥25)

Women

Mexican American ethnicity

Postmenopausal status

Current smoking

Low household income

High carbohydrate intake

No alcohol consumption

Physical inactivity

Note.   National Health and Nutrition Examination Survey (NHANES) III (1988–
1994) and NHANES IV (1999–2000) data.
Source.   Adapted from Ford et al. 2002, 2004; Park et al. 2003.

percent of the sample met the NCEP-ATP III criteria, indicating that the metabolic syndrome is as alarmingly prevalent in patients with bipolar disorder as it is
in the general population. Depression is associated with the metabolic syndrome
as well, at least in females. In a population sample (*N*=3,003) of individuals who
underwent a medical examination and completed the depression module from
the Diagnostic Interview Schedule, Kinder et al. (2004) found that women with
a history of major depressive episode were twice as likely to have the metabolic
syndrome as those with no history of depression. This relationship remained the
same even after adjustment for age, race, education, smoking, physical inactivity,
carbohydrate consumption, and alcohol use.

CLINICAL SIGNIFICANCE

Even with the lack of a universally accepted definition for the metabolic syndrome,
there is a wealth of well-designed studies that indicate patients with this syndrome
are at increased risk for premature death as well as the development of CAD and
diabetes. Individuals with the metabolic syndrome also are susceptible to other
conditions, notably polycystic ovary syndrome, fatty liver, cholesterol gallstones,
asthma, sleep disturbances, and some forms of cancer (Grundy et al. 2004b). Girman et al. (2004) conducted two large clinical trials that showed patients with the
metabolic syndrome have a 50% increased chance of having a major coronary
event when compared with those without the syndrome. After adjusting for age,
cholesterol level, and smoking, Hu et al. (2004) found that nondiabetic patients
with the metabolic syndrome had an increased risk for all-cause death—mainly
from CAD. Lakka and colleagues followed middle-aged Finnish men with no base-

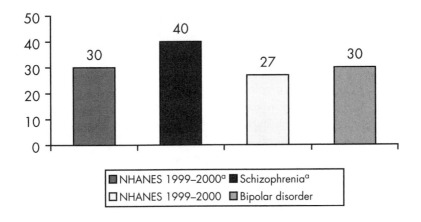

FIGURE 2–2. Prevalence of the metabolic syndrome in mental health populations compared with National Health and Nutrition Examination Survey IV (1999–2000).

[a]Reflects modified National Cholesterol Education Program–Adult Treatment Panel III definition using a fasting glucose cutoff of 100 mg/dL or more.

Source. Fagiolini et al. 2005; Ford et al. 2004; McEvoy et al. 2005.

line diabetes or CAD for more than 11 years. The authors reported a two- to three-fold increase in cardiovascular mortality among patients with the metabolic syndrome as defined by the NCEP-ATP III and WHO (Lakka et al. 2002). Data from the NHANES III also showed a higher prevalence of CAD among people with the metabolic syndrome compared with those without the diagnosis. This result was even more pronounced when diabetes was present (Ford et al. 2002).

People with the metabolic syndrome also have an increased all-cause (cardiac- and noncardiac-related) mortality rate. Men in the Kuopio Ischemic Heart Disease Risk Factor Study met WHO criteria for metabolic syndrome and were followed for more than 13 consecutive years (Lakka et al. 2002). At the end of the study, patients with the metabolic syndrome had a 16% mortality rate, and those without the syndrome had a mortality rate of 10%. A study done by Isomaa et al. (2001) in Sweden and Finland demonstrated a similar difference, with mortality rates of 18% and 4.6% for those with the metabolic syndrome and those without, respectively.

Although many of the studies in this area have been done with men, similar results are found in women. Ridker et al. (2003) monitored 14,719 healthy (without diabetes or CAD) female participants from the Women's Health Study over an 8-year period. Patients with the metabolic syndrome had a 2.5-fold increase in risk of cardiovascular events when compared with those without the metabolic syndrome. In this case, a commonly used marker for increased inflammation, C-reactive protein, added predictive value when cardiovascular risk was being assessed.

Psychiatric patients are at high risk for the development of the metabolic syndrome, CAD, and diabetes, with resultant increased overall mortality. Patients with schizophrenia have a 20% shorter life span than the general population (Casey 2005). Similarly, people with mood disorders have high standardized mortality rates (higher by a factor of 2.0 for bipolar disorder and 1.6 for depressed patients; Osby et al. 2001). Unfortunately, the quality of preventive medical care for psychiatric patients is generally poor, because they often have limited access to primary care practitioners and therefore are less likely to be screened for common "silent diseases" such as hypertension, dyslipidemia, diabetes, and CAD (Druss and Rosenheck 1998; Druss et al. 2002).

There are numerous studies indicating high rates of glucose dysregulation, insulin resistance, central obesity, and CAD in patients with schizophrenia. These conditions persist both in patients taking antipsychotic medications and in psychotropic-naïve patients. As early as 1879, Sir Henry Maudsley wrote in his book *The Pathology of Mind*, "Diabetes is a disease which often shows itself in families in which insanity prevails" (Holt et al. 2004). In recent times, many studies have shown that glucose intolerance and diabetes are increased by a factor of two to three in patients with schizophrenia. Ryan et al. (2003) found that first-episode psychotropic-naïve patients with schizophrenia had a higher prevalence of impaired fasting glucose, higher insulin resistance, and increased levels of insulin concentration when compared with nonschizophrenic control subjects. Another study that used computed tomography found that psychotropic drug–naïve schizophrenic patients had more than three times as much visceral or intraabdominal fat when compared with matched control subjects (Thakore et al. 2002). Patients who take atypical antipsychotics have increased risk for the development of prediabetes, diabetes, and dyslipidemia. This discovery resulted in well-defined, strict guidelines used to decrease the onset of metabolic abnormalities within this patient population (American Diabetes Association 2004a).

There is also evidence of increased metabolic anomalies and central obesity in patients with major depressive disorder. Three large, randomized studies showed that depressive symptoms can predict a future diagnosis of diabetes (Arroyo et al. 2004; Eaton et al. 1996; Golden et al. 2004). Many depressed patients (particularly those with sedentary lifestyles) have increased central obesity. One small study involving antidepressant-naïve depressed women showed increased visceral fat on computed tomography scans compared with nondepressed control subjects (Thakore et al. 1997).

Patients with major depressive disorder often have elevated proinflammatory markers, including C-reactive protein, tumor necrosis factor, interleukin-1, and white blood cell count (Ford and Erlinger 2004; Panagiotakos et al. 2004; Penninx et al. 2003). It is postulated that the increase in visceral obesity seen in depressed people is largely responsible for the release of these markers as well as many others. This heightened proinflammatory state is likely to be at least partially responsible for the two- to fourfold increase in mortality found with depressed patients after a myocardial infarction (Frasure-Smith et al. 1993; Ladwig et al. 1991).

A CRITICAL APPRAISAL

In September 2005, the American Diabetes Association and the European Association for the Study of Diabetes published a joint statement questioning the clinical significance of the metabolic syndrome (Kahn et al. 2005). Specifically, this report suggested that "providers should avoid labeling patients with the term metabolic syndrome, as this might create the impression that the metabolic syndrome denotes a greater risk than its components, or that it is more serious than other cardiovascular disease (CVD) risk factors, or that the underlying pathophysiology is clear" (p. 2299). In addition to the lack of a clearly defined and universally accepted definition for this syndrome, two other key issues regarding its clinical utility include 1) whether the construct of the metabolic syndrome is useful in predicting CAD risk relative to the widely used Framingham risk score and 2) whether the treatment of the syndrome differs from the treatment of its individual components.

An ICD-9 diagnosis of the metabolic syndrome is generally thought to be useful as a predictor for CAD and diabetes as well as an increasingly popular means to increase awareness of risk for cardiac disease. Although the recent increased presence of the metabolic syndrome in the medical literature is evident, the predictive quality of this syndrome relative to other established assessment tools is debatable. Stern et al. (2004) followed 1,709 nondiabetic San Antonio Heart Study patients over a 7.5-year period and 1,353 nondiabetic patients from the Mexico City Diabetes Study for a 6.5-year period. All of the subjects had a diagnosis of diabetes or a cardiovascular event as their primary endpoints. When compared with the Diabetes Risk Score (DRS) in predicting a future diagnosis of diabetes in San Antonio participants, use of the metabolic syndrome resulted in a sensitivity of 66.2% and a false-positive rate of 27.8%. At this same false-positive rate, the DRS had an increased sensitivity of 75.9%. Moreover, the combined use of the DRS and the NCEP definition of the metabolic syndrome had a less favorable outcome than use of the DRS alone. Data from the Mexico City group showed similar results.

The use of the metabolic syndrome to predict cardiac ischemic events was also inferior when compared with established prediction tools. In the San Antonio Heart Study (Stern et al. 2004), the metabolic syndrome had a 67.3% sensitivity, with a specificity of 65.8%. At this same specificity, the Framingham risk score, a commonly used method to predict CAD risk, had a sensitivity of 81.4%.

In sum, it does not appear that the metabolic syndrome is more accurate than existing valid tools used to predict diabetes and cardiac ischemic events. It is also uncertain as to whether the collective CAD risk from this syndrome is greater than the sum of the individual components.

Because there is no definitive etiology for the metabolic syndrome, there is no related single treatment. Currently, treatment of the syndrome is simply directed toward treating the individual components. Those who criticize the usefulness of the metabolic syndrome diagnosis argue that prevention and treatment of the individual diseases composing the syndrome is sufficient and that there is no clinical need for the syndrome itself.

The Metabolic Tetrad

The metabolic tetrad—or core components—of the metabolic syndrome comprises glucose dysregulation, hypertension, dyslipidemia, and central obesity (predominantly visceral obesity). All of these entities are highly prevalent, easily assessed, potentially deadly, often preventable, and usually treatable. Unfortunately, commonly used definitions of the metabolic syndrome have different abnormal "cutoff points" for these components. Moreover, preventive guidelines for the individual factors are often not emphasized in the metabolic syndrome literature. The following discussion is a brief overview of current diagnostic criteria and preventive guidelines for the individual components of the metabolic tetrad.

GLUCOSE DYSREGULATION

Diabetes is no longer a risk factor for the development of CAD—it is a risk equivalent. In other words, once patients are diagnosed with diabetes, it is extremely likely they have established vascular disease (Expert Panel on Detection, Evaluation, and Treatment of High Blood Cholesterol in Adults 2001). An estimated 9% of adults in the United States have diabetes and are therefore predisposed to heart disease, cerebrovascular accidents, blindness, renal disease, and peripheral vascular disease (American Diabetes Association 2004b). Unfortunately, one-third of people with diabetes are often asymptomatic and their condition is undiagnosed.

More than 90% of patients with diabetes are free of symptoms during the early course of the disease, thus prompting the need for screening. Although no data definitively demonstrate a benefit from screening asymptomatic adults, expert consensus strongly suggests checking a fasting plasma glucose (FPG; plasma glucose collected after no caloric intake for at least 8 hours) every 3 years beginning at age 45. Patients presenting with comorbid cardiac risk factors or a history of polycystic ovary disease, first-degree relatives with diabetes, habitual inactivity, or impaired FPG (100–125 mg/dL) should be screened at an earlier age and on a more frequent schedule (American Diabetes Association 2004b).

Like other risk assessments for cardiac disease, recent changes in diagnostic criteria for diabetes now include patients who were once deemed to be in the "normal" range and free from disease. There are three ways to diagnose diabetes, but only the measurement of an FPG is recommended for asymptomatic patients, because it is cost-effective and generally more convenient. An FPG of less than 100 mg/dL is normal, and a value of 100–125 mg/dL is consistent with prediabetes or impaired fasting glucose. If a patient has an FPG of 126 mg/dL or more, then a provisional diagnosis of diabetes is made and a follow-up test on another day must be done to confirm the diagnosis (American Diabetes Association 2004b). Of note, an elevated hemoglobin A_{1c} level is used to measure the effectiveness of treatment over a 3-month period prior to the test and should not be used to establish a diagnosis of diabetes.

Psychiatrists should closely monitor patients who have treated or untreated schizophrenia, because studies have shown that the prevalence of diabetes is increased up to three times in those with schizophrenia relative to the general population (Holt et al. 2004). Also, the use of atypical antipsychotics carries an increased risk for the development of both hyperlipidemia and glucose dysregulation. In addition to the diabetes screening guidelines discussed, patients who are on any atypical antipsychotic medication should have a fasting glucose level checked before initiation of the medication, again at week 12, and annually thereafter (American Diabetes Association 2004a).

HYPERTENSION

Hypertension is an important part of the metabolic syndrome, because 50 million Americans have this mainly asymptomatic but potentially deadly disorder. Although awareness and treatment for hypertension has increased since the late 1970s, the number of adults with "controlled" blood pressure (<140/90 mm Hg) is only 35% (Chobanian et al. 2003). The seventh report of the Joint National Committee on Prevention, Detection, Evaluation, and Treatment of High Blood Pressure (Chobanian et al. 2003) stressed the fact that normalizing blood pressure can reduce the incidence of stroke and myocardial infarction by 35% and 25%, respectively. Additionally, the report showed that even individuals who are normotensive at age 55 have a 90% chance of eventually developing hypertension.

These findings prompted the committee to change the standard of care for diagnosing hypertension. Currently, normal blood pressure is a systolic pressure less than 120 mm Hg and a diastolic pressure less than 80 mm Hg. The category of "prehypertension" was introduced and defined as a systolic blood pressure of 120–139 mm Hg or a diastolic blood pressure of 80–89 mm Hg (Table 2–3). According to the U.S. Preventive Services Task Force (McTigue et al. 2003), there is clear evidence to support the measurement of blood pressure during a medical evaluation at least every 2 years. A diagnosis of hypertension should be made after

TABLE 2–3. Joint National Committee on Prevention, Detection, Evaluation, and Treatment of High Blood Pressure VII definitions and management of hypertension for adults age 18 or older

Blood pressure classification	Systolic BP, mm Hg[a]		Diastolic BP, mm Hg[a]	Lifestyle modification	Initial drug therapy	
					Without compelling indication	With compelling indications
Normal	<120	and	<80	Encourage		
Prehypertension	120–139	or	80–89	Yes	No antihypertensive drug indicated	Drug(s) for the compelling indications[b]
Stage 1 hypertension	140–159	or	90–99	Yes	Thiazide-type diuretics for most; may consider ACE inhibitor, angiotensin receptor blocker, β-blocker, calcium channel blocker, or combination	Drug(s) for the compelling indications Other antihypertensive drugs (diuretics, ACE inhibitor, angiotensin receptor blocker, β-blocker, calcium channel blocker) as needed
Stage 2 hypertension	≥160	or	≥100	Yes	Two-drug combination for most (usually thiazide-type diuretic and ACE inhibitor, angiotensin receptor blocker, β-blocker, or calcium channel blocker)[c]	Drug(s) for the compelling indications Other antihypertensive drugs (diuretics, ACE inhibitor, angiotensin receptor blocker, β-blocker, calcium channel blocker) as needed

Note. ACE=angiotensin-converting enzyme; BP=blood pressure.
[a]Treatment determined by highest blood pressure category. [b]Treat patients with chronic kidney disease or diabetes to blood pressure goal of less than 130/80 mm Hg. [c]Initial combined therapy should be used cautiously in those at risk for orthostatic hypotension.
Source. Chobanian et al. 2003.

two abnormal readings on separate office visits. If unable to measure blood pressure in the office setting, psychiatrists should provide referrals for primary medical care and, at minimum, encourage their patients to monitor blood pressure using reliable over-the-counter measuring devices.

DYSLIPIDEMIA

In terms of decreasing morbidity related to the metabolic syndrome, dyslipidemia is one of the most important modifiable risk factors. The role of aggressive primary preventive measures, involving lifestyle changes with diet and exercise as well as use of lipid-lowering agents, is indisputable. For example, every 10% reduction in serum cholesterol results in a 10%–15% drop in cardiovascular-related mortality (Gould et al. 1998). Data from the large, prospective Framingham heart study showed a 25% increase in myocardial infarctions with each decrease in HDL by 5 mg/dL below the age-based median for men and women (Gordon et al. 1977). Moreover, an elevated serum triglyceride level (>150 mg/dL) not only is a clear indicator for the future development of CAD but also increases the likelihood of an abnormally low HDL.

Elevated low-density lipoprotein (LDL) cholesterol is the other major lipid marker for CAD risk. For every 30-mg/dL change in LDL, the relative risk for CAD is changed proportionately by 30% (Grundy et al. 2004b). The NCEP-ATP III emphasized this problem by classifying LDL as the "primary target of cholesterol lowering therapy," with the suggestion that the therapeutic goal for "very high risk" patients should be lowered from less than 100 mg/dL to less than 70 mg/dL. Interestingly, most of the commonly used definitions of the metabolic syndrome do not include total cholesterol or LDL as part of the diagnostic criteria.

The diagnosis of lipid abnormalities is fairly straightforward (Expert Panel on Detection, Evaluation, and Treatment of High Blood Cholesterol in Adults 2001). Serum cholesterol is within normal limits at a level of less than 200 mg/dL. HDL is normal at levels greater than 40 mg/dL and cardioprotective when greater than 60 mg/dL. Patients with less than one risk factor for CAD have a goal LDL level of less than 160 mg/dL. Any history of diabetes, symptomatic carotid artery disease, peripheral vascular disease, CAD, or abdominal aortic aneurysm will lower the therapeutic goal to less than 100 mg/dL, with the optional goal of less than 70 mg/dL. Those who have intermediate risk have a target goal of less than 130 mg/dL. Secondary causes of dyslipidemia, such as hypothyroidism, must be considered before starting lipid-lowering medications.

Although many recommendations for cholesterol screening exist, it is best to check a fasting lipid profile or serum cholesterol, LDL, HDL, and triglyceride levels beginning at age 20 and about every 5 years thereafter (Expert Panel on Detection, Evaluation, and Treatment of High Blood Cholesterol in Adults 2001). If the patient has intermediate or high risk for CAD or is being treated for dyslipidemia, the frequency of monitoring should increase and be based on clinical judgment.

OBESITY

Obesity is defined as excess body fat relative to lean body mass. The best indicator of obesity is the BMI. Obesity is currently defined as a BMI of 30 kg/m^2 or greater; BMI of 25–29.9 kg/m^2 is considered overweight. More than 30% of adults in the United States are now obese, with about 65% of adults being either obese or overweight (McTigue et al. 2003).

Obesity is an independent risk factor for heart disease and is associated with type 2 diabetes, hypertension, stroke, hyperlipidemia, osteoarthritis, sleep apnea, and increased death rates for most cancers. Central obesity, as defined by a large waist circumference or high waist-to-hip ratio, is felt to represent visceral adiposity (see Figure 2–3). Central obesity and visceral fat have been associated with increased cardiovascular risk as compared with noncentral obesity (McTigue et al. 2003). A pattern of upper-body obesity is more strongly associated with insulin resistance and the metabolic syndrome than is lower-body obesity (Grundy et al. 2005).

Thus obesity plays a central role in many features of the metabolic syndrome, and BMI or waist circumference is a part of the diagnostic criteria for metabolic syndrome. It is clear, however, that non-obese patients can also develop metabolic syndrome, so obesity alone is only one of multiple factors influencing the development of the syndrome.

Pathogenesis

The pathogenesis of the metabolic syndrome is complex, poorly understood, and based almost entirely on theory. Although much is known about the individual components composing the syndrome, it is unclear whether all entities are mechanistically related. The complicated interaction between metabolically active visceral adipose tissue and resultant insulin resistance is the most widely accepted theory and is discussed briefly here (see Figure 2–4).

The presence of visceral obesity is thought to be atherogenic due to increased lipolysis and release of nonesterified FFAs. The elevated hepatic and plasma FFA concentrations result in abnormal gluconeogenesis or glucose dysregulation. Also, the increased levels of FFAs can increase vasoconstriction and increase systemic blood pressure. Other by-products of lipolysis include proinflammatory markers that damage the vascular system, such as angiotensinogen, adipsin, adiponectin, leptin, interleukin-6, and tumor necrosis factor–α (TNF-α) (Fernandez-Real and Ricart 2003; Sutherland et al. 2004; Weisberg et al. 2003). In addition to causing direct endothelial dysfunction, TNF-α also decreases the activity of lipoprotein lipase, which causes atherogenic dyslipoproteinemia or elevated triglycerides, decreased HDL, and pathologically small LDL particle size.

Measuring the waist: To define the level at which waist circumference is measured: the patient stands, and the clinician palpates the upper hip bone to locate the iliac crest. Just above the uppermost lateral border of the iliac crest, a horizontal mark is drawn, then crossed with a vertical mark on the midaxillary line. The measuring tape is placed in a horizontal plane around the abdomen at the level of this marked point and is parallel to the floor; it is snug but does not compress the skin. The measurement is made at a normal respiration.

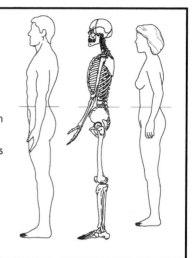

FIGURE 2–3.   Instructions for measuring waist circumference.
Source.   U.S. Department of Health and Human Services 1996.

As visceral obesity increases, so does the likelihood of developing insulin resistance. An insulin-resistant state will worsen proinflammatory lipolysis, blood pressure, and lipid metabolism. Like TNF-α, insulin resistance decreases lipoprotein lipase activity and results in dyslipidemia, with a heightened risk for CAD. Also, hyperinsulinemia increases renal sodium reabsorption as well as the activity of the sympathetic nervous system, which can increase blood pressure. As resistance to insulin progresses, insulin loses its ability to effect vasodilation, which can further increase blood pressure.

Management of the Metabolic Syndrome

The greatest risk to patients with the metabolic syndrome is vascular-related diseases, including fatal and nonfatal stroke and coronary heart disease. Thus the primary goal of managing the metabolic syndrome is to reduce the risk of these events. Given the multiple manifestations of metabolic syndrome, it is no surprise that its treatment is also multifaceted. Treating all CAD risk factors that a patient may have (hypertension, diabetes, dyslipidemia, obesity, and cigarette abuse) is a cornerstone of therapy. In patients with the metabolic syndrome who have not yet developed diabetes, some interventions prevent its development. In addition, some interventions can resolve metabolic syndrome (see Table 2–4).

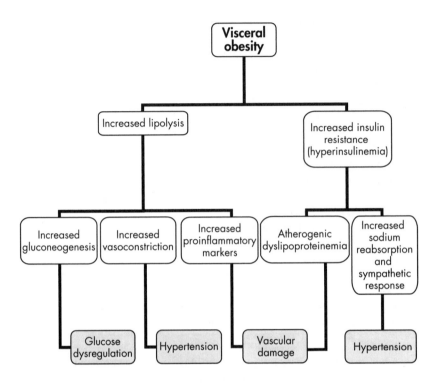

FIGURE 2–4. Theoretical pathogenesis explaining the metabolic syndrome.

GLUCOSE DYSREGULATION

Many patients with the metabolic syndrome will eventually have some type of glucose intolerance or diabetes. Intensive glucose control is proven to reduce microvascular complications of diabetes (retinopathy, neuropathy, and nephropathy) and may also decrease cardiovascular events (Diabetes Control and Complications Trial Research Group 1993; Selvin et al. 2004; U.K. Prospective Diabetes Study Group 1998). For most patients with diabetes, the main goal of glucose control is a glycosylated hemoglobin A_{1c} level less than 7.0 mg/dL. Other secondary goals are to have a preprandial plasma glucose of 90–130 mg/dL and 1- to 2-hour postprandial glucose of less than 180 mg/dL (American Diabetes Association 2005). The hemoglobin A_{1c} level is generally monitored every 3–4 months.

Lifestyle modification is a key therapy of diabetes, including diet, regular exercise, and weight loss. To actively participate in any treatment plan, patients with diabetes must be educated about their condition. Diabetes educators are ex-

TABLE 2–4. Treatment goals for patients with metabolic syndrome

Blood pressure	
Without diabetes or chronic kidney disease	<140/90 mm Hg
With diabetes or chronic kidney disease	<130/90 mm Hg
Lipids	
Primary target: low-density lipoprotein	
High-risk[a]	<100 mg/dL
Moderate-risk[b]	<130 mg/dL
Low-risk[c]	<160 mg/dL
Secondary target: Non-high-density lipoprotein	
Triglycerides	<150 mg/dL
High-density lipoprotein	>45 mg/dL
Diabetes	
Hemoglobin A_{1c}	<7.0 mg/dL
Preprandial glucose	90–130 mg/dL
1- to 2-hour postprandial glucose	<180 mg/dL
Obesity	
Reduce body weight 7%–10% in first year	
Achieve body mass index less than 25 kg/m²	
Exercise	
Brisk exercise for at least 30 minutes most days of the week	
Diet	
Reduce saturated and trans fats, cholesterol, and simple sugars	
Increase consumption of fruits, vegetables, and whole grains	
Consider Mediterranean diet	
Other	
Smoking cessation	
Consideration of low-dose aspirin prophylaxis	

[a]High-risk: patients with established cardiovascular disease, diabetes, or 10-year coronary heart disease risk greater than 20%.
[b]Moderate-risk: patients with two or more cardiac risk factors (10-year risk for coronary heart disease 20% or less).
[c]Low-risk: no or one cardiac risk factor (10-year coronary heart disease risk less than 10%).

cellent resources in this regard. Individualized nutrition therapy with a registered dietician should be offered to all patients.

When lifestyle changes alone are ineffective, patients with type 2 diabetes are usually treated with oral agents. First-line drugs are metformin or sulfonylureas, but thiazolidinediones (pioglitazone, rosiglitazone) are also an option. Combination

therapy is often needed to achieve treatment goals. If oral agents alone are not sufficient, insulin therapy is often added to or substituted for the oral hypoglycemic
agents (American Diabetes Association 2004b).

Monitoring for complications of diabetes and preventive care are critical ele-
ments of diabetes care. Patients are monitored for nephropathy (urine micro-
albumin), retinopathy (dilated ophthalmoscopic examination), and peripheral
neuropathy (monofilament testing) annually. All diabetic patients should receive
a pneumococcal vaccine and an annual influenza vaccine.

Aggressive treatment of other cardiovascular risk factors is also warranted, and
lower blood pressure and LDL cholesterol goals are recommended as mentioned
earlier. The LDL cholesterol goal for diabetics is less than 100 mg/dL. Even in
patients with a baseline LDL less than 100 mg/dL, two studies have shown that
therapy with statins reduces cardiovascular events regardless of the starting LDL
value (Colhoun et al. 2005; Heart Protection Study Collaborative Group 2003).

Patients with the metabolic syndrome who have impaired glucose tolerance
but do not meet criteria for the diagnosis of diabetes should focus primarily on
lifestyle modification, particularly weight reduction and increased exercise. This
has been shown to reduce the development of type 2 diabetes and cause regression of the metabolic syndrome (Orchard et al. 2005). Metformin, thiazolidinediones, and acarbose have also lowered the risk of type 2 diabetes in patients with
the metabolic syndrome, but no data exist on whether this approach lessens cardiovascular risks (Grundy et al. 2005).

Hypertension

Treating hypertension reduces the risk of future cardiovascular events, especially
stroke and myocardial infarction (Chobanian et al. 2003). Lifestyle modification
is a core component of therapy and can often control blood pressure in patients
with mild hypertension. Maintaining a normal weight or reducing weight, keep-
ing sodium intake low (<2 g/day), increasing physical activity, and reducing alcohol consumption (two or fewer drinks per day for men, one for women) have all
been shown to cause modest reductions in blood pressure. In addition, a diet rich
in fresh fruits and vegetables, low-fat dairy products, and low fat and saturated fat
has been shown to be beneficial for patients with hypertension (Chobanian et al.
2003).

Many patients with hypertension require pharmacological agents in addition
to lifestyle modifications to achieve adequate control, and two-thirds will need
more than one agent. Usual first-line agents include thiazide-type diuretics, beta-
blockers, calcium channel blockers, and angiotensin-converting enzyme inhibitors.
Certain comorbid conditions (e.g., diabetes, renal disease, CAD) may compel the
use of certain agents over others. In addition, the Joint National Committee on
Prevention, Detection, Evaluation, and Treatment of High Blood Pressure guidelines recommend that patients with stage 2 hypertension (systolic pressure ≥160

mm Hg or diastolic pressure ≥ 100 mm Hg) begin taking two drugs in combination, one of which should usually be a thiazide-type diuretic (Chobanian et al. 2003).

Dyslipidemia

Treatment of hyperlipidemia for primary or secondary prevention reduces risk for CAD and related mortality (Expert Panel on Detection, Evaluation, and Treatment of High Blood Cholesterol in Adults 2001). The current NCEP-ATP III guidelines have different lipid goals based on underlying risk for CAD. LDL cholesterol is the primary target in clinical lipid management, whereas low HDL and high triglycerides are secondary targets.

Lifestyle modification is a key component of the therapy of lipid disorders. A diet low in saturated fats and high in fiber is recommended for all patients, as is regular exercise. Smoking cessation can also raise HDL levels and independently lower overall CAD risk. Dietary therapy alone usually reduces LDL levels by 20%–30%. As such, many patients need pharmacological treatment in addition to lifestyle changes to reach treatment goals. Many pharmacological agents can be used in clinical lipid management. The choice of medication depends on the treatment goal, potential adverse side effects (especially with combinations of agents), and potential important drug–drug interactions.

The primary target is LDL cholesterol. Many patients with the metabolic syndrome will already have diabetes or underlying coronary, cerebral, or peripheral vascular disease. Such patients are considered at high risk for cardiovascular events, and the LDL goal is less than 100 mg/dL, although patients with high-risk CAD may benefit from an LDL goal of less than 70 mg/dL (Grundy et al. 2004b). The LDL goals of all other patients are assessed based upon their estimated 10-year risk of cardiovascular events, which is determined by the individual patient clinical profile.

The first-line agents to lower the LDL cholesterol are 3-hydroxy-3-methylglutaryl coenzyme A (HMG-CoA) reductase inhibitors, or statins, because they have proven to reduce cardiovascular events and death in patients with hyperlipidemia in both primary and secondary prevention trials. These agents reduce LDL by 25%–35% when used at standard dosages. They have a more modest effect on lowering triglycerides and raising HDL, although the more potent agents, atorvastatin and rosuvastatin, have greater triglyceride-lowering effects. All statins are metabolized by the cytochrome P450 system, but there are differences in the isoenzyme that each drug utilizes, which can have important impact on drug–drug interactions The main adverse effects of statins are hepatotoxicity and myopathy, including rhabdomyolysis (Bellosta et al. 2004).

Niacin can improve LDL, lower triglycerides, and increase HDL. It is often relegated to a second choice after statins due to its poor tolerance by patients, especially paroxysms of fascial flushing. Niacin can also increase serum glucose levels, which may be problematic for patients with the metabolic syndrome. Bile acid sequestrants such as cholestyramine are efficacious when used in combination with statins but suffer from poor patient tolerance and potential interruption of absorption of other medications if the timing of dosing is incorrect. Lastly, a newer agent, ezetimibe, can be used as monotherapy to lower LDL in patients unable to tolerate statins and/or niacin. More commonly, ezetimibe is combined with statins to achieve LDL goals when statins alone are not effective.

Many patients achieve LDL goals with statin or niacin therapy alone but have persistent abnormalities of two key components of the metabolic syndrome, triglycerides and HDL. In addition to regularly scheduled exercise, treatment options include an increased statin dose or the addition of a second agent that targets triglycerides and HDL, particularly niacin or fibrates. Combining fibrates and statins increases the risk of myopathy. Fenofibrate has fewer pharmacological interactions with statins than gemfibrozil (Rubins et al. 1999) and seems to have less risk of myopathy when used in combination. Thus, fenofibrate should be the preferred fibrate when used in combination with other agents (Grundy et al. 2004b). The combination of niacin and a statin has an increased risk of myopathy and hepatotoxicity.

Obesity

The three lifestyle risk factors for the metabolic syndrome and for CAD are an atherogenic diet, obesity, and a sedentary lifestyle. Lifestyle modifications addressing these three factors can improve every aspect of the metabolic syndrome. Thus a healthy diet, regular exercise, and weight loss (or maintaining a healthy weight if not overweight) must be a key part of the treatment plan for all patients with the metabolic syndrome (see Chapter 3, "Severe Mental Illness and Obesity, this volume).

Nutrition.   The typical diet in the United States is generally high in calories, fat, saturated fats, and cholesterol, which are associated with increased cardiac events. The NCEP-ATP III guidelines recommend the Therapeutic Lifestyle Changes (TLC) Diet for patients with the metabolic syndrome. This diet is low in saturated fats, trans fats, cholesterol, and simple sugars, with suggested increased consumption of fruits, vegetables, and whole grains. Patients should be referred to registered dieticians to get individualized diet counseling. When necessary, this counseling can target multiple dietary goals that often exist in patients with the metabolic syndrome, including lipid lowering, weight reduction, and/or blood pressure control.

There is evidence that a Mediterranean-style diet may also prevent the metabolic syndrome. This diet includes regular helpings of fish, nuts, low-fat dairy products, fruits, vegetables, legumes, and whole grains. Fats are not restricted as long as they emphasize vegetable oils that are low in saturated fats and partially hydrogenated oils (e.g., canola and olive oils). The Mediterranean diet reduces cardiac mortality and cardiac events after myocardial infarction. This particular diet has also been associated with lower blood pressure, improved lipid profiles, lower homocysteine levels, decreased risk of thrombosis, improved insulin resistance, and improved endothelial function (de Lorgeril et al. 1999; Panagiotakos and Polychronopoulos 2005). When compared with a low-fat diet in patients with metabolic syndrome, the Mediterranean diet has also been shown to improve measures of inflammation, insulin resistance, endothelial function, and weight (Esposito et al. 2004). Patients with the metabolic syndrome who eat a Mediterranean diet also had resolution of the syndrome more frequently (56%) than did those eating a low-fat diet (13%) (Esposito et al. 2004).

There has been recent interest in high-protein, low-carbohydrate diets for weight reduction. Although studies do show weight reduction with these diets, data on long-term maintenance is lacking. Such diets also tend to be higher in fat and lack fruits, vegetables, and whole grains, which may adversely impact CAD risk. Thus these diets are not currently recommended specifically for treatment of the metabolic syndrome (Grundy et al. 2005).

Exercise.   Regular exercise can lower weight, improve the lipid profile (especially in lowering triglycerides and raising HDL), improve blood pressure control, reduce visceral fat and abdominal obesity, and improve insulin resistance. Of course, this also results in a significant decrease in risk for the development of CAD and diabetes.

It is recommended that all patients with the metabolic syndrome maintain a regular exercise regimen with moderate physical activity most days of the week. Current recommendations are for 30 minutes or more of moderate-intensity exercise most, if not all, days of the week (Thompson et al. 2003). More exercise leads to greater benefits, particularly with regard to weight management. This must be tailored to each patient, taking into account age and comorbid conditions such as coronary heart disease, and some high-risk patients will need exercise testing before starting such a program. Examples of brisk activity include brisk walking for 30–40 minutes, swimming laps for 20 minutes, basketball for 15–20 minutes, heavy housecleaning, dancing for 30 minutes, or golfing (carrying clubs or pulling a cart) (Expert Panel on Detection, Evaluation, and Treatment of High Blood Cholesterol in Adults 2001).

Lifestyle modification programs.   Complete lifestyle modification programs that specifically address diet, exercise, and weight reduction have also been evaluated. The Diabetes Prevention Program evaluated 3,234 persons (1,171 participants met the criteria for the metabolic syndrome at the study onset) with impaired glucose tolerance and obesity (Orchard et al. 2005). They were randomly assigned to either intensive lifestyle intervention, designed to achieve and maintain a 7% weight loss and 150 minutes of exercise per week, or no intensive program. For those patients with the metabolic syndrome at the study onset who received the intensive lifestyle intervention, 38% no longer met the criteria for the metabolic syndrome at 3 years, versus only 18% in the placebo group. For all of the patients the lifestyle intervention reduced the incidence of type 2 diabetes by 58% as compared with patients in the placebo group (Knowler et al. 2002). Other trials of patients with impaired glucose tolerance found similar benefits with lifestyle modification programs for preventing diabetes (Lindstrom et al. 2003; Pan et al. 1997).

Medication.   Pharmacological treatment of obesity may be offered to obese patients who have failed to reach weight goals with diet and exercise alone. Options include sibutramine, orlistat, phentermine, diethylpropion, fluoxetine, and bupropion. The choice depends on the side-effect profile of the drugs and patient characteristics. Weight loss achieved with these agents is usually modest (<5 kg at 1 year), and often the weight is regained after the medication is stopped. Although these agents have not been specifically examined in patients with the metabolic syndrome, similar amounts of weight loss in other patient groups have shown improved lipid profiles and blood pressure control and decreased progression to diabetes in obese patients with impaired glucose tolerance (Snow et al. 2005).

Surgery.   Weight reduction surgery can also be a successful obesity treatment but can have significant side effects. Recent guidelines recommend that it be considered for patients with a BMI of 40 kg/m^2 or greater who have failed an adequate lifestyle modification program and who have obesity-related comorbid conditions (i.e., hypertension, diabetes, impaired glucose tolerance, hyperlipidemia, obstructive sleep apnea) (Snow et al. 2005). Surgical weight loss can lead to dramatic improvements in obese patients with the metabolic syndrome. In one study, 337 patients who had the metabolic syndrome and underwent laparoscopic weight reduction surgery had a cure rate of the metabolic syndrome of 96% at 1 year after a mean weight loss of 38 kg (Lee et al. 2004).

In general, an initial goal for weight loss in overweight or obese patients with the metabolic syndrome is 7%–10% over 6–12 months. To produce a 1-lb weight loss per week, a 500 kcal/day deficit is necessary. Although some recommendations to reach this goal are simple (e.g., avoid nondiet sodas, candy bars, and fast foods and reduce portion sizes), working with a clinical nutritionist to develop a specific dietary plan with the patient and family is very helpful. Exercise is also a key component of any weight loss program.

Other Cardiovascular Risk Reduction

All patients with the metabolic syndrome should be counseled to quit smoking, which dramatically reduces cardiovascular-related morbidity. Intensive smoking cessation programs are the most effective, but nicotine replacement and sustained-release bupropion are also effective treatments. Patients at moderate or high risk for CAD should also consider taking cardioprotective low-dose aspirin every day.

Future Considerations

The lack of a universally accepted definition of the metabolic syndrome with an evidenced-based rationale for some abnormal thresholds is clearly a central problem when it comes to utilizing the syndrome in clinical practice. For example, the Joint National Committee on Prevention, Detection, Evaluation, and Treatment of High Blood Pressure (Chobanian et al. 2003) has provided commonly used guidelines for diagnosing abnormal blood pressure. With regard to establishing metabolic syndrome–related hypertension, both the NCEP and WHO criteria deviate not only from each other but from the criteria of the Joint National Committee as well. Further research and consensus on this issue will help practitioners better understand the role of the metabolic syndrome.

At this time, it is unclear whether there is a common mechanistic link for all the individual components of the metabolic syndrome, and thus there is no distinct treatment for this syndrome, per se, which further clouds the clinical utility of a metabolic syndrome diagnosis. Is the primary role of the metabolic syndrome to assess risk for cardiovascular disease and diabetes? If so, valid tools for these purposes already exist. Also, should other established risk factors such as family history of CAD, LDL, and cigarette smoking be included in the diagnostic criteria with the intent of optimizing estimates of future CAD risk? It may be less confusing to just diagnose and treat each of the syndrome components instead of labeling a select group of risk factors as "the metabolic syndrome." Future research will likely sharpen our understanding of the underlying pathology and interactions between the components of the metabolic syndrome, and this should help define its role in the care of our patients and guide future therapy.

KEY CLINICAL CONCEPTS

- Core components of the metabolic syndrome are glucose dysregulation, hypertension, dyslipidemia, and central obesity. This constellation of metabolic disturbances was first described in the medical literature in the 1920s, and the rate appears to be increasing in the U.S. population.

- The metabolic syndrome is associated with type 2 diabetes, cardiovascular disease, and increased risk for all-cause mortality as well as other physical health problems.

- Individuals with mental illness, particularly those with schizophrenia, bipolar disorder, and major depression, may be at high risk for the syndrome.

- The metabolic syndrome can be easily identified in clinical settings by using NCEP-ATP III criteria.

- Early intervention and treatment of the individual components of the metabolic syndrome has been shown to delay and decrease cardiovascular disease and the onset of type 2 diabetes.

References

Alberti KG, Zimmet PZ: Definition, diagnosis and classification of diabetes mellitus and its complications, part 1: diagnosis and classification of diabetes mellitus. Provisional report of a WHO consultation. Diabet Med 15:539–553, 1998

American Diabetes Association: Consensus development conference on antipsychotic drugs and obesity and diabetes. Diabetes Care 27:596–601, 2004a

American Diabetes Association: Screening for type 2 diabetes. Diabetes Care 27(suppl): S11–S14, 2004b

American Diabetes Association: Standards of medical care in diabetes. Diabetes Care 28 (suppl):S4–S36, 2005

American Heart Association: Heart disease and stroke statistics: 2006 update. Circulation January 11, 2006 (epub). Available at: http://circ.ahajournals.org/cgi/content/full/ 113/6/e85. Accessed October 3, 2006.

Arroyo C, Hu FB, Ryan LM, et al: Depressive symptoms and risk of type 2 diabetes in women. Diabetes Care 27:129–133, 2004

Aubert H, Frere C, Aillaud MF, et al: Weak and non-independent association between plasma TAFI antigen levels and the insulin resistance syndrome. J Thromb Haemost 1:791–797, 2003

Bellosta S, Paoletti R, Corsini A: Safety of statins: focus on clinical pharmacokinetics and drug interactions. Circulation 109(suppl):III50–III57, 2004

Casey DE: Metabolic issues and cardiovascular disease in patients with psychiatric disorders. Am J Med 118:15S–22S, 2005

Chobanian AV, Bakris GL, Black HR, et al: The seventh report of the Joint National Committee on Prevention, Detection, Evaluation, and Treatment of High Blood Pressure: the JNC VII report. JAMA 289:2560–2572, 2003

Colhoun HM, Betteridge DJ, Durrington PN, et al: Primary prevention of cardiovascular disease with atorvastatin in type 2 diabetes in the Collaborative Atorvastatin Diabetes Study (CARDS): multicentre randomized placebo-controlled trial. Lancet 364:685–696, 2005

de Lorgeril M, Salen P, Martin JL, et al: Mediterranean diet, traditional risk factors, and the rate of cardiovascular complications after myocardial infarction: final report of the Lyon Diet Heart Study. Circulation 99:779–785, 1999

Diabetes Control and Complications Trial Research Group: The effect of intensive treatment of diabetes on the development and progression of long-term complications in insulin-dependent diabetes mellitus. N Engl J Med 329:977–986, 1993

Druss B, Rosenheck R: Mental disorders and access to medical care in the United States. Am J Psychiatry 155:1775–1777, 1998

Druss BG, Rosenheck RA, Desai MM, et al: Quality of preventive medical care for patients with mental disorders. Med Care 40:129–136, 2002

Eaton WW, Armenian H, Gallo J, et al: Depression and risk for onset of type II diabetes: a prospective population-based study. Diabetes Care 19:1097–1102, 1996

Einhorn D, Reaven GM, Cobin RH, et al: American College of Endocrinology position statement on the insulin resistance syndrome. Endocr Pract 9:237–252, 2003

Esposito K, Marfella R, Ciotola M, et al: Effect of a Mediterranean-style diet on endothelial dysfunction and markers of vascular inflammation in the metabolic syndrome: a randomized trial. JAMA 292:1440–1446, 2004

Expert Panel on Detection, Evaluation, and Treatment of High Blood Cholesterol in Adults: Executive Summary of the Third Report of the National Cholesterol Education Program (NCEP) Expert Panel on Detection, Evaluation, and Treatment of High Blood Cholesterol in Adults (Adult Treatment Panel III). JAMA 285:2486–2497, 2001

Fagiolini A, Frank E, Scott JA, et al: Metabolic syndrome in bipolar disorder: findings from the Bipolar Disorder Center for Pennsylvanians. Bipolar Disord 7:424–430, 2005

Fernandez-Real JM, Ricart W: Insulin resistance and chronic cardiovascular inflammatory syndrome. Endocr Rev 24:278–301, 2003

Flegal KM, Carroll MD, Ogden CL, et al: Prevalence and trends in obesity among U.S. adults, 1999–2000. JAMA 288:1723–1727, 2002

Ford DE, Erlinger TP: Depression and C-reactive protein in U.S. adults: data from the Third National Health and Nutrition Examination Survey. Arch Intern Med 164:1010–1014, 2004

Ford ES, Giles WH, Dietz WH: Prevalence of the metabolic syndrome among U.S. adults: findings from the Third National Health and Nutrition Examination Survey. JAMA 287:356–359, 2002

Ford ES, Giles WH, Mokdad AH: Increasing prevalence of the metabolic syndrome among U.S. adults. Diabetes Care 27:2444–2449, 2004

Frasure-Smith N, Lesperance F, Talajic M: Depression following myocardial infarction: impact on 6-month survival. JAMA 270:1819–1825, 1993

Girman C, Rhodes T, Mercuri M, et al: The metabolic syndrome and risk of major coronary events in the Scandinavian Simvastatin Survival Study (4S) and the Air Force/Texas Coronary Atherosclerosis Prevention Study. Am J Cardiol 93:136–154, 2004

Golden SH, Williams JE, Ford DE, et al: Depressive symptoms and the risk of type 2 diabetes: the Atherosclerosis Risk in Communities Study. Diabetes Care 27:429–435, 2004

Gordon T, Castelli WP, Hjortland MC, et al: High density lipoprotein as a protective factor against coronary artery disease: The Framingham Study. Am J Med 62:707–714, 1977

Gould AL, Rossouw JE, Santanello NC, et al: Cholesterol reduction yields clinical benefits: impact of statin trials. Circulation 97:946–952, 1998

Grundy SM, Brewer HB, Cleeman JI, et al: Definition of metabolic syndrome: report of the National Heart, Lung, and Blood Institute/American Heart Association Conference on Scientific Issues Related to Definition. Circulation 109:433–438, 2004a

Grundy SM, Cleeman JI, Merz CN, et al: Implications of recent clinical trials for the National Cholesterol Education Program Adult Treatment Panel III Guidelines. J Am Coll Cardiol 44:720–732, 2004b

Grundy SM, Cleeman JI, Daniels SR, et al: Diagnosis and management of the metabolic syndrome. Circulation 112:2735–2752, 2005

Heart Protection Study Collaborative Group: MRC/BHF Heart Protection Study of cholesterol-lowering with simvastatin in 5963 people with diabetes: a randomized placebo-controlled trial. Lancet 361:2005–2016, 2003

Holt RIG, Peveler RC, Byrne CD: Schizophrenia, the metabolic syndrome and diabetes. Diabet Med 21:515–523, 2004

Hu G, Qiao Q, Tuomilehto J, et al: Prevalence of the metabolic syndrome and its relation to all-cause and cardiovascular mortality in nondiabetic European men and women. Arch Intern Med 164:1066–1076, 2004

Isomaa B, Almgren P, Tuomi T, et al: Cardiovascular morbidity and mortality associated with the metabolic syndrome. Diabetes Care 24:683–689, 2001

Jensen MD, Haymond MW, Rizza RA, et al: Influence of body fat distribution on free fatty acid metabolism in obesity. J Clin Invest 83:1168–1173, 1989

Kahn R, Buse J, Ferrannini E, et al: The metabolic syndrome: time for a critical appraisal. Diabetes Care 28:2289–2304, 2005

Kinder LS, Carnethon MR, Palaniappan LP, et al: Depression and the metabolic syndrome in young adults: findings from the Third National Health and Nutrition Examination Survey. Psychosom Med 66:316–322, 2004

Knowler WC, Barrett-Connor E, Fowler SE, et al: Reduction in the incidence of type 2 diabetes with lifestyle intervention or metformin. N Engl J Med 346:393–403, 2002

Kylin E: Hypertonie-hyperglykamie-hyperurikamiesyndrom. Zentralblatt fur innere Medizin 44:105–127, 1923

Ladwig KH, Kieser M, Konig J, et al: Affective disorder and survival after acute myocardial infarction: results from the post-infarction late potential study. Eur Heart J 12:959–964, 1991

Lakka HM, Laaksonen DE, Lakka TA, et al: The metabolic syndrome and total cardiovascular disease mortality in middle-aged men. JAMA 288:2709–2716, 2002

Lee WJ, Huang MT, Wang W, et al: Effects of obesity surgery on the metabolic syndrome. Arch Surg 139:1088–1092, 2004

Lindstrom J, Eriksson JG, Valle TT, et al: Prevention of diabetes mellitus in subjects with impaired glucose tolerance in the Finnish Diabetes Prevention Study: results from a randomized clinical trial. J Am Soc Nephrol 14(suppl):S108–S113, 2003

McEvoy JP, Meyer JM, Goff DC, et al: Prevalence of the metabolic syndrome in patients with schizophrenia: baseline results from the Clinical Antipsychotic Trials of Intervention Effectiveness (CATIE) schizophrenia trial and comparison with national estimates from NHANES III. Schizophr Res 80:19–32, 2005

McTigue KM, Harris R, Hemphill B, et al: Screening and interventions for obesity in adults: summary of the evidence for the U.S. Preventive Services Task Force. Ann Intern Med 139:933–949, 2003

National Cholesterol Education Program Expert Panel on Detection, Evaluation, and Treatment of High Blood Cholesterol in Adults: Third report of the National Cholesterol Education Program (NCEP) Expert Panel on Detection, Evaluation, and Treatment of High Blood Cholesterol in Adults (Adult Treatment Panel III): final report. Circulation 106:3143–3421, 2002

Orchard TJ, Temprosa M, Goldberg R, et al: The effect of metformin and intensive lifestyle intervention on the metabolic syndrome: the Diabetes Prevention Program randomized trial. Ann Intern Med 142:611–619, 2005

Ösby U, Brandt L, Correia N, et al: Excess mortality in bipolar and unipolar disorder in Sweden. Arch Gen Psychiatry 58:844–850, 2001

Pan XR, Li GW, Hu YH, et al: Effects of diet and exercise in preventing NIDDM in people with impaired glucose tolerance: The Da Qing IGT and Diabetes Study. Diabetes Care 20:537–544, 1997

Panagiotakos DB, Polychronopoulos D: The role of Mediterranean diet in the epidemiology of metabolic syndrome: converting epidemiology to clinical practice. Lipids Health Dis 4:7–12, 2005

Panagiotakos DB, Pitsavos C, Chrysohoou C, et al: Inflammation, coagulation, and depressive symptomatology in cardiovascular disease-free people: the ATTICA study. Eur Heart J 25:492–499, 2004

Park YW, Zhu S, Palaniappan L, et al: The metabolic syndrome: prevalence and associated risk factor findings in the U.S. population from the Third National Health and Nutrition Examination Survey, 1988–1994. Arch Intern Med 163:427–433, 2003

Penninx B, Kritchevsky SB, Yaffe K, et al: Inflammatory markers and depressed mood in older persons: results from the Health, Aging and Body Composition Study. Biol Psychiatry 54:566–572, 2003

Reaven GM: Banting lecture 1988: role of insulin resistance in human disease. Diabetes 37: 1595–1607, 1988

Ridker PM, Buring JE, Cook NR, et al: C-reactive protein, the metabolism, and risk of incident cardiovascular events: an 8-year follow-up of 14,719 initially healthy American women. Circulation 107:391–397, 2003

Rubins HB, Robins SJ, Collins D, et al: Gemfibrozil for the secondary prevention of coronary heart disease in men with low HDL-cholesterol. N Engl J Med 341:410–418, 1999

Ryan MC, Collins P, Thakore JH: Impaired fasting glucose tolerance in first-episode, drug naïve patients with schizophrenia. Am J Psychiatry 160:284–289, 2003

Selvin E, Marinopoulos S, Berkenblit G, et al: Meta-analysis: glycosylated hemoglobin and cardiovascular disease in diabetes mellitus. Ann Intern Med 141:421–431, 2004

Snow V, Barry P, Fitterman N, et al: Pharmacologic and surgical management of obesity in primary care: a clinical practice guideline from the American College of Physicians. Ann Intern Med 142:525–531, 2005

Stern MP, Williams K, Gonzalez-Villalpando C, et al: Does the metabolic syndrome improve identification of individuals at risk of type 2 diabetes and/or cardiovascular disease? Diabetes Care 27:2676–2681, 2004

Sutherland J, McKinnley B, Eckel RH: The metabolic syndrome and inflammation. Metabolic Syndrome Related Disorders 2:82–104, 2004

Thakore JH, Richards PJ, Reznek RH, et al: Increased intra-abdominal fat deposition in patients with major depressive illness as measured by computed tomography. Biol Psychiatry 41:1140–1142, 1997

Thakore JH, Mann JN, Vlahos I, et al: Increased visceral fat distribution in drug-naïve and drug-free patients with schizophrenia. Int J Obes Relat Metab Disord 26:137–141, 2002

Thompson PD, Buchner D, Pina IL, et al: Exercise and physical activity in the prevention and treatment of atherosclerotic cardiovascular disease: a statement from the Council on Clinical Cardiology. Circulation 107:3109–3116, 2003

U.K. Prospective Diabetes Study Group: Effect of intensive blood-glucose control with metformin on complications in overweight patients with type 2 diabetes (UKPDS 34). Lancet 352:854–865, 1998

U.S. Department of Health and Human Services: NHANES III Anthropometric Procedures (video). U.S. Government Printing Office Stock Number 017–022–01335–5. Washington, DC, Government Printing Office, 1996

Weisberg SP, McCann D, Desai M, et al: Obesity is associated with macrophage accumulation in adipose tissue. J Clin Invest 112:1796–1808, 2003

World Health Organization: Appropriate body-mass index for Asian populations and its implications for policy and intervention strategies. Lancet 363:157–163, 2004

Chapter 3

SEVERE MENTAL ILLNESS AND OBESITY

Susan L. McElroy, M.D.
Anna Guerdjikova, Ph.D.
Renu Kotwal, M.D.
Paul E. Keck Jr., M.D.

Severe mental illness and obesity are each important public health problems that overlap to a significant degree, especially in clinical populations (McElroy et al. 2006a). The degree, nature, and causes of this overlap, however, are not well understood. Indeed, no major epidemiological study has yet evaluated the co-occurrence of obesity, as assessed using the definitions of the National Institutes of Health (NIH) (National Institutes of Health 1998), with the full range of psychotic and mood disorders, as defined by DSM-IV-TR (American Psychiatric Association 2000) or other widely accepted operational diagnostic criteria. Also, the treatment of patients with both severe mental illness and obesity has received little empirical study. Therefore, to elucidate present knowledge about the relationship between obesity and severe mental illness, we first present an overview of obesity and the obesity-related conditions: overweight, abdominal obesity, and the metabolic syndrome. Next, we review the relationship between severe mental disorders, especially psychotic and mood disorders, and obesity. We then review psychiatric, behavioral, medical, and surgical treatments available for the obese patient with a severe mental disorder.

Overview of Obesity

As obesity becomes an increasingly severe public health problem (Flegal et al. 1998, 2002; Manson et al. 2004; Mokdad et al. 1999, 2000, 2001, 2003; Ogden et al. 2006), it is imperative that mental health professionals understand the definition, etiology, complications, and treatment of obesity and its related conditions. It is likely that mental health professionals will be playing a larger role in the management of this global epidemic (Devlin et al. 2000).

DEFINITION AND EPIDEMIOLOGY

Obesity is an excess of adipose tissue relative to lean body mass (Table 3–1; Heymsfield et al. 2004). Adipose tissue consists of adipocytes (fat cells), collagenous and elastic fibers, capillaries, and extracellular fluid. It is classified into two main types, subcutaneous and internal; internal adipose tissue can be further classified into visceral and nonvisceral. Growing research indicates that there are important metabolic differences between visceral and subcutaneous adipose tissue.

Overweight and obesity are most often defined clinically in terms of the body mass index (BMI), which is calculated by dividing weight (in kilograms) by the square of height (in meters). Guidelines developed by the NIH define overweight as a BMI of 25–29.9 kg/m^2 (National Institutes of Health 1998). A BMI of 30–34.9 kg/m^2 is classified as class I obesity, 35–39.9 kg/m^2 as class II obesity, and 40 kg/m^2 or more as class III or extreme obesity. Normal weight is a BMI of 18.5–24.9 kg/m^2 and underweight is a BMI of less than 18.5 kg/m^2 (Table 3–2).

Overweight and obesity are both highly prevalent in the general population (Figure 3–1). In the Behavioral Risk Factor Surveillance System, a national survey in which participants reported their weights, it was estimated that the combined incidence of obesity and overweight among adults in the United States increased from 12% and 45%, respectively, in 1991 to 21% and 58% in 2001 (Mokdad et al. 2003). The prevalence of extreme obesity (BMI≥40) increased from 0.9% in 1991 to 2.3% in 2001. Data from the National Health and Nutrition Examination Surveys (NHANES), in which respondents were weighed, show that obesity and overweight increased in prevalence from 22.9% and 55.9%, respectively, in 1988–1994 to 30.5% and 64.5% in 1999–2000 (Flegal et al. 2002). Among adults aged at least 20 years in 2001–2002, 65.7% were overweight or obese, 30.6% were obese, and 5.1% were extremely obese (Hedley et al. 2004); in 2003–2004, 66.3% were overweight or obese, 32.2% were obese, and 4.8% were extremely obese (Ogden et al. 2006).

Obesity has also increased in children and adolescents (obesity is usually defined in this population as ≥95th percentile of the sex-specific BMI for age growth charts). Although the percentages of obese children and adolescents were relatively stable during NHANES I (1971–1974) and II (1976–1980), they doubled to 11% during NHANES III (1988–1994), increased to 15.5% during NHANES IV (1999–2000) (Ogden et al. 2002) and increased again to 17.1% during NHANES 2003–2004 (Ogden et al. 2006).

TABLE 3–1. Important definitions related to obesity

Term	Definition
Obesity	An excess of adipose tissue relative to lean body mass. Obesity is generally measured as being 20% or more above the individual's ideal body weight. Obesity is most often defined clinically in terms of the body mass index (see Table 3–2).
Adipose tissue (fat)	Adipose tissue is composed of fat cells (adipocytes), collagen and elastic fibers, capillaries, and extracellular fluid. The main role of adipose tissue is to store energy in the form of fat. Different compartments of adipose tissue are defined in the literature, including *subcutaneous* and *internal*.
Subcutaneous adipose tissue	The primary location for adipose tissue (80%) is below the skin, where it accumulates in the subcutaneous layer. In this location, a large function of adipose tissue is to provide an insulator function for changes in temperature. Total subcutaneous adipose tissue can be further subdivided into abdominal subcutaneous and nonabdominal subcutaneous adipose tissue compartments.
Internal adipose tissue	Total internal adipose tissue is usually divided into intraabdominal internal (visceral) and nonabdominal internal (nonvisceral) adipose tissue. Intraabdominal fat is drained by the portal vein and can be further subdivided into mesenteric and omental. A number of studies have concluded that typical complications of obesity (dyslipidemia, insulin resistance, type 2 diabetes) are closely correlated with visceral obesity. Nonabdominal internal adipose tissue is not associated with the complications of obesity; this includes, for example, adipose tissue between muscle planes.
Android obesity	Traditionally thought of as "male obesity." This is fat accumulation in the upper body or in the subcutaneous abdominal area. Other terms include central obesity and "apple-shaped" obesity. Obese men tend to distribute weight in this fashion, and obese females can accumulate fat centrally as well.
Gynoid obesity	Obese women traditionally accumulate subcutaneous fat in the lower part of the abdominal wall and the gluteofemoral region. This female type of obesity is referred to as peripheral, gynoid, or "pear-shaped" obesity. The link between gender and regional obesity is not absolute. There are many obese men who have peripheral fat distribution.

TABLE 3–2.   Obesity clinical classes for children, adolescents, and adults

	Body mass index (BMI) definition	
Class	Adult, kg/m^2	Child/Adolescent (percentile)[a]
Healthy weight	18.5–24.9	5th–85th
Overweight	25.0–29.9	85th–95th
Obesity	30.0 and above	95th and above
Class I	30.0–34.9	
Class II	35.0–39.9	
Class III	40.0 and above	
Abdominal obesity		
Men	Waist circumference > 102 cm (40 in)	
Women	Waist circumference > 88 cm (35 in)	

[a]BMI is calculated and then plotted on the Centers for Disease Control and Prevention BMI-for-age growth charts (for either girls or boys) to obtain a percentile ranking.

ETIOLOGY

Obesity is now viewed as a chronic medical disease resulting from a persistent imbalance between energy intake and energy expenditure. In most cases, this imbalance is thought to be due to genetic factors interacting adversely with an "obesigenic" environment—an environment characterized by increased access to highly palatable, energy-dense food and decreased access to physical activity (Friedman 2003, 2004).

CONSEQUENCES

People with obesity are at increased risk for a number of general medical conditions (Table 3–3; Bray and Bouchard 2004; Bray et al. 2003; Klein et al. 2004; National Institutes of Health 1998). These include type 2 diabetes (T2DM), cardiovascular disease (e.g., coronary heart disease, stroke, and peripheral vascular disease), dyslipidemias (e.g., increased total cholesterol, low-density lipoprotein [LDL] cholesterol, and triglycerides and decreased high-density lipoprotein [HDL] cholesterol), hypertension, and certain cancers (e.g., breast, uterus, cervix, colon, esophagus, pancreas, kidney, and prostate). Other complications include pulmonary disease (e.g., hypoventilation syndromes and obstructive sleep apnea), nonalcoholic fatty liver disease (e.g., steatosis, steatohepatitis, and cirrhosis), gall bladder disease, severe pancreatitis, gynecological abnormalities (e.g., abnormal menses, infer-

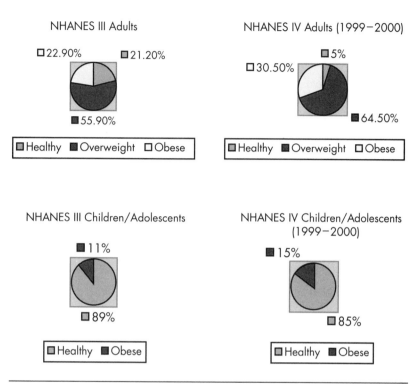

FIGURE 3–1. Increasing burden of obesity in the United States.

Source. National Health and Nutrition Examination Survey (NHANES) data (Flegel et al. 2002; Ogden et al. 2002).

tility, pregnancy complications, and polycystic ovarian syndrome), osteoarthritis, gout, idiopathic intracranial hypertension, phlebitis, and dermatological problems. In addition, obese people, especially those with BMIs of 35 or more, have increased mortality compared with individuals of normal weight (although the precise number of deaths due to obesity is controversial) (Flegal et al. 2005).

A link in particular has been demonstrated between abdominal obesity and coronary artery disease, dyslipidemias, hypertension, and T2DM. Abdominal obesity is defined by the NIH as a waist circumference of more than 102 cm (40 in) in men and more than 88 cm (35 in) in women (National Institutes of Health 1998). The metabolic syndrome, also known as "syndrome X," the "insulin resistance syndrome," and the "deadly quartet," is a constellation of metabolic disturbances that are all risk factors for cardiovascular disease (see Chapter 5, "Cardiovascular Disease," this volume). The metabolic abnormalities include abdominal obesity, glucose intolerance (e.g., T2DM, impaired glucose tolerance, or impaired fasting glycemia), insulin resistance, dysliplidemias, and hypertension. When grouped together, these abnormalities are associated with a greater risk for cardiovascular disease than when they exist alone (Lakka et al. 2002; Sacks 2004).

TABLE 3–3.   Physical health complications of obesity

Cancers	Breast
	Uterine
	Cervical
	Colon
	Esophageal
	Pancreatic
	Kidney
	Prostate
Cardiovascular disorders	Coronary heart disease
	Stroke
	Peripheral vascular disease
Dermatological problems	Skin infections (candidiasis)
	Dermatitis
	Pressure ulcers
Endocrine disorders	Type 2 diabetes
	Dyslipidemia
	Metabolic syndrome
Gynecological problems	Abnormal menses
	Infertility
	Polycystic ovary syndrome
	Pregnancy complications
Pulmonary disease	Hypoventilation syndromes
	Obstructive sleep apnea
Other conditions	Osteoarthritis
	Gout
	Gall bladder disease
	Nonalcoholic fatty liver disease
	Hypertension
	Phlebitis
	Severe pancreatitis

The metabolic syndrome is viewed as an increasingly common metabolic disorder due in part to the increasing prevalence of obesity. There are presently three sets of operationalized definitions for the metabolic syndrome (see Chapter 2, "The Metabolic Syndrome"). Definitions agree on the essential components of obesity, glucose intolerance, hypertension, and dyslipidemias but differ in details and criteria (Eckel et al. 2005). General population rates vary depending on the study design and definition used, but the metabolic syndrome tends to be more common in urban than rural populations, in women than men, and in older than younger age groups. In the United States, Ford et al. (2002), using National Cholesterol Education Program–Adult Treatment Panel (NCEP-ATP III) criteria (Expert Panel on Detection, Evaluation, and Treatment of High Blood Cholesterol in Adults 2001), found metabolic syndrome in 23.7% of the general population.

In addition to medical complications, obese persons are more likely to experience impaired quality of life (Lean et al. 1999) and are at risk for stigmatization and possibly discrimination (Puhl and Brownell 2001). Whether people with obesity have elevated rates of severe mental disorders, however, continues to be a matter of debate. Nonetheless, several lines of evidence suggest that obese persons may have increased rates of mood disorders (McElroy et al. 2004b; Stunkard et al. 2003).

In the first line of evidence, studies using operationalized diagnostic criteria and structured clinical interviews have consistently found high rates of depressive and bipolar disorders in persons of all ages and both genders seeking treatment for obesity, especially severe obesity (Black et al. 1992; Britz et al. 2000; Kotwal et al. 2005).

A second line evidence, comprising findings from community studies using operationalized diagnostic criteria and structured assessments, suggests an association between obesity (usually defined as a BMI≥30) and major depressive episodes (usually defined by DSM criteria), although this association appears to be affected by various factors, especially gender and definition of obesity (K.M. Carpenter et al. 2000; Onyike et al. 2003; Roberts et al. 2003; Stunkard et al. 2003). Thus major depressive episodes are more likely to occur in women with obesity (BMI≥30) and in men and women with severe obesity (BMI≥40).

A third line of evidence suggesting a relationship between obesity and mood disorders comprises the many clinical and community studies finding high levels of depressive symptoms in persons with obesity (Friedman and Brownell 1995; Johnston et al. 2004; Lee et al. 2005; McElroy et al. 2004b). Moreover, a number of studies differentiating between obesity subtypes have found a stronger association between depressive symptoms and abdominal obesity or visceral adipose tissue than between depressive symptoms and BMI or subcutaneous adipose tissue (Lee et al. 2005; McElroy et al. 2004b; Rosmond and Björntorp 1998a, 1998b; Rosmond et al. 1996; Wing et al. 1991). Such observations have led to the hypothesis that visceral fat deposition, or even the metabolic syndrome, may in part be due to glucocorticoid oversecretion from hypothalamic-pituitary-adrenal axis dysregulation secondary to stress (Rosmond 2005) or depression (Thakore et al. 1997). Indeed, preliminary epidemiological data suggest the metabolic syndrome may be related to major depressive episodes in women. Kinder et al. (2004) evaluated 3,186 men and 3,003 women from the NHANES III survey ages 17–39 years for the presence of a lifetime major depressive episode as defined by DSM-III-R (American Psychiatric Association 1987) criteria based on the Diagnostic Interview Schedule, and for the presence of the metabolic syndrome as defined by NCEP-ATP III. Only subjects free of coronary heart disease and diabetes were analyzed. Women with a lifetime major depressive episode were twice as likely to have the metabolic syndrome as compared with women with no history of depression. This relationship, however, was not present in men.

Growing research also indicates that obesity is associated with binge eating disorder (BED), a recently recognized eating disorder characterized by recurrent episodes of distressing, uncontrollable eating of excessively large amounts of food (binge eating) without the inappropriate compensatory weight loss behaviors of bulimia nervosa or anorexia nervosa (Bulik et al. 2000; Dingemans et al. 2002; Hudson et al. 2006; Smith et al. 1998; Yanovski 2003). BED, in turn, appears to be related to mood disorders; it has been shown to co-occur with depressive and bipolar disorders (McElroy et al. 2005a; Smith et al. 1998; Yanovski et al. 1993) and to co-aggregate significantly in families with bipolar disorder (Hudson et al. 2005). It has also been suggested that binge eating may contribute to overweight and obesity in some patients with mood disorders (McElroy et al. 2002, 2004b). Although the relationship between eating and psychotic disorders has received far less attention, preliminary data suggest that a subset of psychotic patients also binge eat (Ramacciotti et al. 2004) and that binge eating may contribute to weight gain and obesity in these patients (Theisen et al. 2003). It is also well documented that depressive symptoms and episodes are common in patients with schizophrenia (Hafner et al. 2005; Siris 1995); however, the relationship of depressive symptoms with binge eating and body weight in patients with psychotic disorders has not been studied.

TREATMENT OF UNCOMPLICATED OBESITY

The treatment of obesity without psychopathology (uncomplicated obesity) can be viewed as a pyramid with three levels of therapeutic options (Figure 3–2). The first level, often referred to as *behavioral weight management* or *lifestyle modification,* aims to help patients change their lifestyle behaviors to decrease energy intake and increase energy output (National Institutes of Health 1998; Wadden and Butryn 2003; Wadden and Foster 2000; Wing 2004). The second level, *pharmacotherapy,* is a useful adjunct to lifestyle modification for properly selected patients. The third level, *bariatric surgery,* is reserved for patients with severe obesity, often with co-occurring medical complications, who have not responded to lifestyle modification and pharmacotherapy. These three levels of obesity treatment for the obese patient without psychopathology are briefly reviewed in the following sections.

Behavioral Weight Management

Behavioral weight management has three goals: decreasing calorie intake, increasing physical activity, and learning cognitive-behavioral strategies to reinforce positive changes in dietary habits and physical activity. Extensive research indicates that most patients with uncomplicated obesity typically lose 10%–15% of initial body weight with state-of-the-art behavioral treatment. After 6 months, however, weight loss slows down and plateaus. Even for patients who manage to lose a large

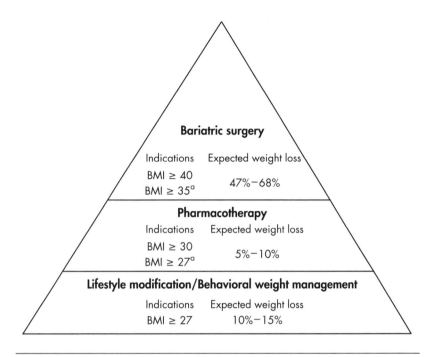

FIGURE 3–2. Pyramid of interventions to treat obesity.

[a]Comorbid obesity-related conditions.

amount of weight initially, many cannot maintain the loss over the long term. A review of 12 of the more recent largest and longest behavioral weight management trials that all employed cognitive-behavioral therapy (most with dietary and/or exercise components) found that participants lost an average of 10.4 kg at 5.6 months, with an average weight loss of 8.1 kg at final follow-up at 17.6 months (Wing 2004).

Importantly, considerable research shows that small weight losses, on the order of 5%–10% of baseline body weight, are associated with significant health improvements, including hypertension, lipoprotein profile, and T2DM (National Institutes of Health 1998). Moreover, behavioral weight management has been shown to reduce by half the incidence of T2DM in persons at high risk to develop the disorder (Tuomilehto and Lindstrom 2003). For example, in the Diabetes Prevention Program, 3,234 nondiabetic persons with elevated fasting and postload plasma glucose concentrations were randomly assigned to placebo, to receive metformin (850 mg twice daily), or to participate in a lifestyle modification program with the goals of at least a 7% body weight loss and at least 150 minutes of physical activity per week (Knowler et al. 2002; Tuomilehto and Lindstrom 2003; Tuomilehto et al. 2001). After a mean follow-up of 2.8 years, the incidence of diabetes was 11.0, 7.8, and 4.8 cases per 100 person-years in the placebo, metformin, and lifestyle groups, respectively. The average weight loss in the three groups was 0.1, 2.1, and 5.6 kg, respectively. Lifestyle modification and metformin were superior to placebo, and lifestyle modification was superior to metformin, in reducing diabetes in persons at high risk to develop the disorder.

Calorie reduction is generally considered the most important component of behavioral weight management for weight loss in uncomplicated obesity (Freedman et al. 2001). In its 1998 review of 25 randomized, controlled trials of low-calorie diets varying in duration from 6 months to 1 year, the NIH concluded that, compared with control subjects, individuals eating low-calorie diets had a mean body weight loss of about 8% (National Institutes of Health 1998).

There is some controversy, however, as to the optimal rate and macronutrient composition of calorie reduction that should occur in dietary therapy for uncomplicated obesity. For example, greater initial weight loss can be achieved with very-low-calorie diets (<800 calories/day) as compared with low-calorie diets (800–1,500 calories/day). Because most studies have shown that there is no difference in weight loss at 1 year between the two strategies due to weight regained, the NIH guidelines recommend that moderate calorie reduction be used to achieve a gradual weight loss (National Institutes of Health 1998).

Regarding optimal macronutrient composition of diet for weight loss and weight maintenance, three recent randomized, controlled trials in obese patients found greater weight loss with a low-carbohydrate diet compared with a calorie- and fat-restricted diet at 6 months (Brehm et al. 2003; Foster et al. 2003; Samaha et al. 2003) but not at 1 year in two extended trials (Samaha et al. 2003; Stern et al. 2004). More recently, Dansinger et al. (2005) compared four popular diets: 160 overweight or obese participants with known hypertension, dyslipidemia, or fasting hyperglycemia were randomized to Atkins, Ornish, Weight Watchers, or Zone diets for 1 year. All four diets resulted in modest, statistically significant weight loss at 1 year, with no statistically significant differences between groups. There was a nonsignificant trend toward a higher discontinuation rate for the more extreme diets (48% for Atkins and 50% for Ornish) than for the moderate diets (35% for Zone and 35% for Weight Watchers). A strong association was found between self-reported dietary adherence and weight loss that was almost identical for each diet. On average, participants in the top percentile of adherence lost 7% of body weight. Cardiac risk factor reductions were associated with weight loss regardless of diet type. The authors concluded that adherence level rather than diet type was the key determinant of clinical benefit.

Regarding physical activity, studies have shown that weight reduction by increased physical activity alone, without also reducing calorie intake, is only modest (National Institutes of Health 1998). However, correlational studies have consistently found an association between weight loss, especially maintenance of weight loss, and increased physical activity (Fogelholm and Kukkonen-Harjula

2000). Experts have attributed these disparate observations to poor adherence with prescribed exercise as well as the prescription of too little exercise (Fogelholm and Kukkonen-Harjula 2000; Jeffery et al. 2003; W.C. Miller and Wadden 2004; Wing 1999).

Importantly, physical activity is divided into two types: programmed and lifestyle. Programmed exercise consists of regularly scheduled periods of relatively high intensity activity (e.g., 20–40 minutes of walking, running, or swimming). Lifestyle activity involves increasing energy expenditure throughout the day by walking whenever possible instead of riding, taking elevators or escalators, and not using energy-saving devices. Controlled studies have shown lifestyle activity to be just as effective as programmed activity in maintaining weight loss and in improving fitness, decreasing blood pressure, and reducing cholesterol (Andersen et al. 1999; Dunn et al. 1999).

Because many obese patients have low exercise tolerance, it is generally recommended that they begin with short bouts of low-intensity activity and gradually increase to frequent bouts of moderate-intensity activity. The NIH guidelines specifically recommend that most patients start walking at a slow pace for 10 minutes three times per week and gradually increase to 30–45 minutes of moderate-intensity physical activity three to five times per week (National Institutes of Health 1998). Progression to 30–60 minutes of moderate-intensity physical activity every day may enhance weight loss and weight maintenance.

Pharmacotherapy

A growing number of antiobesity drugs have been made available for the management of persons with obesity (Bray and Greenway 1999; Haddock et al. 2002; Ioannides-Demos et al. 2005; Kaplan 2005; Shekelle et al. 2004; Yanovski and Yanovski 2002). These drugs can be broadly categorized into agents that reduce food intake by acting on the central nervous system (appetite suppressants) and those that modify fat absorption or otherwise alter metabolism (metabolic agents) (Figure 3–3). The former group includes the noradrenergic agents phentermine, mazindol, and diethylpropion and the monoamine reuptake inhibitor sibutramine, and the latter includes the lipase inhibitor orlistat. Phentermine, mazindol, and diethylpropion are approved by the U.S. Food and Drug Administration (FDA) for short-term use in obesity (e.g., for acute weight loss only), whereas sibutramine and orlistat are also approved for long-term use (e.g., for both acute weight loss and maintenance of weight loss). The NIH recommends that FDA-approved weight loss drugs be used in combination with behavioral weight management for patients with a BMI of 30 or more who have no concomitant obesity-related risk factors or diseases and for patients with a BMI of 27 or more who have concomitant obesity-related risk factors or diseases (National Institutes of Health 1998). Of note, the noradrenergic agent phenylpropanolamine and the serotonergic agonists fenfluramine and dexfenfluramine, once FDA approved for the treatment of obesity, have since been withdrawn from

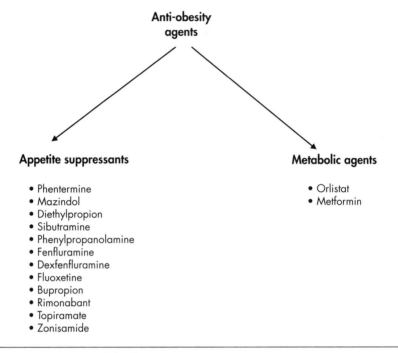

Anti-obesity agents

Appetite suppressants

- Phentermine
- Mazindol
- Diethylpropion
- Sibutramine
- Phenylpropanolamine
- Fenfluramine
- Dexfenfluramine
- Fluoxetine
- Bupropion
- Rimonabant
- Topiramate
- Zonisamide

Metabolic agents

- Orlistat
- Metformin

FIGURE 3–3.   Antiobesity agents.

the market for safety concerns (increased risk of stroke for phenylpropanolamine and an association with valvular heart disease and primary pulmonary hypertension for the fenfluramines) (Ioannides-Demos et al. 2005). These last-mentioned agents therefore receive minimal attention in this chapter.

The amount of weight loss attributed to available antiobesity drugs is modest (typically less than 5 kg at 1 year) but usually of clinical benefit. Recent meta-analyses of controlled studies of these agents in obese patients reported mean differences in weight loss compared with placebo for phentermine of 3.6 kg at 6 months; for sibutramine of 3.4 kg at 6 months and 4.45 kg at 12 months; and for orlistat of 2.9 kg at 12 months (Arterburn et al. 2004; Haddock et al. 2002; Li et al. 2005). Systematic reviews of randomized controlled trials lasting up to 2 years for sibutramine and up to 4 years for orlistat have demonstrated statistically greater weight loss with active drug than with placebo as well as statistically less weight regain during maintenance treatment (Ioannides-Demos et al. 2005). Treatment with sibutramine was associated with modest increases in heart rate and blood pressure, small improvements in HDL cholesterol and triglycerides, and very small improvements in glycemic control among diabetic patients (Shekelle et al. 2004). Treatment with orlistat was associated with an increase in gastrointestinal adverse events (diarrhea, flatulence, and bloating/abdominal pain/

dyspepsia) as well as small but significant improvements in blood pressure, lipid profiles, and fasting blood glucose (O'Meara et al. 2004; Shekelle et al. 2004).

Of note is a growing trend to use certain antidepressants and antiepileptics for weight management in patients with uncomplicated obesity (Appolinario et al. 2004). Antidepressants studied in obesity include several selective serotonin reuptake inhibitors (SSRIs; especially fluoxetine; Bray and Greenway 1999) and bupropion (Anderson et al. 2002; Fava et al. 2005a; Gadde et al. 2001; Jain et al. 2002). A recent meta-analysis of nine fluoxetine studies showed a mean weight loss, compared with placebo, of 4.7 kg at 6 months and 3.1 kg at 12 months (Shekelle et al. 2004). A meta-analysis of three bupropion studies showed a mean weight loss of 2.8 kg at 6–12 months (Shekelle et al. 2004). Fluoxetine was associated with an increase in nervousness, sweating, and tremors; nausea and vomiting; fatigue, asthenia, hypersomnia, and somnolence; insomnia; and diarrhea. Bupropion was associated with dry mouth and insomnia.

Antiepileptics studied in uncomplicated obesity include topiramate and zonisamide. A recent meta-analysis of six studies of topiramate reported that mean weight loss for topiramate at 6 months was 6.5% (Li et al. 2005). The most common side effects associated with topiramate were paresthesias and taste perversion. In the one zonisamide study (Gadde et al. 2003), 60 obese patients were treated for 16 weeks with double-blind zonisamide or placebo. Patients receiving zonisamide lost an average of 5.9 kg (6.0% of baseline body weight) compared with 0.9 kg (1.0% of baseline body weight) for placebo patients ($P<0.001$). Zonisamide was well tolerated, with fatigue being the only side effect more common with zonisamide than with placebo.

Although not FDA approved for the treatment of obesity, the insulin-sensitizing agent metformin has been associated with weight loss in several groups of patients characterized by insulin resistance, including women with polycystic ovarian disease and obese hyperlipidemic men and women with and without T2DM (Harborne et al. 2003; Saenz et al. 2005). Metformin is therefore sometimes used in these populations for weight loss as well as for improvement in metabolic parameters. A recent review, however, concluded that there was little evidence that metformin has significant weight loss properties in overweight or obese patients without T2DM or polycystic ovarian disease (Levri et al. 2005).

Finally, in early 2006 Sanofi-Aventis received an "approvable" letter from the FDA for its cannabinoid-1 receptor blocker rimonabant for weight loss in obesity (AcompliaReport 2006a, 2006b, 2006c). However, the FDA also notified Sanofi-Aventis that it needed more information before it would grant formal approval for rimonabant for this indication. In June 2006, rimonabant was approved for sale in all 25 European Union countries, but as of this writing it has not been approved in the United States. The Phase III Obesity Program for rimonabant involves seven double-blind, placebo-controlled trials with more than 6,600 overweight or obese patients and is designed to explore the drug's role in weight loss, weight management, and treatment of obesity-related risk factors such as dyslipi-demia and diabetes. Published trials ($N= 1,036$; 1,507; and 3,045) have thus far shown that rimonabant 20 mg is superior to placebo at 1 year for weight loss and for improvement in waist circumference, HDL cholesterol, triglycerides, and insulin resistance (Després et al. 2005; Pi-Sunyer et al. 2006; Van Gaal et al. 2005). In the only 2-year study published thus far ($N= 3,045$), patients who con-tinued to take rimonabant 20 mg maintained their weight loss and favorable metabolic changes, whereas those switching to placebo experienced weight regain (Pi-Sunyer et al. 2006). Although the drug was generally well tolerated, psychiat-ric side effects especially were a concern. In the 2-year trial, rimonabant-treated patients experienced psychiatric disorders nearly twice as often as did placebo-treated patients (Pi-Sunyer et al. 2006).

Bariatric Surgery

Bariatric surgery is an option for patients with severe and treatment-resistant obe-sity who are at high risk for obesity-associated morbidity or mortality. It is specif-ically reserved for well-informed and motivated patients with a BMI 40 or higher or those with a BMI 35 or higher who have a comorbid obesity-related medical condition and acceptable operative risks (National Institutes of Health 1998). Surgical procedures may be purely restrictive (e.g., gastric banding or gastroplasty) or involve a gastric bypass (Roux-en-Y) component (e.g., gastric banding or gas-troplasty with gastric bypass).

Weight loss with bariatric surgery can be substantial. The NIH reviewed five randomized trials and found that patients who received bariatric surgery lost 10–159 kg over 12–48 months (National Institutes of Health 1998). A recent meta-analysis of 136 studies of bariatric surgery involving 22,094 patients found that the mean excess weight loss was 61.2% for all patients (Buchwald et al. 2004). Weight loss was greater for patients undergoing gastric bypass (61.6%) or gastro-plasty (68.2%) than gastric banding (47.5%). Importantly, comorbid medical disorders also improved significantly: diabetes resolved in 76.8% of patients, hyper-tension resolved in 61.7% of patients, obstructive sleep apnea resolved in 85.7% of patients, and hyperlipidemia improved in 70% of patients. Operative mortality (death at 30 or less days postsurgery) was 0.1% for the purely restrictive proce-dures, 0.5% for gastric bypass, and 1.1% for biliopancreatic diversion or duode-nal switch.

Obesity and Psychotic Disorders

As noted earlier, there have been no formal epidemiological studies of obesity or obesity-related conditions (overweight, abdominal obesity, or metabolic syn-drome) in persons with psychotic disorders that have used formal assessments of psychiatric diagnoses or anthropometric measure. However, at least 31 studies have evaluated rates of obesity or obesity-related conditions in persons with psychotic or other chronic mental disorders. Twenty six-of these studies used clinical samples and five used community samples. These studies are described in the following section.

CLINICAL AND COMMUNITY STUDIES OF OBESITY IN PSYCHOTIC DISORDERS

The 26 clinical studies of obesity and related conditions in patients with psychotic disorders are difficult to compare because of different methodologies, including the use of different patient populations and different definitions of obesity. They include 20 studies of obesity in primarily antipsychotic-treated patients with psychotic and/or chronic metal disorders (see Table 3–4); 3 studies of visceral fat deposition in antipsychotic-free or antipsychotic-naïve patients with schizophrenia (Ryan et al. 2004; Thakore et al. 2002; Zhang et al. 2004); and 3 studies of metabolic syndrome in patients with schizophrenia or schizoaffective disorder (Basu et al. 2004; Heiskanen et al. 2003; Kato et al. 2004). Rates of obesity, defined as a BMI of 30 or more, ranged from 26% (Kendrick 1996) to 63% (Kato et al. 2005). Rates of abdominal obesity were higher, ranging from 68% (Kato et al. 2005) to 89% (B. Wallace and Tennant 1998). All three studies evaluating metabolic syndrome found elevated rates, ranging from 37% in a group of schizophrenia patients from Finland (Heiskanen et al. 2003) to 42% in a group of American patients with schizoaffective disorder receiving antipsychotics often in combination with mood stabilizers (Basu et al. 2004), to 63% in a group of American outpatients with schizophrenia who were receiving antipsychotics (Kato et al. 2004).

The three studies exploring visceral fat deposition in schizophrenia patients had mixed results. In the first study, Thakore et al. (2002) reported that eight drug-free and seven drug-naïve patients with schizophrenia had greater amounts of visceral fat (determined by abdominal computed tomography [CT]) as well as a higher mean BMI and waist-to-hip ratio (WHR) and higher plasma cortisol levels than 15 age- and sex-matched control subjects. In contrast, Zhang et al. (2004) found no differences in weight, BMI, or fat distribution (determined by WHR and magnetic resonance imaging measurement of subcutaneous and abdominal fat) between 45 antipsychotic-naïve inpatients with first-episode schizophrenia from China and gender- and age-matched healthy control subjects. They also found no differences between the patient and control groups in fasting plasma leptin or insulin levels. However, female patients had significantly higher WHRs and significantly higher fasting insulin levels than female control subjects. In the third study, Ryan et al. (2004) found that 17 patients with drug-naïve, first-episode schizophrenia had a significantly higher amount of intraabdominal fat (as measured by CT) and higher plasma cortisol levels than age- and sex-matched control subjects who were also matched for BMI (BMI for patients, 24.6; for control subjects, 23). These findings

TABLE 3–4.   Clinical studies of obesity and related disorders in patients with psychotic disorders

Study	Patients	Definition of weight categories or anthropomorphic measures	Findings
Dynes 1969	33 Veterans Hospital inpatients with schizophrenia receiving phenothiazines and 22 medical inpatients with diabetes	Not provided	64% were obese compared with 5% of the medical patients.
Gopalaswamy and Morgan 1985	190 chronically mentally disabled inpatients, 74% with schizophrenia	Overweight: BMI ≥ 25.1 for men, ≥ 23.9 for women Obese: ≥ 20% above the upper limit of the acceptable weight range	54% of the entire group were overweight or obese; 45% of male patients were overweight and 15% were obese (compared with 39% and 6% of men in the general population, respectively); 67% of female patients were overweight and 36% were obese (compared with 32% and 8% of women in the general population, respectively).
Silverstone et al. 1988	226 patients, most with chronic schizophrenia, receiving depot antipsychotics	Overweight: BMI 25–29 Obese: BMI 30–39.9 Severely obese: BMI ≥ 40	70% of men were overweight (39%), obese (27%), or severely obese (4%); 58% of women were overweight (21%), obese (33%), or severely obese (6%).
Stedman and Welham 1993	51 female long-term inpatients receiving antipsychotics and other psychotropic drugs; 49% had DSM-III-R schizophrenia	Overweight: BMI 25–30 Obese: BMI > 30 Abdominal obesity: WHR ≥ 0.8	62% were overweight (31%) or obese (31%); 73% were abdominally obese.

TABLE 3–4. Clinical studies of obesity and related disorders in patients with psychotic disorders *(continued)*

Study	Patients	Definition of weight categories or anthropomorphic measures	Findings
Centorrino et al. 1994	44 chronically psychotic outpatients treated with clozapine	Obese: Weight > 200 lb	55% were obese.
Martinez et al. 1994	311 custodial-care inpatients with DSM-III-R schizophrenia; 225 received antipsychotics and 86 received no psychotropics	BMI	Male and female patients receiving antipsychotics had higher mean BMIs (27 and 30, respectively) than male and female patients not receiving antipsychotics (26 and 28, respectively).
Kendrick 1996	101 chronically mentally ill adults	Obese: BMI ≥ 30	26% were obese.
Wallace and Tennant 1998	40 patients (79% with schizophrenia) living in mental health residential services in Australia, 95% taking antipsychotics	Overweight: BMI 25.1–30 Obese: BMI ≥ 30.1 Abdominal obesity: WHR > 0.90 in men and > 0.80 in women	71% were overweight (34%) or obese (37%); 89% were abdominally obese.

TABLE 3–4. Clinical studies of obesity and related disorders in patients with psychotic disorders *(continued)*

Study	Patients	Definition of weight categories or anthropomorphic measures	Findings
Brown et al. 1999	102 outpatients with schizophrenia	Overweight: BMI 26–30 Obese: BMI >30	Rates of overweight and obesity in male patients (42% and 18%) were similar to those in the reference male population (52% and 16%); there was a trend for an increased rate of overweight (47%) but not obesity (23%) in female patients compared with the female reference population (39% and 24%, respectively).
Coodin 2001	183 patients with psychotic disorders receiving hospital-based treatment compared with Canada's 1996–1997 NPHS	Obese: BMI > 30	42% of patients were obese, 3.5 times higher that the 12% of the Canadian general population who were obese according to the NPHS.
Theisen et al. 2001	151 adolescent and young adult inpatients, 109 with ICD-10 schizophrenia spectrum disorders, in a psychiatric rehabilitation center in Germany	Obese: ≥ 90th percentile	45% of male and 59% of female patients were obese; 51% of male and 64% of female patients with schizophrenia spectrum disorders were obese.
Leonard et al. 2002	21 patients receiving clozapine for treatment-resistant schizophrenia	Overweight: BMI 25–30 Obese: BMI > 30	85% were overweight (57%) or obese (29%).

TABLE 3–4. Clinical studies of obesity and related disorders in patients with psychotic disorders *(continued)*

Study	Patients	Definition of weight categories or anthropomorphic measures	Findings
Strassnig et al. 2003	143 outpatients with psychotic disorders	Overweight: BMI 25–29.9 Obese: BMI ≥ 30	82.5% were overweight (22%) or obese (60%).
Arranz et al. 2004	50 antipsychotic-naïve patients with first-episode schizophrenia, 50 antipsychotic-free inpatients with DSM-IV paranoid schizophrenia, and 50 healthy control subjects	BMI	The mean BMI (24.5) of the antipsychotic-free patients was significantly higher than that of the antipsychotic-naïve patients (22) and the healthy control subjects (22; $P=0.002$), but the antipsychotic-free patients were significantly older (35 years) than the antipsychotic-naïve (25 years) and control (30 years) groups ($P=0.000$).
Hsiao et al. 2004	201 Taiwanese outpatients with schizophrenia spectrum disorders receiving antipsychotics	Overweight: BMI 24.2–26.4 Obese: BMI > 26.4 Severely obese: BMI ≥ 28.6	40% of male and 40% females were obese, 23% of males and 28% of females were severely obese; the prevalence of obesity in male and female patients was, respectively, 2.7- and 2.5- fold greater than in the Taiwanese reference population; the prevalence of severe obesity was 4.7- and 3.5-fold greater, respectively, than that in the reference population; the prevalence of severe obesity in male and female patients was, respectively, 4.7- and 3.5-fold greater than in the Taiwanese reference population.

TABLE 3–4. Clinical studies of obesity and related disorders in patients with psychotic disorders *(continued)*

Study	Patients	Definition of weight categories or anthropomorphic measures	Findings
Paton et al. 2004	166 inpatients receiving antipsychotics	Overweight: BMI 25–30 Obese: BMI>30	62% were overweight (29%) or obese (33%).
Kato et al. 2005	62 outpatients with schizophrenia, 69% taking atypical antipsychotics	Obese: BMI ≥ 30; Abdominal obesity: Waist circumference > 102 cm in men and > 88 cm in women	63% were obese and 68% were abdominally obese.
Stahl et al. 2005	258 patients with DSM-IV chronic schizophrenia receiving antipsychotics in various clinical settings	BMI	Mean BMI in men was 26 and mean BMI in women was 29.
Susce et al. 2005	560 patients with severe mental illnesses from inpatient and outpatient facilities in central Kentucky	Overweight: BMI ≥ 25 Obese: BMI ≥ 30 Severely obese: BMI ≥ 40	74% were overweight (15%), obese (46%), or extremely obese (13%).

Note. BMI = body mass index (kg/m²); NPHS = National Population Health Survey; WHR = waist-to-hip ratio.

have led some to suggest that persons with schizophrenia, especially women, have important metabolic disturbances, including abdominal obesity, impaired glucose metabolism, and a predisposition to the metabolic syndrome, and that these disturbances are independent of, but worsened by, exposure to weight-gaining medications (Ryan et al. 2003, 2004; Thakore 2004).

The results of the community studies, which are somewhat mixed, also suggest that a relationship exists between schizophrenia and obesity but that factors affect this relationship. In the first study, Allison et al. (1999a) compared data from two groups of individuals: 1) 150 persons with self-reported schizophrenia and 80,310 persons without schizophrenia from the mental health supplement of the 1989 National Health Interview Survey (NHIS), an annual survey conducted by the National Center for Health Statistics from 1987 to 1996 to assess the health of the U.S. civilian, noninstitutionalized population; and 2) 420 noninstitutionalized individuals with psychotic disorders (schizophrenia or schizoaffective disorder), as defined by DSM-IV (American Psychiatric Association 1994), from a Pfizer, Inc.–supported ziprasidone trial and 17,689 persons without schizophrenia from NHANES III. In the NHIS data set, men with schizophrenia had a mean BMI similar to that of men without schizophrenia (26.1 vs. 25.6, respectively), whereas women with schizophrenia had a significantly higher mean BMI than did women without schizophrenia (27.4 vs. 24.5, respectively; $P < 0.0001$). In the ziprasidone and NHANES III data sets, men and women with schizophrenia each had mean BMIs similar to those of men and women without schizophrenia (26.8 vs. 26.5 for men and 27.3 vs. 27.4 for women, respectively). The authors concluded that individuals with schizophrenia were, on the whole, as obese or more obese than individuals without schizophrenia.

In the second community study, Homel et al. (2002) evaluated BMI levels and the prevalence of overweight and obesity in persons with ($n = 877$) and without ($n = 427,760$) schizophrenia among the Personal Characteristic and Health Condition files of the NHIS. Persons with schizophrenia in general had a higher BMI (mean, 28.0) than persons without schizophrenia (mean, 25.7). This difference was more pronounced for females with schizophrenia (mean BMI, 29.1 vs. 24.9 for females without schizophrenia) than for males with schizophrenia (mean BMI, 27.3 vs. 26.6 for males without schizophrenia). Consistent with other community studies, persons without schizophrenia showed a steady and significant increase in BMI from 1987 to 1996 as a whole and when stratified by gender and age. By contrast, persons with schizophrenia showed little or no evidence of an increase in BMI over time, with one exception: females aged 18–30 years with schizophrenia initially showed similar BMI levels to persons without schizophrenia but then showed significant and dramatic increases in BMI.

In the third community study, Wyatt et al. (2003) compared the height, weight, and BMI of 7,514 U.S. military active-duty personnel hospitalized for either schizophrenia, bipolar disorder, or major depressive disorder and 85,940 healthy subjects matched for date of entry into the service to evaluate the relationship between psychiatric illness and physique. No consistent differences in height, weight, or BMI were found between patients and control subjects or between patient groups. A limitation of this study was that entry criteria (including mental health and weight status) for the U.S. Armed Forces were not described.

In the fourth community study, Weiser et al. (2004) examined the weight before illness onset and initiation of antipsychotic medication for persons who went on to develop schizophrenia. Specifically, the authors analyzed data on height and weight of 203,257 male adolescents obtained by the Israeli draft board and followed the subjects for 2–6 years for later hospitalization for schizophrenia using the Israeli National Psychiatric Hospitalization Case Registry. After exclusion of adolescents with evidence of illness before or within 1 year of draft board assessment, 204 future schizophrenia patients were left for analysis. Compared with the rest of the group, the future patients had significantly lower BMIs (21.2 vs. 21.8; $P=0.03$) and significantly lower body weights (64.2 vs. 66.3 kg; $P=0.01$). The authors concluded that before illness onset, future schizophrenia patients were not heavier than their peers, suggesting that the weight gain and obesity associated with schizophrenia are illness effects, including the effects of antipsychotic medication.

In the fifth community study, Saari et al. (2005) assessed the prevalence of the metabolic syndrome, as defined by NCEP-ATP III criteria, in 5,613 members of a population-based birth cohort born in 1966 in northern Finland who participated in a field study from 1997 to 1998. Cohort subjects were divided into four diagnostic categories: 1) schizophrenia ($n=31$); 2) other functional psychoses ($n=22$); 3) nonpsychotic disorders ($n=105$); and no psychiatric hospital treatment ($n=5,455$, comparison group). The prevalence of the metabolic syndrome was higher in subjects with schizophrenia as compared with the comparison group (19% vs. 6%; $P=0.01$); 84% of the schizophrenia group and none of the comparison group reported receiving antipsychotic medications. By contrast, rates of the metabolic syndrome in patients with other psychoses (4.5%) and those with nonpsychotic disorders (8.6%) did not differ from that of the comparison group; 27% and none, respectively, of these two patient groups were receiving antipsychotics.

Taken together, the clinical and community studies suggest that schizophrenia is associated with obesity but that different stages of the illness may be associated with different aspects of body weight dysregulation. Thus most studies of chronically ill patients, many of whom had been receiving long-term treatment with antipsychotics, found elevated rates of obesity (BMI≥30), abdominal obesity, and the metabolic syndrome. In contrast, studies of those with first-episode or antipsychotic-naïve schizophrenia generally found that patients were of normal weight (Arranz et al. 2004; Weiser et al. 2004; Wyatt et al. 2003). However, two of three studies found that first-episode, treatment-naïve schizophrenic patients had increased visceral fat deposition (Ryan et al. 2004; Thakore et al. 2002; Zhang et al. 2004).

Review of the clinical and community studies also suggests that there are correlates of obesity in patients with psychotic or chronic mental disorders. In particular, considerable evidence indicates that treatment with antipsychotics, especially clozapine and olanzapine, is associated with obesity. For example, Theisen et al. (2001) evaluated rates of obesity among 151 inpatients attending a psychiatric rehabilitation center in Germany, 109 of whom had schizophrenia spectrum disorders. The authors found that prevalence rates of obesity were highest in patients treated with clozapine (64%) followed by other atypical antipsychotics (olanzapine, sulpiride, and risperidone; 56%) and classic antipsychotics (haloperidol, flupentixol, perazine; 30%). Rates of obesity were lowest for the drug-free patients (28%).

These studies further suggest that obesity in patients with schizophrenia is associated with other factors, including several that are associated with obesity in persons in the general population. Such factors have included female gender (Allison et al. 1999a; Homel et al. 2002); unhealthy lifestyle habits such as eating high-fat diets and engaging in low levels of physical activity or exercise (Ryan et al. 2004); impaired physical functioning (Strassnig et al. 2003); and elevated rates of diabetes (Hung et al. 2005). One clinical study found a stronger correlation between waist circumference and cardiovascular risk factors than between BMI and such risk factors (Kato et al. 2005). Other potential correlates of obesity in schizophrenia include long-term illness treatment or duration; treatment with psychotropic combinations (especially antipsychotics with tricyclics); and the presence of binge eating or substance abuse (Daumit et al. 2003; Susce et al. 2005; Theisen et al. 2001).

Obesity and Mood Disorders

At least 21 studies have evaluated rates of obesity or obesity-related conditions in persons with syndromal mood disorders (McElroy et al. 2004b, 2006a, 2006b). Fourteen of these studies used clinical samples, eight used community samples, and five used prospective designs. These studies are described in the following section.

CLINICAL STUDIES OF OBESITY IN MOOD DISORDER

One prospective and 13 cross-sectional studies evaluated obesity (or a related condition) in patients with mood disorders. In the prospective study, Pine et al. (2001) followed two age- and sex-matched groups of children, 6–17 years of age, with major depression ($n=90$) or no psychiatric disorder ($n=87$), for 10–15 years with standardized psychiatric evaluations. Childhood major depression was significantly positively associated with adulthood BMI, and this association persisted after controlling for age, gender, substance use, social class, pregnancy, and medication exposure. Specifically, children with major depression had a higher mean BMI as adults (26.1) than control children (24.2). In addition, a bivariate logistic analysis showed that childhood depression predicted a twofold-increased risk for adult overweight status. Duration of depression between childhood and adulthood was associated with adult BMI, but this was not found for gender, change in eating patterns occurring with depressive episodes, diet, or medication use. Also, BMI did not differ between subjects who were and those who were not currently depressed at the time of the adult assessment.

The 13 cross-sectional studies are difficult to compare because of their different methodologies, including the use of different patient populations and different definitions of obesity and mood disorders. Thus 10 studies reported rates of overweight or obesity, or mean BMIs, in various mood disorder patients (see Table 3–5), whereas 3 studies explored visceral fat deposition in normal-weight women with major depressive disorder. As compared with similar studies in psychotic disorders, the rates of obesity in the 10 cross-sectional studies in mood disorders were more variable: obesity rates ranged from a low of 5.7% in a group of male and female patients with major depressive disorder participating in a phase-IV antidepressant trial (Berlin and Lavergne 2003) to a high of 67% in a group of mixed mood disorder patients, also of both genders, from Germany (Muller-Oerlinghausen et al. 1979). Four of these studies, described next, used comparison groups.

Muller-Oerlinghausen et al. (1979) reported that 49 stable patients with mood disorder (26 with bipolar disorder) receiving lithium maintenance therapy had a significantly higher rate of "severe obesity" (BMI$\geq$30; 12%) than the expected general population rate (5.7%). Elmslie et al. (2000) compared the prevalences of overweight, obesity, and abdominal obesity in 89 euthymic outpatients with bipolar I disorder (87% of whom were receiving pharmacological maintenance treatment) with those of 445 age- and sex-matched community control subjects in New Zealand. Female patients had significantly higher prevalence rates of overweight (BMI=25–29.9) (44% vs. 25%), obesity (BMI$\geq$30) (20% vs. 13%), and abdominal obesity (59% vs. 17%) than female control subjects. Male patients had significantly higher rates of obesity (19% vs. 10%) and abdominal obesity (58% vs. 35%), but the rates of overweight between male patients (29%) and control subjects (43%) were not significantly different. McElroy et al. (2002) assessed the prevalence of overweight and obesity in 644 outpatients with bipolar disorder, types I and II, in both the United States and Europe; 57% of the total group was overweight or obese, with 31% overweight (BMI=25–29.9), 21% obese (BMI 30–39.9), and 5% extremely obese (BMI$\geq$40). Compared with rates from NHANES III, rates of obesity and extreme obesity in female bipolar patients from the United States were higher, but rates of overweight were lower than those in reference women. Male bipolar patients from the United States had higher rates of overweight and obesity, but not extreme obesity, than reference men.

By contrast, in Japan, Shiori et al. (1993) compared the frequency distribution of body weight of 106 patients hospitalized for DSM-III (American Psychiatric Association 1980) major depression with that of a standard group. These authors found significantly more patients in the underweight groups than expected. This was particularly true for women and for patients with melancholia.

Taken together, these four studies suggest that bipolar patients are more likely to be overweight or obese, whereas those with melancholic unipolar depression are more likely to be underweight. Indeed, the only two cross-sectional studies reporting rates of underweight as well as obesity had similar findings. Berlin and Lavergne (2003) found that among 1,694 subjects with DSM-IV major depression participating in a phase-IV antidepressant trial, more subjects were underweight (BMI < 18.5; 8.5%) than were obese (BMI ≥ 30; 5.7%). By contrast, Fagiolini et al. (2002) reported that among 50 patients with bipolar I disorder entering a lithium-based maintenance trial, substantially more patients were obese (BMI ≥ 30; 32%) than underweight (BMI < 18.5; 2%).

Regarding the three studies of visceral fat deposition, in the first study, Thakore et al. (1997) compared the body fat distribution (assessed with abdominal CT) of seven medication-free women (mean age = 36.6 years; mean BMI = 24.4) with DSM-III-R melancholic major depression with that of seven healthy control women (mean age = 32.7 years; mean BMI = 23.6). Although patients and control subjects did not differ regarding weight, BMI, WHR, and total body fat, patients had significantly greater intraabdominal fat stores. Patients also had significantly higher baseline cortisol levels, and their intraabdominal fat stores correlated with both their WHRs and cortisol levels. Similarly, Kahl et al. (2005) found that 36 premenopausal women with major depressive disorder (18 with comorbid borderline personality disorder) had increased visceral fat (assessed with magnetic resonance imaging) compared with 20 healthy control subjects and 12 borderline personality disorder patients without major depression. In contrast, Weber-Hamann et al. (2002) found that visceral fat stores (determined by abdominal CT) did not differ between 22 postmenopausal women with DSM-IV major depression (mean age = 65.1 years; mean BMI = 24.5) and 23 healthy control women (mean age = 64.0; mean BMI = 24.3) or between the hypercortisolemic depressed patients and control subjects. However, hypercortisolemic depressed patients had significantly more visceral fat than normocortisolemic depressed patients.

COMMUNITY STUDIES OF OBESITY IN MOOD DISORDERS

Of the eight studies evaluating body weight in community samples of persons with mood disorders, four used cross-sectional designs and four employed prospective designs (McElroy et al. 2004b, 2006a, 2006b). Kendler et al. (1996) assessed depressive symptoms in a community-based registry of 1,029 female twin pairs and concluded that major depression consisted of at least three etiologically heteroge-

TABLE 3–5. Clinical studies of obesity and related disorders in patients with mood disorders

Study	Patients	Definition of weight categories or anthropomorphic measures	Findings
Muller-Oerlinghausen et al. 1979	49 patients with bipolar disorder (n=26), major depression (n=14), SAD (n=8), and unclassified (n=1)	Obese: For females, BMI=24–30; for males, BMI=25–30 Severely obese: BMI>30	67% were obese (43%) or severely obese (24%).
Berken et al. 1984	40 outpatients with major depression	Not provided	25% were obese prior to TCA therapy.
Shiori et al. 1993	106 Japanese inpatients with DSM-III major depression	Not provided	Patients' body weight distribution on admission had significantly more individuals in the underweight groups compared with a standard distribution from the general population. Also, more patients with melancholia were in the underweight groups than expected. Rates of patients in body weight categories were not provided.
Elmslie et al. 2000	89 euthymic outpatients with bipolar I disorder from New Zealand; 445 community control subjects	Overweight: BMI=25–29.9 Obese: BMI≥30 Abdominal obesity: WHR>0.8 for females and >0.9 for males	Female patients had significantly higher prevalence rates of overweight (44% vs. 25%), obesity (20% vs. 13%), and abdominal obesity (59% vs. 17%). Male patients had significantly higher rates of obesity (19% vs. 10%) and abdominal obesity (58% vs. 35%).

TABLE 3–5. Clinical studies of obesity and related disorders in patients with mood disorders *(continued)*

Study	Patients	Definition of weight categories or anthropomorphic measures	Findings
McElroy et al. 2002	644 outpatients from U.S. and Europe with DSM-IV bipolar I and II disorders	Overweight: BMI = 25–29.9 Obese: BMI = 30–39.9 Extremely obese: BMI≥40	57% were overweight or obese, with 31% overweight, 21% obese, and 5% extremely obese.
Fagiolini et al. 2002	50 outpatients with DSM-IV bipolar I disorder	Overweight: BMI = 25–29.9 Obese: BMI≥30	68% were overweight (36%) or obese (32%).
Fagiolini et al. 2003	175 outpatients with DSM-IV bipolar I disorder	Overweight: BMI = 25–29.9 Obese: BMI≥30	35% were obese.
Berlin and Lavergne 2003	1,694 clinical trial subjects with DSM-IV major depressive disorder	Underweight: BMI = 18.5 or less Overweight: BMI = 25–29.9 Obese BMI≥30	8.5% were underweight, 26.9% were overweight (21.2%) or obese (5.7%)
Hennen et al. 2004	113 inpatients with bipolar I mania in an olanzapine trial	BMI	Mean baseline BMI was 29.
Papakostas et al. 2004	369 outpatients with major depression enrolled in an 8-week trial of fluoxetine	Overweight: BMI = 25–29.9 Obese: BMI≥30	51% were overweight (31%) or obese (20%); 47% of women and 56% of men were overweight, whereas 25% of women and 14% of men were obese.

Note. BMI=body mass index; SAD=schizoaffective disorder; TCA=tricyclic antidepressant; WHR=waist-to-hip ratio.
Source. Copyright 2004. Adapted from "Are Mood Disorders and Obesity Related? A Review for the Mental Health Professional," by McElroy SL, Kotwal R, Malhotra S, et al. *Journal of Clinical Psychiatry* 65:634–651, 2004. Reproduced by permission of Routledge/Taylor & Francis Group, LLC.

neous syndromes: mild typical depression, atypical depression, and severe typical depression. They found that twins with atypical depression were significantly more likely to be obese (BMI > 28.6; 28.9%) than were those with mild typical depression (6.0%) or those with severe typical depression (3.1%).

G.E. Miller et al. (2002) recruited 50 medically healthy persons from the community with a major ($n=32$) or minor ($n=18$) depressive episode according to DSM-IV criteria and 50 matched control subjects free of lifetime psychiatric disorders to explore the relationships between depression and expression of inflammatory risk markers for coronary heart disease. The depressed subjects showed a significantly greater mean BMI (30.5) than control subjects (25.9; $P<0.003$), along with significantly higher levels of C-reactive protein and interleukin-6.

Lamertz et al. (2002) evaluated 3,021 German adolescents and young adults ages 14–24 years for DSM-IV diagnoses, using a modified version of the Composite International Diagnostic Interview, and calculated BMI percentages for age and gender. The authors found no significant associations between mood disorders (or anxiety, substance use, or somatoform disorders) and obesity or BMI. There also were no significant associations between any mental disorder and underweight. These findings were limited by the exclusion of eating disorder subjects, who have elevated rates of mood disorders and weight disturbances (Bulik et al. 2000).

In a study mentioned earlier, Wyatt et al. (2003) compared the height, weight, and BMI of 7,514 U.S. military active-duty personnel hospitalized for bipolar disorder, major depressive disorder, or schizophrenia with those of 85,940 healthy subjects matched for date of service entry and found no consistent differences in height, weight, or BMI between patients and control subjects or between patient groups. However, they found a diagnostic effect on BMI for white males: the mean BMI in patients with bipolar disorder was greater than the mean BMI in control subjects, which was equal to the mean BMI in patients with schizophrenia. The BMI in schizophrenia patients, in turn, was greater than the mean BMI in patients with major depressive disorder.

In the first prospective community study, Pine et al. (1997) evaluated 644 adolescents in 1983 (mean age = 14 years) and again in 1992 (mean age = 22 years) to assess the relationship between major depressive disorder and conduct disorder in youth and obesity in early adulthood. Diagnoses were assessed in 1992 with the Diagnostic Interview Schedule for Children. Univariate analyses showed that a higher BMI in adulthood was associated with increasing depressive and conduct symptoms in adolescence. Also, adulthood obesity was associated with adolescent depression in females, but not in males, and with depression in adulthood in both sexes. However, the latter association was positive in females and negative in males. Multivariate analyses showed that adulthood obesity was predicted by adolescent conduct disorder and the gender × adult depression interaction.

In the second prospective community study, Roberts et al. (2003) evaluated 1,886 survey respondents who were 50 years or older and found that current major depressive episodes were increased in subjects with obesity. Conversely, they also found that the prevalence ratio for obesity among those with a current major depressive episode was increased at 1.65 (95% CI = 1.28–2.13) and concluded that there was a bidirectional association between obesity and depression. Moreover, they reported that depression in 1994 predicted obesity in 1999 (odds ratio [OR] = 1.92; 95% CI = 1.31–2.80), but not after controlling for obesity in 1994 (OR = 1.32; 95% CI = 0.65–2.70).

In the third prospective community study, L.P. Richardson et al. (2003) used data from a longitudinal study of a birth cohort of children (*N* = 1,037) born between April 1, 1972, and March 31, 1973, in Dunedin, New Zealand, to assess relationships between major depression in adolescence and the risk for obesity at age 26 years. Collected data included regular diagnostic mental health interviews and height and weight measurements throughout childhood and adolescence. Major depression occurred in 7% of the cohort during early adolescence (11, 13, and 15 years of age) and in 27% during late adolescence (18 and 21 years of age). Obesity occurred in 12% of the cohort at age 26 years. After adjusting for individuals' baseline BMI, depressed late-adolescent girls were at a greater than twofold increased risk for obesity in adulthood compared with their nondepressed female peers (relative risk = 2.32; 95% CI = 1.29–3.83). Also, a dose-response relationship between the number of depressive episodes during adolescence and the risk for adult obesity was observed in late-adolescent girls but not in boys or early adolescent girls.

In the fourth prospective community study, Hasler et al. (2004) evaluated mood disorders in 591 young adults ages 18–19 years from the general population of Zurich, Switzerland, and followed them until 40 years of age. Nineteen percent were classified as overweight (BMI > 25). Atypical depression was positively associated with overweight in males and females; hypomanic symptoms were associated with overweight in males only. These associations remained significant after controlling for medication, social, and educational variables.

In sum, six of the eight community studies of obesity in persons with mood disorders found positive relationships between the two conditions: two of the four cross-sectional studies found relationships between depression, or a subtype of depression, and elevated body weight; and all four prospective studies found a relationship between a mood disorder or a major depressive episode and the subsequent development of overweight or obesity. Taking the clinical and community studies of obesity in mood disorders together, they suggest that some forms of mood disorders may be associated with overweight or obesity, whereas other forms may be associated with underweight (McElroy et al. 2004a, 2006b). Mood disorder subtypes associated with overweight or obesity might include major depressive disorder with atypical features, major depressive disorder with juvenile onset, depressive disorders in females, and bipolar disorder, especially when depressive features predominate. Mood disorder subtypes associated with underweight might include major depressive disorder with melancholic features and depressive disorders in males. Moreover, major depressive disorder with hypercortisolemia, even when associated with normal or low body weight, may be associated with visceral fat deposition. Importantly, these conclusions are preliminary and need to be verified in epidemiological and longitudinal studies using validated assessments of both mood disorders and anthropometric measures.

As with psychotic disorders, a number of studies have explored correlates of overweight and obesity in mood disorder patients. For bipolar disorder, factors associated with obesity have included treatment with antipsychotics; greater ingestion of carbohydrates; low levels of exercise; co-occurring BED; comorbid hypertension, T2DM, and arthritis; less coffee consumption; and variables suggestive of more severe bipolar illness (Elmslie et al. 2000, 2001; Fagiolini et al. 2003, 2004; McElroy et al. 2002). For example, in a group of 175 consecutive bipolar I patients receiving lithium-based treatment, Fagiolini et al. (2003) reported that, compared with nonobese patients, obese patients (35% of the group) had more previous depressive and manic episodes, had higher baseline scores on the Hamilton Rating Scale for Depression (Ham-D), and required more time in acute treatment to achieve remission. During maintenance treatment, significantly more obese patients experienced a recurrence ($n=25$; 54%) as compared with those who were not obese ($n=28$; 35%). Also, the time to recurrence was significantly shorter for patients who were obese at baseline. When recurrence type was examined, the percentage of patients experiencing depressive recurrences was significantly greater for obese patients ($n=15$; 33%) than for nonobese patients ($n=11$; 14%). In a subsequent study on this group of patients, Fagiolini et al. (2004) reported that higher BMI was significantly associated with more severe bipolar illness and history of a suicide attempt. In a group of 369 outpatients with major depressive disorder receiving an 8-week fluoxetine trial, Papakostas et al. (2004) found that obese patients had worse somatic well-being scores compared with nonobese patients and that greater relative body weight, but not obesity, predicted nonresponse to fluoxetine. Although preliminary, these observations suggest that increasing BMI, overweight, or obesity may be associated with poorer outcome and less favorable treatment response in mood disorder patients.

Treatment of the Severely Mentally Ill Patient With Obesity

Many of the medications used to treat patients with severe mental disorders are associated with weight gain (Aronne and Segal 2003; Baptista et al. 2004; Keck and McElroy 2003). These include many antipsychotics and mood stabilizers and some antidepressants (see Figure 3–4). Importantly, emerging data indicate the

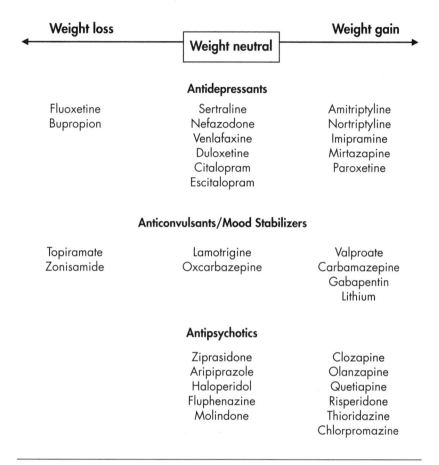

FIGURE 3–4.	Weight liability of psychotropic agents.

potential of psychotropics within classes to induce weight gain varies among the different compounds. Thus, for antipsychotics, a meta-analysis by Allison et al. (1999b) showed that clozapine and olanzapine were associated with the greatest weight gain, followed by thioridazine, sertindole, risperidone, and ziprasidone; molindone was associated with a small weight loss. Available data on quetiapine indicate that the weight gain associated with this drug is somewhere between that associated with olanzapine and risperidone (Lieberman et al. 2005; Wirshing 2004). An 18-month effectiveness trial comparing five antipsychotics in 1,460 patients with schizophrenia found that olanzapine was associated with the most weight gain (mean, 2 lb/month), followed by quetiapine and risperidone (mean, 0.5 and 0.4 lb/month, respectively); perphenazine and ziprasidone were associated with a mean weight loss of 0.2 and 0.3 lb/month, respectively. Data for aripiprazole show that it is associated with minimal weight gain, less than that associated with olanzapine and comparable with that associated with ziprasidone (Baptista et al. 2004; Lieberman 2004; McQuade et al. 2004; Wirshing 2004). For mood stabilizers, available comparative data suggest that olanzapine is associated with the greatest weight gain, followed by valproate, lithium, and carbamazepine; lamotrigine appears to be weight neutral or possibly associated with weight loss (Keck and McElroy 2003).

Antidepressants that cause weight gain include tricyclics (tertiary amines more so than secondary amines), monoamine oxidase inhibitors, the novel antidepressant mirtazapine, and possibly some SSRIs (Fava 2000; Kraus et al. 2002). Paroxetine in particular may be more likely than other SSRIs to be associated with weight gain (Fava et al. 2000). Antidepressants that are weight neutral or may even reduce body weight, at least over the short term, include the novel noradrenergic/dopaminergic agent bupropion, the serotonin-norepinephrine selective reuptake inhibitor venlafaxine, and some SSRIs (especially fluoxetine) (Croft et al. 2002; Edwards and Anderson 1999; Fava 2000; Goldstein et al. 1997; Harto et al. 1988; Harto-Traux et al. 1983; Kraus et al. 2002; McGuirk and Silverstone 1990; McIntyre et al. 2002; Rudolph et al. 1998). For SSRIs, controlled data indicate that this weight loss may not be sustained over the long term, but data are mixed as to whether there is weight gain above that associated with placebo (Michelson et al. 1999). Nefazodone appears to be weight neutral (Sussman et al. 2001). As noted earlier, fluoxetine and bupropion have been shown to have weight loss effects in patients with uncomplicated obesity (Shekelle et al. 2004).

Importantly, medications associated with weight gain may also be associated with the medical complications associated with obesity, including dyslipidemias, hyperglycemia and T2DM, and hypertension. Thus, of the atypical antipsychotics, the two agents most likely to cause weight gain, clozapine and olanzapine, are most likely to be associated with hyperglycemia, diabetes, hypercholesterolemia, and hypertriglyceridemia (Lieberman et al. 2005; Newcomer 2004). Whether these agents cause such metabolic disturbances by mechanisms other than increasing adiposity is presently unknown but is an area of active research (Bergman and Ader 2005).

The general approach to treating severely mentally ill patients with obesity is to choose pharmacological agents that are efficacious for the patient's primary mental disorder and also weight neutral or associated with weight loss, thus attempting to minimize or prevent further weight gain (Figure 3–5; Keck and McElroy 2003; Keck et al. 2003; Wirshing 2004). However, some patients will require medications that also cause weight gain for adequate control of their severe mental disorders. Growing data indicate that clozapine, although consistently shown to cause more weight gain, and, to a lesser extent, olanzapine are more effective than other antipsychotics or mood stabilizers for severely ill patients with schizophrenia (Davis et al. 2003; Kane et al. 1988, 2001; Lieberman et al. 2005) and bipolar disorder (Calabrese et al. 1996; Suppes et al. 1999; Tohen et al. 2002, 2003a). Indeed, many studies (Ascher-Svanum et al. 2005; Czobor et al. 2002; Hennen et al. 2004; Klett

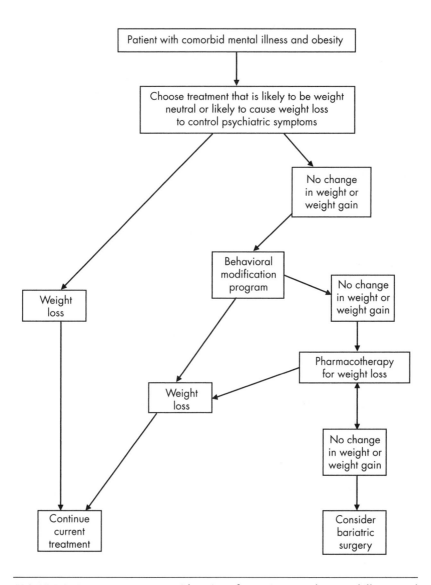

FIGURE 3–5.   Treatment considerations for patients with mental illness and comorbid obesity.

and Caffey 1960), although not all (Bustillo et al. 1996), suggest weight gain is associated with favorable therapeutic response to clozapine—and to a lesser extent olanzapine, haloperidol, and chlorpromazine—in patients with schizophrenia spectrum disorders and bipolar I disorder. The obese patient with a psychotic or mood disorder who requires a medication with weight-gaining properties for adequate treatment of his or her mental disorder will therefore require management of at least two chronic diseases: severe mental illness and obesity, along with any obesity-related medical comorbidities.

Guidelines for the medical monitoring of such patients have been provided by Keck et al. (2003), the American Diabetes Association et al. (2004), the American Psychiatric Association (Marder et al. 2004), and Goff et al. (2005). For patients with psychotic disorders receiving second-generation antipsychotics, most of these guidelines recommend regular monitoring of BMI, waist circumference, and fasting plasma glucose level and lipid profile. Specific recommendations made in the American Psychiatric Association guidelines include recording the patient's BMI before medication initiation or change and at every visit for the first 6 months thereafter; subsequently the BMI can be determined quarterly as long as it remains stable. These guidelines also specify that, unless the patient is underweight, a weight gain of 1 BMI unit indicates the need for an intervention. Suggested interventions include closer monitoring of the patient's weight, a change in the patient's antipsychotic medication to an agent with less weight gain liability, engagement of the patient in a weight management program, and the use of an adjunctive medication to reduce or maintain weight.

With regard to switching antipsychotic medication for weight loss, clinical data suggest that patients may successfully be switched from olanzapine to risperidone (Ried et al. 2003) or quetiapine (Koponen and Larmo 2003) and from various antipsychotics to either ziprasidone (Weiden et al. 2003) or aripiprazole (Casey et al. 2003). In addition to weight loss, patients switched to ziprasidone or aripiprazole may also have improvement in metabolic measures such as hyperlipidemia (Ball et al. 2005; Lieberman et al. 2005). However, there are also reports of clozapine-treated patients who destabilized upon switching to other atypical antipsychotics with less weight-gaining liability (Ball et al. 2005).

The last two options, behavioral weight management and adjunctive pharmacotherapy, are reviewed in the following sections. Regarding adjunctive pharmacotherapy for weight loss, the psychotropic and weight loss effects of increasingly used and potentially useful drug candidates are evaluated. Bariatric surgery, which is rarely used for obese patients with severe mental illness, is mentioned as an option of last resort.

BEHAVIORAL WEIGHT MANAGEMENT

No prospective study has yet evaluated behavioral weight management in a group of obese patients with syndromal mood disorders, including patients whose mood disorders were stabilized by antidepressants or mood stabilizers. Five controlled trials, however, have evaluated behavioral weight management paradigms in psychotic or chronically mentally ill patients with obesity or related conditions (usually antipsychotic-associated weight gain) who are receiving antipsychotic medication. These studies suggest behavioral weight management is safe and effective in controlling weight gain and obesity in some patients with psychotic disorders, particularly when administered in conjunction with adjunctive psychosocial treatment strategies (Faulkner et al. 2003; C.R. Richardson et al. 2005; Werneke et al. 2003).

In an early study, Rotatori et al. (1980) randomly assigned 14 chronically ill psychiatric patients living in a "semi-independent" residential facility to a 14-week behavioral program that focused on techniques to reduce calorie intake ($n=7$) or a waiting list control group ($n=7$). Both individual and group reinforcement contingencies were used throughout the behavioral program. The seven patients randomly assigned to behavioral treatment displayed a mean 7.3-lb weight loss compared with a 5.6-lb mean gain in the control group. There were no dropouts.

Ball et al. (2001) evaluated a Weight Watchers program for 11 outpatients with schizophrenia or schizoaffective disorder and olanzapine-related weight gain (baseline mean BMI=31.9). Eleven patients matched on olanzapine use and weight gain who did not participate in the program but who continued their usual olanzapine treatment constituted the control group. The program consisted of 10 weekly Weight Watchers meetings held at an outpatient research program. Exercise sessions (the primary mode was walking) were scheduled three times a week. A parent or caregiver was asked to supervise each patient's diet and exercise at home. Adherence to diet and exercise was reinforced with tokens.

Participants who completed the Weight Watchers program ($n=11$) lost more weight (mean=5.1 lb) than comparison group participants (mean=0.5 lb), but the difference was not statistically significant. However, there was a significant sex × group × time interaction for BMI ($P=0.05$). All seven male participants lost weight (mean=7.3 lb), whereas three of the four female participants gained weight (mean not reported). No significant correlation was found between exercise participation and weight loss. Psychiatric rating scales showed that patients remained clinically stable during the study, and no adverse events were observed with either the diet or the exercise program.

Menza et al. (2004) evaluated a 52-week multimodal weight control program in 31 patients with schizophrenia ($n=20$) or schizoaffective disorder ($n=11$) receiving antipsychotic medication and participating in two day-treatment programs. A comparison group consisted of 20 "usual care" patients who were contemporaneously treated in the same clinics. The weight control program incorporated nutritional counseling, exercise, and behavioral modification and consisted of four phases: 1) an assessment phase; 2) an intensive 12-week weight control program with group meetings twice per week and one 15-minute individual session per week; 3) a 12-week, step-down, less-intensive weight control program with one group meeting per week and one 15-minute individual session per month; and 4) a 6-month weight-maintenance extension program with a group meeting once per week and one 15-minute individual session per month. Behavioral strategies used included self-monitoring of eating and physical activity, stress management, stimulus control, problem solving, and social support. Techniques aimed at enhancing patients' confidence in their ability to cope with obstacles and to succeed in change were employed. Special teaching approaches for people with cognitive deficits, such as repetition, homework, and the use of visual materials, were also used.

Twenty-seven (87.1%) of the 31 patients completed the 12-week intensive program and lost a mean of 2.7 kg and a mean of 1.0 BMI units compared with a mean gain of 2.9 kg and 1.2 BMI units in the control group. Twenty (64.5%) patients completed the entire 52-week program. Statistically significant posttreatment improvements in weight, BMI, glycosylated hemoglobin, diastolic and systolic blood pressure, exercise level, and nutrition knowledge were seen in the intervention group. Weight and BMI also decreased significantly in the intervention group compared with the usual care group, who gained weight.

Brar et al. (2005) conducted a 14-week multicenter, open-label, rater-blinded, randomized study comparing group-based behavioral therapy for weight loss with usual care in stable patients with schizophrenia or schizoaffective disorder. Patients had been treated with risperidone for 6 weeks after having their medication switched from olanzapine and had BMIs greater than 26. (After switching to risperidone, patients showed no weight loss.) Behavior therapy included 20 sessions over the 14-week period and focused on learning healthy eating habits; there was no exercise component. Members of the usual care group were encouraged to lose weight on their own without specific instructions but received monthly anthropometric assessments. Of 70 patients randomly assigned, 50 (71.4%) completed the program. Both groups lost weight, but the between-group difference was not statistically significant (–2.0 kg vs. –1.1 kg for group behavior therapy and usual care, respectively). However, there was a trend for more patients in the behavior therapy group than in the usual care group to have lost 5% or more of their body weight at endpoint (26.5% vs. 10.8%). Also, post hoc analysis of patients attending at least one behavior therapy session showed that significantly more patients in the behavior therapy than the usual care group had lost 5% or more of their body weight at endpoint (32.1% vs. 10.8%) and at week 14 (40.9% vs. 14.3%).

Littrell et al. (2003) randomized 70 patients with schizophrenia or schizoaffective disorder to an intervention group receiving Eli Lilly's "Solutions for Wellness" program or to a standard-of-care control group to determine whether behavioral weight management could prevent psychotropic-associated weight gain. All patients began olanzapine at study onset, and body weights were recorded monthly over 6 months. The intervention group received 1-hour weekly seminars over 16 weeks related to dietary guidelines, developing support systems, and education about exercise. Patients in the intervention group showed no significant weight changes at 4 and 6 months (0.8 and –0.1 lb, respectively), whereas weight gain occurred in the control group (7.1 and 9.6 lb, respectively). This study is important because, taken together with the findings of relatively low amounts of weight loss in studies of behavioral weight management among obese, severely mentally ill patients, it suggests that behavioral weight management may be more effective for preventing psychotropic-associated weight gain than for reversing it once it has developed.

Of note, two important components of behavioral weight management, dietary therapy and physical activity, have received relatively little empirical study in patients with severe mental disorders. Indeed, dietary therapy has largely been neglected in the management of severe mental illness, despite preliminary data suggesting that dietary composition may be important in the etiology of schizophrenia, bipolar disorder, and major depressive disorder (Peet 2004a, 2004b; Young and Conquer 2005). Thus epidemiological evidence suggests low fish consumption may be associated with increased risk of developing mood disorders and depressive symptoms and with poorer outcome of schizophrenia (Hibbeln 1998; Peet 2004a, 2004b). Also, double-blind, placebo-controlled studies suggest omega-3 supplements may be effective adjunctive treatments for medication-resistant schizophrenia, bipolar disorder, and major depression (Peet and Stokes 2005; Stoll et al. 1999).

Moreover, the effects of various diets on severe mental disorders are unknown. For example, although the ketogenic diet (a high-fat, low-carbohydrate, low-protein diet) has anticonvulsant properties (Vining et al. 1998) and has been hypothesized to have mood-stabilizing effects (El-Mallakh and Paskitti 2001), it has not been systematically tested in obese patients with severe mental disorders. Such diets have been reported to have mood-elevating properties in patients with uncomplicated obesity (Rosen et al. 1985). There is one report of a lean bipolar woman who followed the classic ketogenic diet for 2 weeks for continuous mood cycling but showed no clinical improvement, no weight loss, and no urinary ketosis (Yaroslavsky et al. 2002). There is also one report of a patient with bipolar I disorder developing a manic episode while losing weight on the Atkins diet despite taking valproate, quetiapine, and clonazepam (Junig and Lehrmann 2005). His mania resolved with discontinuation of the diet and weight gain. Thus, until further data are available, we discourage use of such diets in severely mentally ill persons in favor of high-carbohydrate, low-fat diets.

Although exercise has received empirical study in the treatment of depression, there are no controlled trials of exercise in patients with severe mental disorders (Craft and Perna 2004; Faulkner et al. 2003; C.R. Richardson et al. 2005). Preliminary studies conducted to date in patients with schizophrenia suggest exercise is safe and may promote weight loss but is associated with poor adherence unless there is substantial psychosocial support. In one pilot study, 10 of 20 stable patients with schizophrenia or schizoaffective disorder treated with olanzapine for at least 4 weeks were randomized to receive free access to a YMCA fitness facility for 6 months (Archie et al. 2003). Nine patients had dropped out at 6 months because of poor attendance. The main reason given for poor attendance was lack of motivation. The mean weight change in the YMCA group was a gain of 2 kg; mean weight change in the other group was not assessed. The one patient who completed the program and met criteria for full attendance lost 15 kg. In another pilot study, 10 outpatients with schizophrenia were evaluated in a 16-week walking program (Beebe et al. 2005). Compared with a control group not participating in the program during the same 16-week period, participants showed greater reductions in body fat and BMIs, greater aerobic fitness, and fewer psychiatric symptoms at the end of the program. However, only the body fat reduction was statistically significant ($P=0.03$).

Regarding exercise in depression, D.A. Lawlor and Hopker (2001) conducted a meta-analysis of 14 randomized, controlled trials of exercise in clinically depressed patients and concluded that exercise was more effective than no treatment and comparable with cognitive-behavioral therapy in reducing depressive symptoms. However, they noted that all 14 studies had important methodological weaknesses, and because of these weaknesses they also concluded that the effectiveness of exercise in depression could not be adequately determined. Dunn et al. (2005) recently conducted a study addressing many of the limitations of these earlier trials. They randomly assigned 80 adults ages 20–45 years with mild to moderate DSM-IV major depressive disorder to one of four aerobic exercise groups or exercise placebo control (3 days per week of flexibility exercise). The four exercise groups varied in total energy expenditure (7.0 or 17.5 kcal/kg/week) and exercise frequency (three or five days per week). The 17.5 kcal/kg/week expenditure corresponded to the "public health dose," whereas the 7.0 kcal/kg/week expenditure represented the "low dose." The primary outcome was change in depressive symptoms as assessed with the Ham-D. Participants randomized to the public health dose, but not the low dose, of aerobic exercise showed a significant reduction in depressive symptoms as compared with the placebo group. Ham-D scores were decreased 47% from baseline for the public health dose compared with 30% for the low dose and 25% for the placebo. There was no main effect of exercise frequency at 12 weeks. Thus, just as exercise may have a dose-response relationship with weight loss for obesity, it may also have a dose-response relationship with depressive symptoms for major depressive disorder.

PHARMACOTHERAPY

Antidepressants

As reviewed earlier, fluoxetine and bupropion have been shown to be associated with weight loss in patients with uncomplicated obesity (Appolinario et al. 2004; Ioannides-Demos et al. 2005; Li et al. 2005). In a single-blind comparator trial in 36 outpatients with bipolar I depression, adjunctive bupropion and topiramate each decreased both depressed symptoms and body weight after 8 weeks of treatment (McIntyre et al. 2002). Specifically, bupropion- and topiramate-treated patients showed similar rates of antidepressant responses (59% vs. 56%), but bupropion was associated with less weight loss (1.2 kg vs. 5.8 kg).

Several SSRIs have also been shown to be superior to placebo in reducing binge eating in BED in double-blind, placebo-controlled, short-term (6–9 week) monotherapy trials (Appolinario and McElroy 2004; Carter et al. 2003). In the BED studies, all SSRIs assessed were associated with statistically significant weight loss. However, fluoxetine was ineffective for binge eating and weight loss in two controlled studies that compared it with cognitive-behavioral therapy (Devlin et al. 2005; Grilo et al. 2005b). Thus far, to our knowledge, no studies have evaluated an SSRI or other antidepressant in an obese, severely mentally ill population with comorbid binge eating. Bupropion has also been shown superior to placebo for smoking cessation and is FDA approved for this use (Hays and Ebbert 2003). In the smoking trials, bupropion was shown to mitigate the weight gain associated with smoking cessation.

The SSRIs do not appear to be effective in olanzapine-associated weight gain. In an 8-week clinical trial comparing olanzapine monotherapy with the combination of olanzapine and fluoxetine in patients with bipolar depression, both groups showed comparable weight gain that was significantly greater than placebo (Tohen et al. 2003b). Similarly, a small, double-blind, placebo-controlled study showed that coadministration of fluoxetine at 20 mg/day with olanzapine (10 mg/day) for 8 weeks was ineffective in preventing weight gain in 30 first-episode hospitalized patients with schizophrenia (Poyurovsky et al. 2002). In a placebo-controlled study of 31 patients with schizophrenia who had gained 3% or more of their baseline weight in the first 8 weeks of olanzapine treatment, fluoxetine, at the higher dosage of 60 mg/day, again showed no weight loss effects (Bustillo et al. 2003). Of note, patients' psychopathology responded differently to the combination of olanzapine plus fluoxetine in the three different studies. The bipolar depressed patients showed significant improvement in both depressive and manic symptoms on the olanzapine-fluoxetine combination (Tohen et al. 2003b); the first-episode schizophrenia patients receiving the combination showed significantly less improvement in positive and disorganized symptoms than those receiving olanzapine monotherapy (Poyurovsky et al. 2002); and the schizophrenic outpatients receiving the combination showed no differential effects in psychopathology compared with those receiving placebo (Bustillo et al. 2003).

There are no controlled studies of bupropion in psychotropic-associated weight gain. However, the selective norepinephrine reuptake inhibitor antidepressant reboxetine, which promotes noradrenergic neurotransmission (as bupropion is thought to do), was shown to attenuate olanzapine-associated weight gain in a controlled study of 26 patients with schizophrenia (Poyurovsky et al. 2003). Patients receiving olanzapine with reboxetine 4 mg/day displayed a statistically significant lower increase in body weight (mean = 2.5 kg) than those receiving olanzapine with placebo (mean = 5.5 kg) after 6 weeks of treatment. Significantly fewer patients in the olanzapine/reboxetine group (20%) gained at least 7% of their initial weight than in the olanzapine/placebo group (70%). The reboxetine-treated patients also showed a statistically significantly greater reduction in depressive symptoms (as measured by the Ham-D).

Antiepileptics

Topiramate and zonisamide are novel antiepileptics with documented weight loss properties in patients with uncomplicated obesity (Bray 2003; Gadde et al. 2003; Ioannides-Demos et al. 2005; Li et al. 2005; Wilding et al. 2004). In a growing number of open-label reports, topiramate has been used successfully to treat obesity or psychotropic-associated weight gain in patients with schizophrenia who are receiving antipsychotics (Dursun and Devarajan 2000; Levy et al. 2002), patients with bipolar disorder receiving mood stabilizers and antipsychotics (McElroy et al. 2000; McIntyre et al. 2005; Woods et al. 2004), and patients with treatment-resistant major depression receiving antidepressants (L.L. Carpenter et al. 2002; Dursun and Devarajan 2001). Similarly, zonisamide has been used successfully to treat obesity in patients with bipolar disorder who are receiving mood stabilizers and antipsychotics (McElroy et al. 2004a). Only two studies, however, have been double-blind and placebo-controlled. In one study, 66 inpatients with schizophrenia receiving antipsychotic medication and "carrying excess weight" were randomized to topiramate 100 mg/day, topiramate 200 mg/day, or placebo for 12 weeks (Ko et al. 2005). In the topiramate 200-mg/day group, body weight, BMI, and waist and hip circumferences decreased significantly compared with the topiramate 100-mg/day and placebo groups. The WHR did not change in any group. Scores on the Clinical Global Impression—Severity and the Brief Psychiatric Rating Scale also significantly decreased over the 12-week period, but the decrease was not thought to be clinically meaningful. In the other study, 43 women with mood or psychotic disorders who had gained weight while receiving olanzapine therapy were randomized to topiramate ($n=25$) or placebo ($n=18$) for 10 weeks (Nickel et al. 2005). Weight loss was significantly greater in the topiramate-treatment group by 5.6 kg. Patients receiving topiramate also experienced significantly greater improvement in measures of health-related quality of life and psychological impairments.

In the open studies, the weight loss associated with topiramate was sometimes long term and associated with improvement in metabolic indices (Chengappa et al. 2001). Three open-label, prospective trials found that initiating treatment with the combination of topiramate with either risperidone or olanzapine successfully stabilized mood in patients with bipolar disorder while preventing weight gain (Vieta et al. 2003, 2004). The mechanism(s) of the anorectic and weight loss effects of these drugs are unknown, but topiramate's may be related to its anti-glutamatergic action, whereas zonisamide's has been hypothesized to be due to its dual effects on serotonin and dopamine.

Topiramate and zonisamide may also have therapeutic psychotropic properties in patients with severe mental disorders. In a double-blind, placebo-controlled, 12-week crossover trial in 26 patients with treatment-resistant schizophrenia, adjunctive topiramate was superior to placebo in reducing general pathological symptoms but not in decreasing positive or negative symptoms (as assessed by the Positive and Negative Syndrome Scale) (Tiihonen et al. 2005). Controlled studies of topiramate monotherapy in acute bipolar mania in adults did not demonstrate separation from placebo on mania ratings (Kusher et al. 2006; McElroy and Keck 2004). However, the drug was superior to placebo in a prematurely terminated study in adolescent mania (Delbello et al. 2005), comparable with bupropion in reducing depressive symptoms in a single-blind comparator trial in bipolar I depression (as noted earlier; McIntyre et al. 2002), and superior to placebo in reducing symptoms of depression and anger in women with mild-to-moderate recurrent major depressive disorder. In addition, numerous open-label studies report that topiramate (McElroy et al. 2000; McIntyre et al. 2005) and, to a lesser extent, zonisamide (Anand et al. 2005; Baldassano et al. 2004; McElroy et al. 2004a) have antimanic, antidepressant, and/or mood-stabilizing properties in patients with bipolar spectrum disorders when used adjunctively with antipsychotics, mood stabilizers, and/or antidepressants.

Topiramate has also been shown in double-blind, placebo-controlled trials to be effective in a number of the conditions that co-occur in patients with psychotic and mood disorders. These include BED (McElroy et al. 2003, 2004c), bulimia nervosa (Hoopes et al. 2003), alcohol dependence (Johnson et al. 2003), and cocaine dependence (Kampman et al. 2004). There are case reports of topiramate being used to successfully treat comorbid eating and substance use disorders in patients with severe mental disorders (McElroy and Keck 2004). Open data suggest that zonisamide may reduce binge eating and induce weight loss in patients with BED (McElroy et al. 2005b).

Stimulants, Alerting Agents, and Dopamine Agonists

Virtually all stimulants are associated with appetite suppression and weight loss. Modafinil, indicated by the FDA to improve wakefulness in patients with narcolepsy, obstructive sleep apnea/hypopnea syndrome, and shift work sleep disorder, was associated with mild weight loss in a short-term monotherapy study in healthy persons (Makris et al. 2004), an 8-week adjunctive therapy study in 311 patients with major depressive disorder (Fava et al. 2005b), and two clinical trials in children with attention-deficit hyperactivity disorder (ADHD) (Biederman et al. 2005; Greenhill et al. 2006) but not in the disorders for which it is presently indicated (Czeisler et al. 2005; Dinges and Weaver 2003; Moldofsky et al. 2000; U.S. Modafinil in Narcolepsy Multicenter Study Group 2000). Atomoxetine, a highly selective norepinephrine reuptake inhibitor approved for use in ADHD, has been associated with anorexia and weight loss in children and adults (Michelson et al. 2003; Wernicke and Kratochvil 2002). It has also been shown to reduce food consumption in animal models of feeding (Gehlert et al. 1998) and to significantly reduce body weight as compared with placebo in a preliminary 12-week study in 30 women with uncomplicated obesity (Gadde et al. 2006). Regarding dopamine agonists, bromocriptine (at a dosage of 1.6–2.4 mg/day) was shown superior to placebo in reducing weight and improving glucose tolerance in an 18-week study in 17 obese patients (Cincotta and Meier 1996). Bromocriptine was also shown to improve glycemic control and glucose tolerance in a placebo-controlled, 16-week study of 22 obese patients with T2DM who were prescribed a weight-maintaining diet (Pijl et al. 2000). The appetite suppressant and weight loss effects of these drugs have been attributed to their enhancement of brain catecholamine function, which includes promotion of dopamine and/or norepinephrine release or blockade of dopamine and/or norepinephrine reuptake (Bray and Greenway 1999); however, with the exception of the stimulants noted earlier (phentermine, mazindol, and diethylpropion), none of these drugs is approved as a weight loss agent.

Although no stimulant or dopamine agonist is approved by the FDA for the treatment of a psychotic or mood disorder, these agents are relatively commonly used in patients with severe mental illness for several reasons. First, stimulants and dopamine agonists, when used adjunctively with antipsychotics, may have therapeutic effects on negative or cognitive symptoms in some patients with schizophrenia. An evaluation of four short studies of amphetamines in a total of 83 schizophrenia patients found that amphetamines significantly reduced negative, but not positive, symptoms (Nolte et al. 2004). Also, a small, double-blind, placebo-controlled study showed that d-amphetamine significantly improved cognitive function in 10 schizophrenia patients taking typical antipsychotics (Barch and Carter 2005). Similarly, open studies suggest dopamine agonists (pramipexole, roxindole, and talipexole) may improve negative symptoms in patients with schizophrenia who are receiving antipsychotics (Benkert et al. 1995; Kasper et al. 1997). However, a controlled study of mazindol augmentation for negative symptoms in antipsychotic-treated schizophrenia patients failed to show separation between drug and placebo (W.T. Carpenter et al. 2000). Also, there are a number of open-label reports of stimulants and dopamine agonists apparently exacerbating psychotic symptoms in patients with severe mental disorders, especially when these agents are administered without concomitant antipsychotic medication (Cleare 1996; Devan 1990; Krumholz and White 1970; Rubin 1964; West 1974).

Second, these agents may be effective in various depressive syndromes, including those in patients with severe mental disorders (Chiarello and Cole 1987; Klein 1995). A review of 10 early controlled studies suggested stimulant monotherapy was not superior to placebo in the short-term treatment of outpatient major depression (Satel and Nelson 1989), but many of these studies had methodological limitations, including unclear entry criteria and high placebo response rates. Since then, mounting reports, including a number of controlled trials, have found several stimulants, modafinil, and the dopamine agonists amantadine and pramipexole to be effective in treating a range of depressive syndromes, especially when used as adjunctive therapy. Thus *d*-amphetamine was shown to be superior to placebo in reducing anxious-depressive symptoms in obese patients (Rickels et al. 1976); methylphenidate was found to be superior to placebo in older, depressed, medically ill patients (A.E. Wallace et al. 1995); and modafinil was shown to be superior to placebo when used adjunctively with antidepressants to treat residual fatigue symptoms in two studies in patients with major depressive disorder (DeBattista et al. 2003; Fava et al. 2005b). Pramipexole was shown superior to placebo and comparable with fluoxetine as monotherapy in reducing depressive symptoms in an 8-week study of major depression (*N*=174; Corrigan et al. 2000) and in two small 6-week studies as adjunctive therapy in bipolar depression (*N*=22 [Goldberg et al. 2004] and *N*=21 [Zarate et al. 2004]). In a small controlled study of modafinil in patients with schizophrenia and schizoaffective disorder, fatigue improved significantly over time with both modafinil and placebo (Sevy et al. 2005). There have also been reports of the successful use of various stimulants, dopamine agonists, and modafinil to augment antidepressants and mood stabilizers in patients with treatment-resistant mood or psychotic disorders (Carlson et al. 2004; Fawcett et al. 1991; Fernandes and Petty 2003; Huber et al. 1999; Nierenberg et al. 1988; Stryjer et al. 2003). Further supporting the possibility that these agents have antidepressant properties are reports that they may induce manic syndromes; they should therefore be used cautiously in patients with bipolar disorder or manic symptoms (Raison and Klein 1997).

A third reason stimulants are commonly used in severely mentally ill patients is that some of the conditions for which they are approved, especially ADHD and obstructive sleep apnea, often co-occur with severe mental disorders (Scheffer et al. 2005; Tossell et al. 2004). Moreover, there are reports that some of these agents may be effective in treating other conditions that co-occur with psychotic and mood disorders. Thus methylphenidate has been reported to reduce binge eating and purging in bulimia nervosa, including in patients with antidepressant-resistant illness (Drimmer 2003; Schweickert et al. 1997; Sokol et al. 1999).

Finally, although most of the studies of these agents in psychotic or mood disorders did not report effects on weight, some of these medications have been used to treat obesity or weight gain in patients with severe mental disorders. Several double-blind, placebo-controlled studies of *d*-amphetamine (Modell and Hussar 1965), chlorphentermine and phenmetrazine (Sletten et al. 1967), and phenylpropanolamine (Borovicka et al. 2002) in schizophrenic patients with obesity or weight gain showed these agents were not associated with weight loss. In contrast, Goodall et al. (1988) found dexfenfluramine was associated with significantly more weight loss than placebo in a 12-week trial in 33 antipsychotic-treated outpatients.

Several open studies (Correa et al. 1987; Floris et al. 2001; Gracious et al. 2002) and two controlled trials (Deberdt et al. 2005; Graham et al. 2005) suggest amantadine may attenuate antipsychotic-associated weight gain in patients with severe mental disorders. In the first controlled trial, Deberdt et al. (2005) randomized 125 patients with schizophrenia, schizoaffective disorder, or bipolar disorder who were not acutely psychotic or manic, had been treated with olanzapine for 1–24 months, and had gained 5% or more of their initial body weight to treatment with amantadine 100–300 mg/day ($n=60$) or placebo ($n=65$). Weight change from baseline in the olanzapine plus amantadine group was significantly different from that of the olanzapine plus placebo group at weeks 8, 12, and 16. Specifically, at week 16, the amantadine group had lost a mean of 0.2 kg, whereas the placebo group had gained a mean of 1.3 kg. Mean Brief Psychiatric Rating Scale total, positive subscale, and anxiety-depression scores improved comparably in both groups, and the Montgomery-Åsberg Depression Rating Scale total score improved in the amantadine group. In the second controlled trial, Graham et al. (2005) randomly assigned 21 patients with schizophrenia, schizoaffective disorder, or bipolar disorder who had gained 5 lb or more while taking olanzapine to amantadine ($n=12$) or placebo ($n=9$) for 12 weeks. Significantly fewer patients taking amantadine gained weight, with a mean change in BMI of -0.07 kg/m^2 for the amantadine group and 1.24 kg/m^2 for the placebo group. Positive and Negative Syndrome Scale scores remained stable, and there were no changes in metabolic parameters.

Two placebo-controlled studies of adjunctive modafinil in patients with major depressive disorder reported no change in weight (DeBattista et al. 2003) and a small weight loss (0.6 kg with modafinil vs. 0.4 kg gain with placebo) (Fava et al. 2005b). There is a case report of a patient with schizoaffective disorder and obesity who had a 40-lb weight loss and a BMI reduction from 35.5 to 30.4 kg/m^2 over the course of 1 year after modafinil was added to his clozapine (Henderson et al. 2005b). After 3 years of combined clozapine-modafinil treatment, the patient's BMI stabilized at 29.6 kg/m^2. When modafinil was discontinued, he gained 30 lb over a 6-month period. Reinstitution of modafinil resulted in a 10-lb weight loss over a 6-week period.

Appetite Suppressants

Preliminary data suggest sibutramine is effective over the short term for obesity associated with psychotropic use in patients with severe mental illness. In a double-blind, 12-week study, sibutramine was found to be superior to placebo for weight loss in 37 overweight or obese patients with schizophrenia or schizoaffective disorder who received olanzapine (Henderson et al. 2005a). Sibutramine was also associated with greater decreases in waist circumference and glycosylated hemoglobin. Although well tolerated, the drug was associated with a 2.1-mm Hg mean increase in systolic blood pressure and at least twice the rate of anticholinergic side effects and insomnia as compared with placebo.

Although there are no published studies of sibutramine use in patients with mood disorders, sibutramine has displayed antidepressant properties in animal models of depression (Buckett et al. 1988). The drug was shown to be superior to placebo in reducing binge eating behavior and body weight in two 12-week trials of obese patients with BED (Appolinario et al. 2003; Milano et al. 2005). In one of these studies, the drug also significantly reduced depressive symptoms compared with placebo (Appolinario et al. 2003). Further supporting the possibility that sibutramine may have antidepressant properties are reports of it inducing mania and manic symptoms (Cordeiro and Vallada 2002). The drug has also been reported to induce psychotic episodes (Taflinski and Chojnacka 2000). Thus, as with antidepressants and stimulants, sibutramine should be used cautiously in patients with severe mental disorders.

Metabolic Agents

There have been no controlled studies of orlistat in obese patients with severe mental disorders. Cases of patients with schizophrenia, bipolar disorder, and major depression successfully receiving orlistat for psychotropic-associated weight gain have been described (Anghelescu et al. 2000; Hilger et al. 2002; Schwartz et al. 2004). In one report, orlistat promoted varying degrees of weight loss (1%–8.7% of body weight) over an 8-week period, with minimal changes in psychotropic drug plasma levels (Hilger et al. 2002). However, there is a case report of one patient with bipolar II disorder who developed depression after addition of orlistat to venlafaxine upon three successive occasions (Benazzi 2000).

Orlistat has also been shown, in two controlled, 12-week trials (one in combination with cognitive-behavioral therapy), to be superior to placebo in reducing body weight in patients with BED (Golay et al. 2005; Grilo et al. 2005a). However, there are also case reports of eating disorder patients abusing the drug (Cochrane and Malcolm 2002; Malhotra and McElroy 2002). Thus our group will use orlistat in obese patients with comorbid eating pathology (including those with severe mental disorders), but we monitor the patient's eating behavior and use of the drug. We tend to avoid using orlistat in patients with purging behavior or poor insight into their pathological eating behaviors.

One open-label study suggested that the insulin-sensitizing agent metformin may reduce weight in severely mentally ill adolescents receiving antipsychotics (Morrison et al. 2002). However, in a single-blind, 12-week trial in which five antipsychotic-treated women with chronic schizophrenia received 4 weeks of placebo followed by 8 weeks of metformin, body weight loss was greater during placebo treatment (3.3 kg) than during treatment with metformin (1.3 kg) (Baptista et al. 2001).

BARIATRIC SURGERY

Relatively little is known about bariatric surgery for the severely mentally ill patient with extreme obesity. Reports in the literature indicate that obese patients undergoing bariatric surgery often report decreased depressive symptoms with weight loss after surgery, but it is often unclear whether their depressive symptoms were in fact due to severe mood disorders because their psychiatric diagnoses were usually not provided (Dixon et al. 2003). Also, several groups have documented return of patients' depressive symptoms approximately 2 years postsurgery, when weight loss plateaued or weight gain occurred (Hsu et al. 1998; Waters et al. 1991). In the recent meta-analysis of bariatric surgery noted earlier involving 22,094 patients, 17.4% of patients were reported to have "depression," but the outcome of their depression after surgery was not reported (Buchwald et al. 2004).

There are case reports of severely mentally disordered patients with obesity undergoing successful bariatric surgery without destabilization of their illness, but there are also cases of such patients developing postsurgical relapses (Fuller et al. 1986; Kaltsounis and DeLeon 2000). For example, B.A. Lawlor and Rand (1986) described six obese patients with schizophrenia who underwent gastric restrictive surgery between 1980 and 1985 and lost an average of 42.0 kg after 1 year (range, 34.5–55 kg). No patient was psychotic at the time of surgery. The five patients who had had their antipsychotic medications maintained up to 24 hours before surgery, and had received parenteral antipsychotics for 24–48 hours following surgery, remained "fairly stable" (two patients had mild psychotic symptom recurrences but did not require hospitalization). The sixth patient, whose antipsychotic medication was withdrawn and discontinued for 2 weeks before surgery, became psychotic after surgery, requiring a 6-week hospitalization.

Hamoui et al. (2004) described five patients with schizophrenia that was well controlled with antipsychotics, extreme obesity (median BMI 54), and obesity-related medical comorbidities who all underwent successful bariatric surgical procedures after treatment with standard weight reduction methods failed. All patients remained on antipsychotic medication until 24 hours before surgery, and these medications were resumed several days postsurgery. Median percent excess weight loss at 6 months was comparable to that achieved in a nonpsychiatrically ill control group. Only one patient had a brief relapse of psychotic symptoms occurring before her antipsychotic medication was resumed; no patients required psychiatric hospitalization following surgery.

Of note, there is a case report of successful oral haloperidol absorption after gastric bypass in a woman with schizophrenia and obesity (Fuller et al. 1986). There is also a case of the successful use of intravenous valproate for the treatment of manic symptoms that developed in a patient with schizoaffective disorder, bipolar type, after bariatric surgery (Kaltsounis and DeLeon 2000). The patient was eventually stabilized with oral valproate 5,000 mg/day (with a serum concentration of 123 mg/mL) and clozapine 325 mg/day, indicating he was absorbing at least the valproate.

Conclusion

Severe mental illness and obesity are each serious public health problems that over-lap to a clinically significant degree. Many psychotropic medications have adverse or therapeutic effects on appetite, weight, binge eating, and even primary obesity. Conversely, some antiobesity agents may have adverse or possibly therapeutic effects on psychopathology. In managing the patient with a severe mental disorder and obesity, therefore, it is imperative to know the complete therapeutic profile of available psychotropic and antiobesity agents, including the potential effects of psychotropics on appetite, body weight, and metabolic parameters and the potential effects of antiobesity agents on psychotic, manic, and depressive symptoms.

For patients with severe mental illness and obesity, first-line treatments include psychotropics with maximal efficacy for their mental disorder that also possess appetite suppressant, weight loss, or anti–binge eating properties as well as optimal tolerability and safety. If such a drug is not available for a patient's particular psychopathology, drugs that are weight neutral, followed by drugs that have lower weight-gaining liabilities, could be chosen, provided that the drugs have comparable efficacy, tolerability, and safety. However, because some of the most effective drugs for severe mental disorders are associated with the greatest weight-gaining liabilities, it is inevitable that a sizable number of severely mentally ill patients will need to be treated with such agents. Those patients with severe mental disorders and obesity, especially those requiring weight-gaining medication(s), will therefore need to be viewed as having at least two chronic illnesses requiring long-term management: severe mental illness, obesity, and any obesity-related medical conditions. A thorough understanding of the relationships among mental disorders and obesity; the adverse and therapeutic effects of psychotropic drugs on appetite, binge eating, weight, and metabolism; and the effects of anti-obesity agents on eating behavior and psychopathology should enable optimal medical treatment of the obese mentally ill patient's psychopathology while minimizing weight gain or, ideally, promoting weight loss and improving metabolic health.

KEY CLINICAL CONCEPTS

- Obesity and mental illness are public health problems that have significant overlap.
- There are standard classifications for obesity with which mental health providers should be familiar.
- There are numerous complications associated with obesity, ranging from physical disorders to mental health conditions (primarily mood disorders) to stigmatization.
- Treatment of uncomplicated obesity consists of three levels of intervention: 1) behavioral weight management, 2) pharmacotherapy, and 3) bariatric surgery.

- Modest weight loss can reverse many of the physical complications of obesity.
- Patients with psychotic disorders and mood disorders may be at increased risk for obesity.
- Factors that predict obesity in the general population, including female gender, unhealthy lifestyle, and impaired physical functioning, predispose individuals with mental illness to obesity.
- Preliminary evidence suggests that obesity may correlate with less-favorable treatment outcomes in patients with mental illness.
- Weight management in patients with obesity and mental illness should incorporate weight-neutral agents to manage psychiatric symptoms, assessment of associated obesity comorbidity and risk factors, behavioral management strategies, and pharmacotherapy for weight loss.

References

AcompliaReport: Sanofi Update on FDA and Acomplia: March 22nd? Available online at http://www.acompliareport.com/News/news-031806.htm. Accessed April 17, 2006.

AompliaReport: Diet drug Acomplia approved in Europe; diet pill will go on sale in July. Available online at http://www.acompliareport.com/News/news-062106.htm. Accessed October 3, 2006.

AompliaReport: Sanofi optimism on diet drug Acomplia takes hit from FDA rejection of Multaq. Available online at http://www.acompliareport.com/News/news-090106.htm. Accessed October 3, 2006.

Allison DB, Fontaine KR, Heo M, et al: The distribution of body mass index among individuals with and without schizophrenia. J Clin Psychiatry 60:215–220, 1999a

Allison DB, Mentore JL, Heo M, et al: Antipsychotic-induced weight gain: a comprehensive research synthesis. Am J Psychiatry 156:1686–1696, 1999b

American Diabetes Association, American Psychiatric Association, American Association of Clinical Endocrinologists, North American Association for the Study of Obesity: Consensus development conference on antipsychotic drugs and obesity and diabetes. J Clin Psychiatry 65:267–272, 2004

American Psychiatric Association: Diagnostic and Statistical Manual of Mental Disorders, 3rd Edition. Washington, DC, American Psychiatric Association, 1980

American Psychiatric Association: Diagnostic and Statistical Manual of Mental Disorders, 3rd Edition Revised. Washington, DC, American Psychiatric Association, 1987

American Psychiatric Association: Diagnostic and Statistical Manual of Mental Disorders, 4th Edition. Washington, DC, American Psychiatric Association, 1994

American Psychiatric Association: Diagnostic and Statistical Manual of Mental Disorders, 4th Edition, Text Revision. Washington, DC, American Psychiatric Association, 2000

Anand A, Bukhari L, Jennings SA, et al: A preliminary open-label study of zonisamide treatment of bipolar depression in 10 patients. J Clin Psychiatry 66:195–198, 2005

Andersen RE, Wadden TA, Bartlett SJ, et al: Effects of lifestyle activity vs structured aerobic exercise in obese women: a randomized trial. JAMA 281:335–340, 1999

Anderson JW, Greenway FL, Fujioka K, et al: Bupropion SR enhances weight loss: a 48-week double-blind, placebo-controlled trial. Obes Res 10:633–641, 2002

Anghelescu I, Klawe C, Benkert O: Orlistat in the treatment of psychopharmacologically induced weight gain. J Clin Psychopharmacol 20:716–717, 2000

Appolinario JC, McElroy SL: Pharmacological approaches in the treatment of binge eating disorder. Curr Drug Targets 5:301–307, 2004

Appolinario JC, Bacaltchuk J, Sichieri R, et al: A randomized, double-blind, placebo-controlled study of sibutramine in the treatment of binge-eating disorder. Arch Gen Psychiatry 60:1109–1116, 2003

Appolinario JC, Bueno JR, Coutinho W: Psychotropic drugs in the treatment of obesity: what promise? CNS Drugs 18:629–651, 2004

Archie S, Wilson JH, Osborne S, et al: Pilot study: access to fitness facility and exercise levels in olanzapine-treated patients. Can J Psychiatry 48:628–632, 2003

Aronne LJ, Segal KR: Weight gain in the treatment of mood disorders. J Clin Psychiatry 64(suppl):22–29, 2003

Arranz B, Rosel P, Ramirez N, et al: Insulin resistance and increased leptin concentrations in noncompliant schizophrenia patients but not in antipsychotic-naïve first-episode schizophrenia patients. J Clin Psychiatry 65:1335–1342, 2004

Arterburn DE, Crane PK, Veenstra DL: The efficacy and safety of sibutramine for weight loss: a systematic review. Arch Intern Med 164:994–1003, 2004

Ascher-Svanum H, Stensland M, Zhao Z, et al: Acute weight gain, gender, and therapeutic response to antipsychotics in the treatment of patients with schizophrenia. BMC Psychiatry 5:3, 2005

Baldassano CF, Ghaemi SN, Chang A, et al: Acute treatment of bipolar depression with adjunctive zonisamide: a retrospective chart review. Bipolar Disord 6:432–434, 2004

Ball MP, Coons VB, Buchanan RW: A program for treating olanzapine-related weight gain. Psychiatr Serv 52:967–969, 2001

Ball MP, Hooper ET, Skipwith DF, et al: Clozapine-induced hyperlipidemia resolved after switch to aripiprazole therapy. Ann Pharmacother 39:1570–1572, 2005

Baptista T, Hernandez L, Prieto LA, et al: Metformin in obesity associated with antipsychotic drug administration: a pilot study. J Clin Psychiatry 62:653–655, 2001

Baptista T, Zarate J, Joober R, et al: Drug-induced weight gain, an impediment to successful pharmacotherapy: focus on antipsychotics. Curr Drug Targets 5:279–299, 2004

Barch DM, Carter CS: Amphetamine improves cognitive function in medicated individuals with schizophrenia and in healthy volunteers. Schizophr Res 77:43–58, 2005

Basu R, Brar JS, Chengappa KN, et al: The prevalence of metabolic syndrome in patients with schizoaffective disorder—bipolar subtype. Bipolar Disord 6:314–318, 2004

Beebe LH, Tian L, Morris N, et al: Effects of exercise on mental and physical health parameters of persons with schizophrenia. Issues Ment Health Nurs 26:661–676, 2005

Benazzi F: Depression induced by orlistat (Xenical). Can J Psychiatry 45:87, 2000

Benkert O, Müller-Siecheneder F, Wetzel H: Dopamine agonists in schizophrenia: a review. Eur Neuropsychopharmacol 5(suppl):43–53, 1995

Bergman RN, Ader M: Atypical antipsychotics and glucose homeostasis. J Clin Psychiatry 66:504–514, 2005

Berken GH, Weinstein DO, Stern WC: Weight gain: a side-effect of tricyclic antidepressants. J Affect Disord 7:133–138, 1984

Berlin I, Lavergne F: Relationship between body-mass index and depressive symptoms in patients with major depression. Eur Psychiatry 18:85–88, 2003

Biederman J, Swanson JM, Wigal SB, et al: Efficacy and safety of modafinil film coated tablets in children and adolescents with attention-deficit/hyperactivity disorder: results of a randomized, double-blind, placebo-controlled, flexible-dose study. Pediatrics 116: e777–e784, 2005

Black DW, Goldstein RB, Mason EE: Prevalence of mental disorder in 88 morbidly obese bariatric clinic patients. Am J Psychiatry 149:227–234, 1992

Borovicka MC, Fuller MA, Konicki PE, et al: Phenylpronolamine appears not to promote weight loss in patients with schizophrenia who have gained weight during clozapine treatment. J Clin Psychiatry 63:345–348, 2002

Brar JS, Ganguli R, Pandina G, et al: Effects of behavioral therapy on weight loss in overweight and obese patients with schizophrenia or schizoaffective disorder. J Clin Psychiatry 66:205–212, 2005

Bray GA: Risks of obesity. Endocrinol Metab Clin North Am 32:787–804, 2003

Bray GA, Bouchard C (eds): Handbook of Obesity: Etiology and Pathophysiology, 2nd Edition. New York, Marcel Dekker, 2004

Bray GA, Greenway FL: Current and potential drugs for treatment of obesity. Endocr Rev 20:805–875, 1999

Bray GA, Hollander P, Klein S, et al: A 6-month randomized, placebo-controlled, dose-ranging trial of topiramate for weight loss in obesity. Obes Res 11:722–733, 2003

Brehm BJ, Seeley RJ, Daniels SR, et al: A randomized trial comparing a very low carbohydrate diet and a caloric-restricted low fat diet on body weight and cardiovascular risk factors in healthy women. J Clin Endocrinol Metab 88:1617–1623, 2003

Britz B, Siegfried W, Ziegler A, et al: Rates of psychiatric disorders in a clinical study group of adolescents with extreme obesity and in obese adolescents ascertained via a population based study. Int J Obes Relat Metab Disord 24:1707–1714, 2000

Brown S, Birtwistle J, Roe L, et al: The unhealthy lifestyle of people with schizophrenia. Psychol Med 29:697–701, 1999

Buchwald H, Avidor Y, Braunwald E, et al: Bariatric surgery: a systematic review and meta-analysis. JAMA 292:1724–1737, 2004

Buckett WR, Thomas PC, Luscombe GP: The pharmacology of sibutramine hydrochloride (BTS 54 524), a new antidepressant which induces rapid noradrenergic down-regulation. Prog Neuro Psychopharmacol Biol Psychiatry 12:575–584, 1988

Bulik CM, Sullivan PF, Kendler KS: An empirical study of the classification of eating disorders. Am J Psychiatry 157:886–895, 2000

Bustillo JR, Buchanan RW, Irish D, et al: Differential effect of clozapine on weight: a controlled study. Am J Psychiatry 153:817–819, 1996

Bustillo JR, Lauriello J, Parker K, et al: Treatment of weight gain with fluoxetine in olanzapine-treated schizophrenic outpatients. Neuropsychopharmacology 28:527–529, 2003

Calabrese JR, Kimmel SE, Woyshville MJ, et al: Clozapine for treatment-refractory mania. Am J Psychiatry 153:759–764, 1996

Carlson PJ, Merlock MC, Suppes T: Adjunctive stimulant use in patients with bipolar disorder: treatment of residual depression and sedation. Bipolar Disord 6:416–420, 2004

Carpenter KM, Hasin DS, Allison DB, et al: Relationships between obesity and DSM-IV major depressive disorder, suicide ideation, and suicide attempts: results from a general population study. Am J Public Health 90:251–257, 2000

Carpenter LL, Leon Z, Yasmin S, et al: Do obese depressed patients respond to topiramate? A retrospective chart review. J Affect Disord 69:251–255, 2002

Carpenter WT Jr, Breier A, Buchanan RW, et al: Mazindol treatment of negative symptoms. Neuropsychopharmacology 23:365–374, 2000

Carter WP, Hudson JI, Lalonde JK, et al: Pharmacologic treatment of binge eating disorder. Int J Eat Disord 34(suppl):S74–S88, 2003

Casey DE, Carson WH, Saha AR, et al: Switching patients to aripiprazole from other antipsychotic agents: a multicenter randomized study. Psychopharmacol (Berl) 166:391–399, 2003

Centorrino F, Baldessarini RJ, Kando JC, et al: Clozapine and metabolites: concentrations in serum and clinical findings during treatment of chronically psychotic patients. J Clin Psychopharmacol 14:119–125, 1994

Chengappa KN, Levine J, Rathore D, et al: Long-term effects of topiramate on bipolar mood instability, weight change and glycemic control: a case series. Eur Psychiatry 16:186–190, 2001

Chiarello RJ, Cole JO: The use of psychostimulants in general psychiatry: a reconsideration. Arch Gen Psychiatry 44:286–295, 1987

Cincotta AH, Meier AH: Bromocriptine (Ergoset) reduces body weight and improves glucose tolerance in obese subjects. Diabetes Care 19:667–670, 1996

Cleare AJ: Phentermine, psychosis, and family history (letter). J Clin Psychopharmacol 16:470–471, 1996

Cochrane C, Malcolm R: Case report of abuse of orlistat. Eating Behav 3:167–169, 2002

Coodin S: Body mass index in persons with schizophrenia. Can J Psychiatry 46:549–555, 2001

Cordeiro Q, Vallada H: Sibutramine-induced mania episode in a bipolar patient. Int J Neuropsychopharmacol 5:283–284, 2002

Correa N, Opler LA, Kay SR et al: Amantadine in the treatment of neuroendocrine side effects of neuroleptics. J Clin Psychopharmacol 7:91–95, 1987

Corrigan MH, Denahan AQ, Wright CE, et al: Comparison of pramipexole, fluoxetine, and placebo in patients with major depression. Depress Anxiety 11:58–65, 2000

Craft LL, Perna FM: The benefits of exercise for the clinically depressed. Prim Care Companion J Clin Psychiatry 6:104–111, 2004

Croft H, Houser TL, Jamerson BD, et al: Effect on body weight of bupropion sustained-release in patients with major depression treated for 52 weeks. Clin Ther 24:662–672, 2002

Czeisler CA, Walsh JK, Roth T, et al: Modafinil for excessive sleepiness associated with shift-work sleep disorder. N Engl J Med 353:476–486, 2005

Czobor P, Volavka J, Sheitman B, et al: Antipsychotic-induced weight gain and therapeutic response: a differential association. J Clin Psychopharmacol 22:244–251, 2002

Dansinger ML, Gleason JA, Griffith JL, et al: Comparison of the Atkins, Ornish, Weight Watchers, and Zone diets for weight loss and heart disease reduction: a randomized trial. JAMA 293:43–53, 2005

Daumit GL, Clark JM, Steinwachs DM, et al: Prevalence and correlates of obesity in a community sample of individuals with severe and persistent mental illness. J Nerv Ment Dis 191:799–805, 2003

Davis JM, Chen N, Glick ID: A meta-analysis of the efficacy of second generation antipsychotics. Arch Gen Psychiatry 60:553–564, 2003

DeBattista C, Doghramji K, Menza MA, et al: Adjunct modafinil for the short term treatment of fatigue and sleepiness in patients with major depressive disorder: a preliminary double-blind, placebo-controlled study. J Clin Psychiatry 64:1057–1064, 2003

Deberdt W, Winokur A, Cavazzoni PA, et al: Amantadine for weight gain associated with olanzapine treatment. Eur Neuropsychopharmacol 15:13–21, 2005

Delbello MP, Findling RL, Kushner S, et al: A pilot controlled trial of topiramate for mania in children and adolescents with bipolar disorder. J Am Acad Child Adolesc Psychiatry 44:539–547, 2005

Després J-P, Golay A, Sjöström L, et al: Effects of rimonabant on metabolic risk factors in overweight patients with dyslipidemia. N Engl J Med 353:2121–2134, 2005

Devan GS: Phentermine and psychosis. Br J Psychiatry 156:442–443, 1990

Devlin MJ, Yanovski SZ, Wilson GT: Obesity: what mental health professionals need to know. Am J Psychiatry 157:854–866, 2000

Devlin MJ, Goldfein JA, Petkova E, et al: Cognitive behavioral therapy and fluoxetine as adjuncts to group behavioral therapy for binge eating disorder. Obes Res 13:1077–1088, 2005

Dingemans AE, Bruna MJ, van Furth EF: Binge eating disorder: a review. Int J Obes Relat Metab Disord 26:299–307, 2002

Dinges DF, Weaver TE: Effects of modafinil on sustained attention performance and quality of life in OSA patients with residual sleepiness while being treated with nCPAP. Sleep Med 4:393–402, 2003

Dixon JB, Dixon ME, O'Brien PE: Depression in association with severe obesity: changes with weight loss. Arch Intern Med 163:2058–2065, 2003

Drimmer EJ: Stimulant treatment of bulimia nervosa with and without attention-deficit disorder: three case reports. Nutrition 19:76–77, 2003

Dunn AL, Marcus BH, Kampert JB, et al: Comparison of lifestyle and structured interventions to increase physical activity and cardiorespiratory fitness: a randomized trial. JAMA 281:327–334, 1999

Dunn AL, Trivedi MH, Kampert JB, et al: Exercise treatment for depression: efficacy and dose response. Am J Prev Med 28:1–8, 2005

Dursun SM, Devarajan S: Clozapine weight gain, plus topiramate weight loss. Can J Psychiatry 45:198, 2000

Dursun SM, Devarajan S: Accelerated weight loss after treating refractory depression with fluoxetine plus topiramate: possible mechanisms of action? Can J Psychiatry 46:287–288, 2001

Dynes JB: Diabetes in schizophrenia and diabetes in nonpsychotic medical patients. Dis Nerv Sys 30:341–344, 1969

Eckel RH, Grundy SM, Zimmet PZ: The metabolic syndrome. Lancet 365:1415–1428, 2005

Edwards JG, Anderson I: Systemic review and guide to selection of selective serotonin reuptake inhibitors. Drugs 57:507–533, 1999

El-Mallakh RS, Paskitti ME: The ketogenic diet may have mood-stabilizing properties. Med Hypotheses 57:724–726, 2001

Elmslie JL, Silverstone JT, Mann JI, et al: Prevalence of overweight and obesity in bipolar patients. J Clin Psychiatry 61:179–184, 2000

Elmslie JL, Mann JI, Silverstone JT, et al: Determinants of overweight and obesity in patients with bipolar disorder. J Clin Psychiatry 62:486–491, 2001

Expert Panel on Detection, Evaluation, and Treatment of High Blood Cholesterol in Adults: Executive Summary of the third report of the National Cholesterol Education Program (NCEP) Expert Panel on Detection, Evaluation, And Treatment of High Blood Cholesterol in Adults (Adult Treatment Panel III). JAMA 285:2486–2497, 2001

Fagiolini A, Frank E, Houck PR, et al: Prevalence of obesity and weight change during treatment in patients with bipolar I disorder. J Clin Psychiatry 63:528–533, 2002

Fagiolini A, Kupfer DJ, Houck PR, et al: Obesity as a correlate of outcome in patients with bipolar I disorder. Am J Psychiatry 160:112–117, 2003

Fagiolini A, Kupfer DJ, Rucci P, et al: Suicide attempts and ideation in patients with bipolar I disorder. J Clin Psychiatry 65:509–514, 2004

Faulkner G, Soundy AA, Lloyd K: Schizophrenia and weight management: a systematic review of interventions to control weight. Acta Psychiatr Scand 108:324–332, 2003

Fava M: Weight gain and antidepressants. J Clin Psychiatry 61(suppl):37–41, 2000

Fava M, Judge R, Hoog SL, et al: Fluoxetine versus sertraline and paroxetine in major depressive disorder: changes in weight with long-term treatment. J Clin Psychiatry 61:863–867, 2000

Fava M, Rush AJ, Thase ME, et al: 15 years of clinical experience with bupropion HCI: from bupropion to bupropion SR to bupropion XL. Prim Care Companion J Clin Psychiatry 7:106–113, 2005a

Fava M, Thase ME, DeBattista C: A multicenter, placebo-controlled study of modafinil augmentation in partial responders to selective serotonin reuptake inhibitors with persistent fatigue and sleepiness. J Clin Psychiatry 66:85–93, 2005b

Fawcett J, Kravitz HM, Zajecka JM, et al: CNS stimulant potentiation of monoamine oxidase inhibitors in treatment-refractory depression. J Clin Psychopharmacol 11:127–132, 1991

Fernandes PP, Petty F: Modafinil for remitted bipolar depression with hypersomnia. Ann Pharmacother 37:1807–1809, 2003

Flegal KM, Carroll MD, Kuczmarski RJ, et al: Overweight and obesity in the United States: prevalence and trends, 1960–1994. Int J Obes Relat Metab Disord 22:39–47, 1998

Flegal KM, Carroll MD, Ogden CL, et al: Prevalence and trends in obesity among US adults, 1999–2000. JAMA 288:1723–1727, 2002

Flegal KM, Graubard BI, Williamson DF, et al: Excess deaths associated with underweight, overweight, and obesity. JAMA 293:1861–1867, 2005

Floris M, Lejeune J, Deberdt W: Effect of amantadine on weight gain during olanzapine treatment. Eur Neuropsychopharmacol 11:181–182, 2001

Fogelholm M, Kukkonen-Harjula K: Does physical activity prevent weight gain: a systematic review. Obes Rev 1:95–111, 2000

Ford ES, Giles WH, Dietz WH: Prevalence of the metabolic syndrome among U.S. adults: findings from the Third National Health and Nutrition Examination Survey. JAMA 287:356–359, 2002

Foster GD, Wyatt HR, Hill JO, et al: A randomized trial of a low-carbohydrate diet for obesity. N Engl J Med 348:2082–2090, 2003

Freedman MR, King J, Kennedy E: Popular diets: a scientific review. Obes Res 9(suppl):1S–40S, 2001

Friedman JM: A war on obesity, not the obese. Science 299:856–858, 2003

Friedman JM: Modern science versus the stigma of obesity. Nat Med 10:563–569, 2004

Friedman MA, Brownell KD: Psychological correlates of obesity: moving to the next research generation. Psychol Bull 117:3–20, 1995

Fuller AK, Tingle D, DeVane CL, et al: Haloperidol pharmacokinetics following gastric bypass surgery. J Clin Psychopharmacol 6:376–378, 1986

Gadde KM, Parker CB, Maner LG, et al: Bupropion for weight loss: an investigation of efficacy and tolerability in overweight and obese women. Obes Res 9:544–551, 2001

Gadde KM, Franciscy DM, Wagner HR 2nd, et al: Zonisamide for weight loss in obese adults: a randomized controlled trial. JAMA 289:1820–1825, 2003

Gadde KM, Yonish GM, Wagner HR, et al: Atomoxetine for weight reduction in obese women: a preliminary randomised controlled trial. Int J Obesity 30:1138–1142, 2006

Gehlert DR, Dreshfield L, Tinsley F, et al: The selective norepinephrine reuptake inhibitor, LY368975, reduces food consumption in animal models of feeding. J Pharmacol Exp Ther 287:122–127, 1998

Goff DC, Cather C, Evins AE, et al: Medical morbidity and mortality in schizophrenia: guidelines for psychiatrists. J Clin Psychiatry 66:183–194, 2005

Golay A, Laurent-Jaccard A, Habicht F, et al: Effect of orlistat in obese patients with binge eating disorder. Obes Res 13:1701–1708, 2005

Goldberg JF, Burdick KE, Endick CJ: Preliminary randomized, double-blind, placebo-controlled trial of pramipexole added to mood stabilizers for treatment-resistant bipolar depression. Am J Psychiatry 161:564–566, 2004

Goldstein DJ, Hamilton SH, Masica DN, et al: Fluoxetine in medically stable, depressed geriatric patients: effects on weight. J Clin Psychopharmacol 17:365–369, 1997

Goodall E, Oxtoby C, Richards R, et al: A clinical trial of the efficacy and acceptability of D-fenfluramine in the treatment of neuroleptic-induced obesity. Br J Psychiatry 153:208–213, 1988

Gopalaswamy AK, Morgan R: Too many chronic mentally disabled patients are too fat. Acta Psychiatr Scand 72:254–258, 1985

Gracious BL, Krysiak TE, Youngstrom EA: Amantadine treatment of psychotropic-induced weight gain in children and adolescents: case series. J Child Adolesc Psychopharmacol 12:249–257, 2002

Graham KA, Gu H, Lieberman JA: Double-blind, placebo-controlled investigation of amantadine for weight loss in subjects who gained weight with olanzapine. Am J Psychiatry 162:1744–1746, 2005

Greenhill LL, Biederman J, Boellner SW, et al: A randomized, double-blind, placebo-controlled study of modafinil film-coated tablets in children and adolescents with attention-deficit/hyperactivity disorder. J Am Acad Child Adolesc Psychiatry 45:503–511, 2006

Grilo CM, Masheb RM, Salant SL: Cognitive behavioral therapy guided self-help and orlistat for the treatment of binge eating disorder: a randomized, double-blind, placebo-controlled trial. Biol Psychiatry 57:1193–1201, 2005a

Grilo CM, Masheb RM, Wilson GT: Efficacy of cognitive behavioral therapy and fluoxetine for the treatment of binge eating disorder: a randomized double-blind placebo-controlled comparison. Biol Psychiatry 57:301–309, 2005b

Haddock CK, Poston WS, Dill PL, et al: Pharmacotherapy for obesity: a quantitative analysis of four decades of published randomized clinical trials. Int J Obes Relat Metab Disord 26:262–273, 2002

Hafner H, Maurer K, Trendler G, et al: Schizophrenia and depression: challenging the paradigm of two separate diseases—a controlled study of schizophrenia, depression and healthy controls. Schizophr Res 77:11–24, 2005

Hamoui N, Kingsbury S, Anthone GJ, et al: Surgical treatment of morbid obesity in schizophrenic patients. Obes Surg 14:349–352, 2004

Harborne L, Fleming R, Lyall H, et al: Descriptive review of the evidence for the use of metformin in polycystic ovary syndrome. Lancet 361:1894–1901, 2003

Harto NE, Spera KF, Branconnier RJ: Fluoxetine-induced reduction of body mass in patients with major depressive disorder. Psychopharmacol Bull 24:220–223, 1988

Harto-Traux N, Stern WC, Miller LL, et al: Effects of bupropion on body weight. J Clin Psychiatry 44:183–186, 1983

Hasler G, Pine DS, Gamma A, et al: The associations between psychopathology and being overweight: a 20-year prospective study. Psychol Med 34:1047–1057, 2004

Hays JT, Ebbert JO: Bupropion sustained release for treatment of tobacco dependence. Mayo Clin Proc 78:1020–1024, 2003

Hedley AA, Ogden CL, Johnson CL, et al: Prevalence of overweight and obesity among U.S. children, adolescents, and adults, 1999–2002. JAMA 291:2847–2850, 2004

Heiskanen T, Niskanen L, Lyytikainen R, et al: Metabolic syndrome in patients with schizophrenia. J Clin Psychiatry 64:575–579, 2003

Henderson DC, Copeland PM, Daley TB, et al: A double-blind, placebo-controlled trial of sibutramine for olanzapine-associated weight gain. Am J Psychiatry 162:954–962, 2005a

Henderson DC, Louie PM, Koul P, et al: Modafinil-associated weight loss in a clozapine-treated schizoaffective disorder patient. Ann Clin Psychiatry 17: 95–97, 2005b

Hennen J, Perlis RH, Sachs G, et al: Weight gain during treatment of bipolar I patients with olanzapine. J Clin Psychiatry 65:1679–1687, 2004

Heymsfield SB, Shen W, Wang Z, et al: Evaluation of total and regional adiposity, in Handbook of Obesity: Etiology and Pathophysiology, 2nd Edition. Edited by Bray GA, Bouchard C. New York, Marcel Dekker, 2004, pp 33–79

Hibbeln JR: Fish consumption and major depression. Lancet 351:1213, 1998

Hilger E, Quiner S, Ginzel I, et al: The effect of orlistat on plasma levels of psychotropic drugs in patients with long-term psychopharmacotherapy. J Clin Psychopharmacol 22:68–70, 2002

Homel P, Casey D, Allison DB: Changes in body mass index for individuals with and without schizophrenia, 1987–1996. Schizophr Res 55:277–284, 2002

Hoopes SP, Reimherr FW, Hedges DW, et al: Treatment of bulimia nervosa with topiramate in a randomized, double-blind, placebo-controlled trial, part 1: improvement in binge and purge measures. J Clin Psychiatry 64:1335–1341, 2003

Hsiao CC, Ree SC, Chiang YL, et al: Obesity in schizophrenic outpatients receiving antipsychotics in Taiwan. Psychiatry Clin Neurosci 58:403–409, 2004

Hsu LK, Benotti PN, Dwyer J, et al: Nonsurgical factors that influence the outcome of bariatric surgery: a review. Psychosom Med 60:338–346, 1998

Huber TJ, Dietrich DE, Emrich HM: Possible use of amantadine in depression. Pharmacopsychiatry 32:47–55, 1999

Hudson JI, Lalonde JK, Berry JM, et al: Familial factors for binge eating disorder. Biol Psychiatry 57:141S, 2005

Hudson JI, Lalonde JK, Berry JM, et al: Binge eating disorder as a distinct familial phenotype in obese individuals. Arch Gen Psychiatry 63:313–319, 2006

Hung CF, Wu CK, Lin PY: Diabetes mellitus in patients with schizophrenia in Taiwan. Prog Neuropsychopharmacol Biol Psychiatry 29:523–527, 2005

Ioannides-Demos LL, Proietto J, McNeil JJ: Pharmacotherapy for obesity. Drugs 65:1391–1418, 2005

Jain AK, Kaplan RA, Gadde KM, et al: Bupropion SR vs placebo for weight loss in obese patients with depressive symptoms. Obes Res 10:1049–1056, 2002

Jeffery RW, Wing RR, Sherwood NE, et al: Physical activity and weight loss: does prescribing higher physical activity goals improve outcome? Am J Clin Nutr 78:684–689, 2003

Johnson BA, Ait-Daoud N, Bowden CL, et al: Oral topiramate for treatment of alcohol dependence: a randomized controlled trial. Lancet 361:1677–1685, 2003

Johnston E, Johnson S, McLeod P, et al: The relation of body mass index to depressive symptoms. Can J Public Health 95:179–183, 2004

Junig JT, Lehrmann JA: A psychotic episode associated with the Atkins diet in a patient with bipolar disorder. Bipolar Disord 7:305–306, 2005

Kahl KG, Bester M, Greggersen W, et al: Visceral fat deposition and insulin sensitivity in depressed women with and without comorbid borderline personality disorder. Psychosom Med 67:407–412, 2005

Kaltsounis J, De Leon OA: Intravenous valproate treatment of severe manic symptoms after gastric bypass surgery: a case report. Psychosomatics 41:454–456, 2000

Kampman KM, Pettinati H, Lynch KG, et al: A pilot trial of topiramate for the treatment of cocaine dependence. Drug Alcohol Depend 75:233–240, 2004

Kane J, Honigfeld G, Singer J, et al: Clozapine for the treatment-resistant schizophrenic: a double-blind comparison with chlorpromazine. Arch Gen Psychiatry 45:789–796, 1988

Kane JM, Marder SR, Schooler NR, et al: Clozapine and haloperidol in moderately refractory schizophrenia: a 6-month randomized and double-blind comparison. Arch Gen Psychiatry 58:965–972, 2001

Kaplan LM: Pharmacological therapies for obesity. Gastroenterol Clin North Am 34:91–104, 2005

Kasper S, Barnas C, Heiden A, et al: Pramipexole as adjunct to haloperidol in schizophrenia: safety and efficacy. Eur Neuropsychopharmacol 7:65–70, 1997

Kato MM, Currier MB, Gomez CM, et al: Prevalence of metabolic syndrome in Hispanic and non-Hispanic patients with schizophrenia. Prim Care Companion J Clin Psychiatry 6:74–77, 2004

Kato MM, Currier MB, Villaverde O, et al: The relation between body fat distribution and cardiovascular risk factors in patients with schizophrenia: a cross-sectional pilot study. Prim Care Companion J Clin Psychiatry 7:115–118, 2005

Keck PE Jr, McElroy SL: Bipolar disorder, obesity, and pharmacotherapy-associated weight gain. J Clin Psychiatry 64:1426–1435, 2003

Keck PE Jr, Buse JB, Dagogo-Jack S, et al: Managing Metabolic Concerns in Patients With Severe Mental Illness. Minneapolis, MN, Postgraduate Medicine, McGraw-Hill, 2003

Kendler KS, Eaves LJ, Walters EE, et al: The identification and validation of distinct depressive syndromes in a population-based sample of female twins. Arch Gen Psychiatry 53:391–399, 1996

Kendrick T: Cardiovascular and respiratory risk factors and symptoms among general practice patients with long-term mental illness. Br J Psychiatry 169:733–739, 1996

Kinder LS, Carnethon MR, Palaniappan LP, et al: Depression and the metabolic syndrome in young adults: findings from the Third National Health and Nutrition Examination Survey. Psychosom Med 66:316–322, 2004

Klein RG: The role of methylphenidate in psychiatry. Arch Gen Psychiatry 52:429–433, 1995

Klein S, Burke LE, Bray GA, et al: Clinical implication of obesity with specific focus on cardiovascular disease: a statement for professionals from the American Heart Association Council on Nutrition, Physical Activity, and Metabolism: endorsed by the American College of Cardiology Foundation. Circulation 110:2952–2967, 2004

Klett CJ, Caffey EM Jr: Weight changes during treatment with phenothiazine derivatives. J Neuropsychiatr 2:102–108, 1960

Knowler WC, Barrett-Connor E, Fowler SE, et al: Reduction in the incidence of type 2 diabetes with lifestyle intervention or metformin. N Engl J Med 346:393–403, 2002

Ko YH, Joe SH, Jung IK, et al: Topiramate as an adjuvant treatment with atypical antipsychotics in schizophrenic patients experiencing weight gain. Clin Neuropharmacol 28:169–175, 2005

Koponen H, Larmo I: Reversal of antipsychotic-induced weight gain during quetiapine treatment. Int Clin Psychopharmacol 18:355–356, 2003

Kotwal R, Guerjikova A, King KH, et al: Bipolar spectrum comorbidity in a weight management clinic. Bipolar Disord 7(suppl):69, 2005

Kraus T, Haack M, Schuld A, et al: Body weight, the tumor necrosis factor system, and leptin production during treatment with mirtazapine or venlafaxine. Pharmacopsychiatry 35:220–225, 2002

Krumholz WV, White L: Clinical evaluation of mazindol in chronic schizophrenics. Curr Ther Res Clin Exp 12:609–610, 1970

Kusher SF, Khan A, Lane R, et al: Topiramate monotherapy in the management of acute mania: results of four double-blind, placebo-controlled trials. Bipolar Disord 8:15–27, 2006

Lakka HM, Laaksonen DE, Lakka TA, et al: The metabolic syndrome and total and cardiovascular disease mortality in middle-aged men. JAMA 288:2709–2716, 2002

Lamertz CM, Jacobi C, Yassouridis A, et al: Are obese adolescents and young adults at higher risk for mental disorders? A community survey. Obes Res 10:1152–1160, 2002

Lawlor BA, Rand CS: Schizophrenia and gastric surgery for obesity. Am J Psychiatry 143:1321, 1986

Lawlor DA, Hopker SW: The effectiveness of exercise as an intervention in the management of depression: systematic review and meta-regression analysis of randomised controlled trials. BMJ 322:763–767, 2001

Lean ME, Han TS, Seidell JC: Impairment of health and quality of life using new U.S. federal guidelines for the identification of obesity. Arch Intern Med 159:837–843, 1999

Lee ES, Kim YH, Beck SH, et al: Depressive mood and abdominal fat distribution in overweight premenopausal women. Obes Res 13:320–325, 2005

Leonard P, Halley A, Browne S: Prevalence of obesity, lipid and glucose abnormalities in outpatients prescribed clozapine. Ir Med J 95:119–120, 2002

Levri KM, Slaymaker E, Last A, et al: Metformin as treatment for overweight and obese adults: a systematic review. Ann Fam Med 3:457–461, 2005

Levy E, Margolese HC, Chouinard G: Topiramate produced weight loss following olanzapine-induced weight gain in schizophrenia. J Clin Psychiatry 63:1045, 2002

Li Z, Maglione M, Tu W, et al: Meta-analysis: pharmacologic treatment of obesity. Ann Intern Med 142:532–546, 2005

Lieberman JA: Dopamine partial agonists. a new class of antipsychotic. CNS Drugs 18:251–267, 2004

Lieberman JA, Stroup TS, McEvoy JP, et al: Effectiveness of antipsychotic drugs in patients with chronic schizophrenia. N Engl J Med 353:1209–1223, 2005

Littrell KH, Hilligoss NM, Kirshner CD, et al: The effects of an educational intervention on antipsychotic-induced weight gain. J Nurs Scholarsh 35:237–241, 2003

Makris AP, Rush CR, Frederich RC, et al: Wake-promoting agents with different mechanisms of action: comparison of effects of modafinil and amphetamine on food intake and cardiovascular activity. Appetite 42:185–195, 2004

Malhotra S, McElroy SL: Orlistat misuse in bulimia nervosa. Am J Psychiatry 159:492–493, 2002

Manson JE, Skerrett PJ, Greenland P, et al: The escalating pandemics of obesity and sedentary lifestyle: a call to action for clinicians. Arch Intern Med 164:249–258, 2004

Marder SR, Essock SM, Miller AL, et al: Physical health monitoring of patients with schizophrenia. Am J Psychiatry 161:1334–1349, 2004

Martinez JA, Velasco JJ, Urbistondo MD: Effects of pharmacological therapy on anthropometric and biochemical status of male and female institutionalized psychiatric patients. J Am Coll Nutr 13:192–197, 1994

McElroy SL, Keck PE Jr: Topiramate, in American Psychiatric Publishing Textbook of Psychopharmacology, 3rd Edition. Edited by Schatzberg AF, Nemeroff CB. Washington, DC, American Psychiatric Publishing, 2004, pp 627–636

McElroy SL, Suppes T, Keck PE, et al: Open-label adjunctive topiramate in the treatment of bipolar disorders. Biol Psychiatry 47:1025–1033, 2000

McElroy SL, Frye MA, Suppes T, et al: Correlates of overweight and obesity in 644 patients with bipolar disorder. J Clin Psychiatry 63:207–213, 2002

McElroy SL, Arnold LM, Shapira NA, et al: Topiramate in the treatment of binge eating disorder associated with obesity: a randomized, placebo-controlled trial. Am J Psychiatry 160:255–261, 2003

McElroy SL, Kotwal R, Hudson JI, et al: Zonisamide in the treatment of binge-eating disorder: an open-label, prospective trial. J Clin Psychiatry 65:50–56, 2004a

McElroy SL, Kotwal R, Malhotra S, et al: Are mood disorders and obesity related? A review for the mental health professional. J Clin Psychiatry 65:634–651, 2004b

McElroy SL, Shapira NA, Arnold LM, et al: Topiramate in the long-term treatment of binge-eating disorder associated with obesity. J Clin Psychiatry 65:1463–1469, 2004c

McElroy SL, Kotwal R, Keck PE Jr, et al: Comorbidity of bipolar and eating disorders: distinct or related disorders with shared dysregulations? J Affect Disord 86:107–127, 2005a

McElroy SL, Suppes T, Keck PE Jr, et al: Open-label adjunctive zonisamide in the treatment of bipolar disorders: a prospective trial. J Clin Psychiatry 66:617–624, 2005b

McElroy SL, Allison DA, Bray GA (eds): Obesity and Mental Disorders. New York, Taylor and Francis Group, 2006a

McElroy SL, Kotwal R, Malhotra S, et al: Obesity and mood disorders, in Obesity and Mental Disorders. Edited by McElroy SL, Allison DA, Bray GA. New York, Taylor and Francis Group, 2006b, pp 41–92

McGuirk J, Silverstone T: The effect of the 5-HT re-uptake inhibitor fluoxetine on food intake and body weight in healthy male subjects. Int J Obes 14:361–372, 1990

McIntyre RS, Mancini DA, McCann S, et al: Topiramate versus bupropion SR when added to mood stabilizer therapy for the depressive phase of bipolar disorder: a preliminary single-blind study. Bipolar Disord 4:207–213, 2002

McIntyre RS, Riccardelli R, Binder C, et al: Open-label adjunctive topiramate in the treatment of unstable bipolar disorder. Can J Psychiatry 50:415–422, 2005

McQuade RD, Stock E, Marcus R, et al: A comparison of weight change during treatment with olanzapine or aripiprazole: results from a randomized, double-blind study. J Clin Psychiatry 65(suppl):47–56, 2004

Menza M, Vreeland B, Minsky S, et al: Managing atypical antipsychotic-associated weight gain: 12-month data on a multimodal weight control program. J Clin Psychiatry 65:471–477, 2004

Michelson D, Amsterdam JD, Quitkin FM, et al: Changes in weight during a 1-year trial of fluoxetine. Am J Psychiatry 156:1170–1176, 1999

Michelson D, Adler L, Spencer T, et al: Atomoxetine in adults with ADHD: two randomized, placebo-controlled studies. Biol Psychiatry 53:112–120, 2003

Milano W, Petrella C, Casella A, et al. Use of sibutramine, an inhibitor of the reuptake of serotonin and noradrenaline, in the treatment of binge eating disorder: a placebo-controlled study. Adv Ther 22:25–31, 2005

Miller GE, Stetler CA, Carney RM, et al: Clinical depression and inflammatory risk markers for coronary heart disease. Am J Cardiol 90:1279–1283, 2002

Miller WC, Wadden TA: Exercise as a treatment for obesity, in Handbook of Obesity: Clinical Applications, 2nd Edition. Edited by Bray GA, Bouchard C. New York, Marcel Dekker, 2004, pp 169–183

Modell W, Hussar AE: Failure of dextroamphetamine to influence eating and sleeping patterns in obese schizophrenic patients: clinical and pharmacological significance. JAMA 193:275–278, 1965

Mokdad AH, Serdula MK, Dietz WH, et al: The spread of the obesity epidemic in the United States, 1991–1998. JAMA 282:1519–1522, 1999

Mokdad AH, Serdula MK, Dietz WH, et al: The continuing epidemic of obesity in the United States. JAMA 284:1650–1651, 2000

Mokdad AH, Bowman BA, Ford ES, et al: The continuing epidemics of obesity and diabetes in the United States. JAMA 286:1195–1200, 2001

Mokdad AH, Ford ES, Bowman BA, et al: Prevalence of obesity, diabetes, and obesity-related health risk factors, 2001. JAMA 289:76–79, 2003

Moldofsky H, Broughton RJ, Hill JD: A randomized trial of the long-term, continued efficacy and safety of modafinil in narcolepsy. Sleep Med 1:109–116, 2000

Morrison JA, Cottingham EM, Barton BA: Metformin for weight loss in pediatric patients taking psychotropic drugs. Am J Psychiatry 159:655–657, 2002

Muller-Oerlinghausen B, Passoth PM, Poser W, et al: Impaired glucose tolerance in long-term lithium-treated patients. Int Pharmacopsychiatry 14:350–362, 1979

National Institutes of Health, National Heart, Lung and Blood Institute: Clinical Guidelines on the Identification, Evaluation and Treatment of Overweight and Obesity in Adults: The Evidence Report. Bethesda, MD, National Institutes of Health, 1998

Newcomer JW: Metabolic risk during antipsychotic treatment. Clin Ther 26:1936–1946, 2004

Nickel MK, Nickel CN, Muehlbacher M, et al: Influence of topiramate on olanzapine-related adiposity in women: a random, double-blind, placebo-controlled study. J Clin Psychopharmacol 25:211–217, 2005

Nierenberg AA, Dougherty D, Rosenbaun JF: Dopaminergic agents and stimulants as antidepressant augmentation strategies. J Clin Psychiatry 59(suppl):60–63, 1988

Nolte S, Wong D, Lachford G: Amphetamines for schizophrenia. Cochrane Database Syst Rev Oct 18; CD004964, 2004

Ogden CL, Flegal KM, Carroll MD, et al: Prevalence and trends in overweight among U.S. children and adolescents, 1999–2000. JAMA 288:1728–1732, 2002

Ogden CL, Carroll MD, Curtin LR, et al: Prevalence of overweight and obesity in the United States, 1999–2004. JAMA 295:1549–1555, 2006

O'Meara S, Riemsma R, Shirran L, et al: A systematic review of the clinical effectiveness of orlistat used for the management of obesity. Obes Rev 5:51–68, 2004

Onyike CU, Crum RM, Lee HB, et al: Is obesity associated with major depression? Results from the Third National Health and Nutrition Examination Survey. Am J Epidemiol 158:1139–1147, 2003

Papakostas GI, Petersen T, Iosifescu DV, et al: Obesity among outpatients with major depressive disorder. Int J Neuropsychopharmacol 8:59–63, 2004

Paton C, Esop R, Young C, et al: Obesity, dyslipidaemias and smoking in an inpatient population treated with antipsychotic drugs. Acta Psychiatr Scand 110:299–305, 2004

Peet M: International variations in the outcome of schizophrenia and the prevalence of depression in relation to national dietary practices: an ecological analysis. Br J Psychiatry 184:404–408, 2004a

Peet M: Nutrition and schizophrenia: beyond omega-3 fatty acids. Prostaglandins Leukot Essent Fatty Acids 70:417–422, 2004b

Peet M, Stokes C: Omega-3 fatty acids in the treatment of psychiatric disorders. Drugs 65:1051–1059, 2005

Pijl H, Ohashi S, Matsuda M, et al: Bromocriptine: a novel approach to the treatment of type 2 diabetes. Diabetes Care 23:1154–1161, 2000

Pine DS, Cohen P, Brook J, et al: Psychiatric symptoms in adolescence as predictors of obesity in early adulthood: a longitudinal study. Am J Public Health 87:1303–1310, 1997

Pine DS, Goldstein RB, Wolk S, et al: The association between childhood depression and adulthood body mass index. Pediatrics 107:1049–1056, 2001

Pi-Sunyer FX, Aronne LJ, Heshmati HM, et al: Effect of rimonabant, a cannabinoid-1 receptor blocker, on weight and cardiometabolic risk factors in overweight and obese patients. RIO-North America: a randomized controlled trial. JAMA 295:761–775, 2006

Poyurovsky M, Pashinian A, Gil-Ad I, et al: Olanzapine-induced weight gain in patients with first episode schizophrenia: a double-blind, placebo-controlled study of fluoxetine addition. Am J Psychiatry 159:1058–1060, 2002

Poyurovsky M, Isaacs I, Fuchs C, et al: Attenuation of olanzapine-induced weight gain with reboxetine in patients with schizophrenia: a double-blind, placebo-controlled study. Am J Psychiatry 160:297–302, 2003

Puhl R, Brownell KD: Bias, discrimination, and obesity. Obes Res 9:788–805, 2001

Raison CL, Klein HM: Psychotic mania associated with fenfluramine and phentermine use. Am J Psychiatry 154:711, 1997

Ramacciotti CE, Paoli RA, Catena M, et al: Schizophrenia and binge-eating disorders. J Clin Psychiatry 65:1016–1017, 2004

Richardson CR, Faulkner G, McDevitt J, et al: Integrating physical activity into mental health services for persons with serious mental illness. Psychiatr Serv 56:324–331, 2005

Richardson LP, Davis R, Poulton R, et al: A longitudinal evaluation of adolescent depression and adult obesity. Arch Pediatr Adolesc Med 157:739–745, 2003

Rickels K, Hesbacher P, Fisher E, et al: Emotional symptomatology in obese patients treated with fenfluramine and dextroamphetamine. Psychol Med 6:623–630, 1976

Ried LD, Renner BT, Bengtson MA, et al: Weight change after an atypical antipsychotic switch. Ann Pharmacother 37:1381–1386, 2003

Roberts RE, Deleger S, Strawbridge WJ, et al: Prospective association between obesity and depression: evidence from the Alameda County Study. Int J Obes Relat Metab Disord 27:514–521, 2003

Rosen JC, Gross J, Loew D, et al: Mood and appetite during minimal-carbohydrate and carbohydrate-supplemented hypocaloric diets. Am J Clin Nutr 42:371–390, 1985

Rosmond R: Role of stress in the pathogenesis of the metabolic syndrome. Psychoneuroendocrinology 30:1–10, 2005

Rosmond R, Björntorp P: Endocrine and metabolic aberrations in men with abdominal obesity in relation to anxio-depressive infirmity. Metabolism 47:1187–1193, 1998a

Rosmond R, Björntorp P: Psychiatric ill-health of women and its relationship to obesity and body fat distribution. Obes Res 6:338–345, 1998b

Rosmond R, Lapidus L, Marin P, et al: Mental distress, obesity and body fat distribution in middle-aged men. Obes Res 4:245–252, 1996

Rotatori AF, Fox R, Wicks A: Weight loss with psychiatric residents in a behavioral self control program. Psychol Rep 46:483–486, 1980

Rubin RT: Acute psychotic reaction following ingestion of phentermine. Am J Psychiatry 120:1124–1125, 1964

Rudolph RL, Fabre LF, Feighner JP, et al: A randomized, placebo-controlled, dose-response trial of venlafaxine hydrochloride in the treatment of major depression. J Clin Psychiatry 59:116–122, 1998

Ryan MC, Collins P, Thakore JH: Impaired fasting glucose tolerance in first episode, drug-naïve patients with schizophrenia. Am J Psychiatry 160:284–289, 2003

Ryan MC, Flanagan S, Kinsella U, et al: The effects of atypical antipsychotics on visceral fat distribution in first episode, drug-naïve patients with schizophrenia. Life Sci 74:1999–2008, 2004

Saari KM, Lindeman SM, Viilo KM, et al: A 4-fold risk of metabolic syndrome in patients with schizophrenia: the North Finland 1966 Birth Cohort Study. J Clin Psychiatry 66, 559–563, 2005

Sacks FM: Metabolic syndrome: epidemiology and consequences. J Clin Psychiatry 65 (suppl):3–12, 2004

Saenz A, Fernandez-Esteban I, Mataix A, et al: Metformin monotherapy for type 2 diabetes mellitus. Cochrane Database Syst Rev July 20; CD002966, 2005

Samaha FF, Igbal N, Seshadri P, et al: A low-carbohydrate as compared with a low-fat diet in severe obesity. N Engl J Med 348:2074–2081, 2003

Satel SL, Nelson JC: Stimulants in the treatment of depression: a critical overview. J Clin Psychiatry 50:241–249, 1989

Scheffer RE, Kowatch RA, Carmody T, et al: Randomized, placebo-controlled trial of mixed amphetamine salts for symptoms of comorbid ADHD in pediatric bipolar disorder after mood stabilization with divalproex sodium. Am J Psychiatry 162:58–64, 2005

Schwartz TL, Jindal S, Simionescu M, et al: Effectiveness of orlistat versus diet and exercise for weight gain associated with antidepressant use: a pilot study. J Clin Psychopharmacol 24:555–556, 2004

Schweickert LA, Strober M, Moskowitz A: Efficacy of methylphenidate in bulimia nervosa comorbid with attention deficit hyperactivity disorder: a case report. Int J Eating Disord 21:299–301, 1997

Sevy R, Rosenthal MH, Alvir J, et al: Double-blind, placebo-controlled study of modafinil for fatigue and cognition in schizophrenia patients treated with psychotropic medications. J Clin Psychiatry 66:839–843, 2005

Shekelle PG, Morton SC, Maglione MA, et al: Pharmacological and Surgical Treatment of Obesity. Evidence Report/Technology Assessment No.103. Rockville, MD, Agency for Healthcare Research and Quality, 2004

Shiori T, Kato T, Murashita J, et al: Changes in the frequency distribution pattern of body weight in patients with major depression. Acta Psychiatr Scand 88:356–360, 1993

Silverstone T, Smith G, Goodall E: Prevalence of obesity in patients receiving depot antipsychotics. Br J Psychiatry 153:214–217, 1988

Siris SG: Depression and schizophrenia, in Schizophrenia. Edited by Hirsch SR, Weinberger DR. Oxford, England, Blackwell Science, 1995, pp 128–145

Sletten IW, Ognjanov V, Menendez S, et al: Weight reduction with chlorphenetermine and phenmetrazine in obese psychiatric patients during chlorpromazine therapy. Curr Ther Res Clin Exp 9:570–575, 1967

Smith DE, Marcus MD, Lewis CE, et al: Prevalence of binge eating disorder, obesity, and depression in a biracial cohort of young adults. Ann Behav Med 20:227–232, 1998

Sokol MS, Gray NS, Goldstein A, et al: Methylphenidate treatment in bulimia nervosa associated with cluster B personality disorder. Int J Eat Disord 25:233–237, 1999

Stahl Z, Belmaker RH, Friger M, et al: Nutritional and life style determinants of plasma homocysteine in schizophrenia patients. Eur Neuropsychopharmacol 15:291–295, 2005

Stedman T, Welham J: The distribution of adipose tissue in female in-patients receiving psychotropic drugs. Br J Psychiatry 162:249–250, 1993

Stern L, Iqbal N, Seshadri P: The effects of low-carbohydrate versus conventional weight loss diets in severely obese adults: one year follow-up of a randomized trial. Arch Intern Med 140:778–785, 2004

Stoll AL, Severus WE, Freeman MP, et al: Omega 3 fatty acids in bipolar disorder: a preliminary double-blind, placebo-controlled trial. Arch Gen Psychiatry 56:407–412, 1999

Strassnig M, Brar JS, Ganguli R: Body mass index and quality of life in community-dwelling patients with schizophrenia. Schizophr Res 62:73–76, 2003

Stryjer R, Strous RD, Shaked G, et al: Amantadine as augmentation therapy in the management of treatment-resistant depression. Int Clin Psychopharmacol 18:93–96, 2003

Stunkard AJ, Faith MS, Allison KC: Depression and obesity. Biol Psychiatry 54:330–337, 2003

Suppes T, Webb A, Paul B, et al: Clinical outcome in a randomized 1-year trial of clozapine versus treatment as usual for patients with treatment-resistant illness and a history of mania. Am J Psychiatry 156:1164–1169, 1999

Susce MT, Villanueva N, Diaz FJ, et al: Obesity and associated complications in patients with severe mental illnesses: a cross-sectional survey. J Clin Psychiatry 66:167–173, 2005

Sussman N, Ginsberg DL, Bikoff J: Effects of nefazodone on body weight: a pooled analysis of selective serotonin reuptake inhibitor-and imipramine-controlled trials. J Clin Psychiatry 62:256–260, 2001

Taflinski T, Chojnacka J: Sibutramine-associated psychotic episode. Am J Psychiatry 157:2057–2058, 2000

Thakore JH: Metabolic disturbances in first-episode schizophrenia. Br J Psychiatry Suppl 47:S76–S79, 2004

Thakore JH, Richards PJ, Reznek RH, et al: Increased intra-abdominal fat deposition in patients with major depressive illness as measured by computed tomography. Biol Psychiatry 41:1140–1142, 1997

Thakore JH, Mann JN, Vlahos I, et al: Increased visceral fat distribution in drug-naïve and drug-free patients with schizophrenia. Int J Obes Relat Metab Disord 26:137–141, 2002

Theisen FM, Linden A, Geller F, et al: Prevalence of obesity in adolescent and young adult patients with and without schizophrenia and in relationship to antipsychotic medication. J Psychiatr Res 35:339–345, 2001

Theisen FM, Linden A, Konig IR, et al: Spectrum of binge eating symptomatology in patients treated with clozapine and olanzapine. J Neural Transm 110:111–121, 2003

Tiihonen J, Halonen P, Wahlbeck K, et al: Topiramate add-on in treatment-resistant schizophrenia: a randomized, double-blind, placebo-controlled, crossover trial. J Clin Psychiatry 66:1012–1015, 2005

Tohen M, Baker RW, Altshuler LL, et al: Olanzapine versus divalproex in the treatment of acute mania. Am J Psychiatry 159:1011–1017, 2002

Tohen M, Ketter TA, Zarate CA, et al: Olanzapine versus divalproex sodium for the treatment of acute mania and maintenance of remission: a 47-week study. Am J Psychiatry 160:1263–1271, 2003a

Tohen M, Vieta E, Calabrese J, et al: Efficacy of olanzapine and olanzapine-fluoxetine combination in the treatment of bipolar I depression. Arch Gen Psychiatry 60:1079–1088, 2003b

Tossell JW, Greenstein DK, Davidson AL, et al: Stimulant drug treatment in childhood-onset schizophrenia with comorbid ADHD: an open-label case series. J Child Adolesc Psychopharmacol 14:448–454, 2004

Tuomilehto J, Lindstrom J: The major diabetes prevention trials. Curr Diab Rep 3:115–122, 2003

Tuomilehto J, Lindstrom J, Eriksson JG, et al: Prevention of type 2 diabetes mellitus by changes in lifestyle among subjects with impaired glucose tolerance. N Engl J Med 344:1343–1350, 2001

U.S. Modafinil in Narcolepsy Multicenter Study Group: Randomized trial of modafinil as a treatment for the excessive daytime somnolence of narcolepsy. Neurology 54:1166–1175, 2000

Van Gaal LF, Rissanen AM, Scheen AJ, et al: Effects of the cannabinoid-1 receptor blocker rimonabant on weight reduction and cardiovascular risk factors in overweight patients: 1-year experience from the RIO-Europe study. Lancet 365:1389–1397, 2005

Vieta E, Goikolea JM, Olivares JM, et al: 1-year follow-up of patients treated with risperidone and topiramate for a manic episode. J Clin Psychiatry 64:834–839, 2003

Vieta E, Sanchez-Moreno J, Goikolea JM, et al: Effects on weight and outcome of long-term olanzapine-topiramate combination treatment in bipolar disorder. J Clin Psychopharmacol 24:374–378, 2004

Vining EP, Freeman JM, Ballaban-Gil K, et al: A multicenter study of the efficacy of the ketogenic diet. Arch Neurol 55:1433–1437, 1998

Wadden TA, Butryn ML: Behavioral treatment of obesity. Endocrinol Metab Clin North Am 32:981–1003, 2003

Wadden TA, Foster GD: Behavioral treatment of obesity. Med Clin North Am 84:441–461, 2000

Wallace AE, Kofoed LL, West AN: Double-blind, placebo-controlled trial of methylphenidate in older, depressed, medically ill patients. Am J Psychiatry 152:929–931, 1995

Wallace B, Tennant C: Nutrition and obesity in the chronic mentally ill. Aust N Z J Psychiatry 32:82–85, 1998

Waters GS, Pories WJ, Swanson MS, et al: Long-term studies of mental health after the Greenville gastric bypass operation for morbid obesity. Am J Surg 161:154–157, 1991

Weber-Hamann B, Hentscel F, Kniest A, et al: Hypercortisolemic depression is associated with increased intra-abdominal fat. Psychosom Med 64:274–277, 2002

Weiden PJ, Simpson GM, Potkin SG, et al: Effectiveness of switching to ziprasidone for stable but symptomatic outpatients with schizophrenia. J Clin Psychiatry 64:580–588, 2003

Weiser M, Knobler H, Lubin G, et al: Body mass index and future schizophrenia in Israeli male adolescents. J Clin Psychiatry 65:1546–1549, 2004

Werneke U, Taylor D, Sanders TA, et al: Behavioural management of antipsychotic-induced weight gain: a review. Acta Psychiatr Scand 108:252–259, 2003

Wernicke JF, Kratochvil CJ: Safety profile of atomoxetine in the treatment of children and adolescents with ADHD. J Clin Psychiatry 63(suppl):50–55, 2002

West AP: Interaction of low-dose amphetamine use with schizophrenia in outpatients, three case reports. Am J Psychiatry 131:321–323, 1974

Wilding J, Gaal L, Rissanen A, et al: A randomized double-blind placebo-controlled study of the long-term efficacy and safety of topiramate in the treatment of obese subjects. Int J Obes Relat Metab Disord 28:1399–1410, 2004

Wing RR: Physical activity in the treatment of the adulthood overweight and obesity: current evidence and research issues. Med Sci Sports Exerc 31(suppl1):S547–S552, 1999

Wing RR: Behavioral approaches to the treatment of obesity, in Handbook of Obesity: Clinical Applications, 2nd Edition. Edited by Bray GA, Bouchard C. New York, Marcel Dekker, 2004, pp 147–167

Wing RR, Matthews KA, Kuller LH, et al: Waist to hip ratio in middle-aged women: associations with behavioral and psychosocial factors and with changes in cardiovascular risk factors. Arterioscler Thromb 11:1250–1257, 1991

Wirshing DA: Schizophrenia and obesity: impact of antipsychotic medications. J Clin Psychiatry 65(suppl):13–26, 2004

Woods TM, Eichner SF, Franks AS: Weight gain mitigation with topiramate in mood disorders. Ann Pharmacother 38:887–891, 2004

Wyatt RJ, Henter ID, Mojtabai R, et al: Height, weight, and body mass index (BMI) in psychiatrically ill U.S. Armed Forces personnel. Psychol Med 33:363–368, 2003

Yanovski SZ: Binge eating disorder and obesity in 2003: could treating an eating disorder have a positive effect on the obesity epidemic? Int J Eat Disord 34(suppl): S117–S120, 2003

Yanovski SZ, Yanovski JA: Obesity. N Engl J Med 346:591–602, 2002

Yanovski SZ, Nelson JE, Dubbert BK, et al: Association of binge eating disorder and psychiatric comorbidity in obese subjects. Am J Psychiatry 150:1472–1479, 1993

Yaroslavsky Y, Stahl Z, Belmaker RH: Ketogenic diet in bipolar illness. Bipolar Disord 4:75, 2002

Young G, Conquer J: Omega-3 fatty acids and neuropsychiatric disorders. Reprod Nutr Dev 45:1–28, 2005

Zarate CA Jr, Payne JL, Singh J, et al: Pramipexole for bipolar II depression: a placebo-controlled proof of concept study. Biol Psychiatry 56:54–60, 2004

Zhang ZJ, Yao ZJ, Liu W, et al: Effects of antipsychotics on fat deposition and changes in leptin and insulin levels: magnetic resonance imaging study of previously untreated people with schizophrenia. Br J Psychiatry 184:58–62, 2004

Chapter 4

SEVERE MENTAL ILLNESS AND DIABETES MELLITUS

Paul E. Keck Jr., M.D.

Susan L. McElroy, M.D.

Rakesh Kaneria, M.D.

In 1879, Sir Henry Maudsley observed that "diabetes is a disease which often shows itself in families in which insanity prevails" (Maudsley 1879). That patients with severe mental illness, schizophrenia, bipolar disorder, and major depressive disorder are at increased risk for diabetes has been observed for nearly a century and well prior to the modern era of pharmacotherapy of mental illness heralded by John Cade's discovery, in 1949, of lithium's therapeutic effects (Cade 1949).

This association between mental illness and diabetes has been the subject of renewed scientific attention because of concerns that treatment with atypical antipsychotic agents might increase the risk of type 2 diabetes mellitus (T2DM; Keck et al. 2003). However, careful scrutiny of the literature also reveals that similar concerns were raised after the introduction of lithium and typical antipsychotics (neuroleptics; Zimmerman et al. 2003). Thus, in attempting to understand the potential risks associated with treatment of these psychiatric disorders, it is important to discern the risks for diabetes posed by the illnesses themselves. In this chapter, we review the pre–modern era (prior to 1949) literature regarding the risk of diabetes in patients with severe mental illness, subsequent studies in the modern era (1949 and thereafter), and preclinical and clinical data regarding possible mechanisms underlying this risk.

Prevalence of Diabetes in Severe Mental Illness
STUDIES BEFORE 1949

Case-control studies conducted from 1919 to 1946 measuring fasting glucose concentrations (Bowman and Kasanin 1929; Kooy 1919) or glucose concentrations after oral (Barrett and Serre 1924; Cowie et al. 1924; Diethelm 1936; Drury and Farron-Ridge 1921; Henry and Mangan 1925; Kasanin 1926; Lorenz 1922; McCowan and Quastel 1931; McFarland and Goldstein 1939; Raphael and Parsons 1921; Tod 1934, 1937; Whitehorn 1934) and intravenous (Braceland et al. 1945; Freeman 1946; Glidea et al. 1943) glucose tolerance tests reported prevalence rates of diabetes in patients with psychotic and mood disorders ranging from two to four times the prevailing rates of healthy subjects (Table 4–1). Although these studies are noteworthy because they antedated the use of modern medications in the treatment of psychiatric disorders and are thus not confounded by the potential metabolic effects of these agents, there are a number of methodological limitations to these studies that make it difficult to make firm conclusions regarding their findings, even in aggregate. For example, only a few studies included healthy control subjects (Bowman and Kasanin 1929; Braceland et al. 1945; Freeman 1946; Glidea et al. 1943; Kooy 1919; McCowan and Quastel 1931), but even in those studies no data were provided regarding whether the subjects were matched on anthropometric or demographic variables. Important variables affecting risk of diabetes, such as ethnicity, body weight, body mass index (BMI), and family history of diabetes, were also not systematically provided in these studies (Keck et al. 2003). Only one study specifically excluded patients who were obese (Tod 1937). Similar to some contemporary studies, most studies from this era assessed patients who were acutely ill and thus may have had glucose elevations secondary to the stress of that illness. Treatment settings also differed radically from contemporary treatment patterns. In the absence of specific pharmacotherapies for psychotic and mood disorders, many patients in that era remained ill and were hospitalized for long periods of time. Long stays in psychiatric institutions may have led to prolonged periods of reduced activity or inactivity. Diagnostic nomenclature also differed from contemporary nosology, although it is probably reasonable to assume that many patients diagnosed with dementia praecox would have met criteria for schizophrenia, those with manic-depressive illness would have met criteria for bipolar disorder, and those with melancholia would have met criteria for major depressive disorder. The prevalence of catatonia was much higher in these reports than in contemporary inpatient settings, again no doubt reflecting the absence of therapeutic medications. Lastly, some studies provided no diagnostic data at all, instead grouping patients into "inpatient" categories (Bowman and Kasanin 1929; Diethelm 1936; Kasanin 1926; Lorenz 1922; Tod 1934, 1937; Whitehorn 1934).

With these considerable limitations in mind, some consistent findings never-theless emerge from these studies. Elevations in fasting glucose were consistently reported during acute catatonia and melancholia, and in most studies during manic episodes. In fact, only one small study of five patients described as cyclothymic found no evidence of glucose elevations during manic or hypomanic episodes (Newcomer 1922). Separating out the studies with the most rigorous methodological approaches may be more informative. For example, Bowman and Kasanin (1929) reported a 14% prevalence rate of diabetes, defined as repeated fasting glucose concentrations of more than 120 mg/dL, among 295 inpatients compared with 0% in 41 healthy control subjects. Similarly, Whitehorn (1934) reported a 13% prevalence of diabetes, defined as fasting glucose concentration of more than 140 mg/dL, among 951 "excited" inpatients. This prevalence rate was significantly higher than the prevalence rate in the general U.S. population in 1934.

Two studies utilized metabolic challenges to examine glucose metabolism. Braceland et al. (1945) tested insulin sensitivity in 29 patients with schizophrenia and 25 healthy control subjects by measuring glucose disposition following infu-sion of insulin 0.1 U/kg. They found that patients with schizophrenia had im-paired insulin sensitivity compared with the healthy control subjects. Freeman (1946) replicated these observations using the same paradigm, but in patients with schizo-phrenia and manic-depressive illness.

Even when interpretation is restricted to data from these latter, more rigorous studies, the findings continued to suggest that patients with psychotic and mood disorders were at increased risk for developing diabetes compared with the gen-eral population or healthy control subjects.

STUDIES SINCE 1949

In the following review, we include studies published since 1949 that examined the prevalence of diabetes in patients with schizophrenia and other chronic psy-chotic disorders, bipolar disorder, and major depressive disorder. We exclude stud-ies of patients receiving atypical antipsychotics but include studies in which patients were receiving typical antipsychotics, lithium, tricyclic antidepressants (TCAs), or monoamine oxidase inhibitor (MAOI) antidepressants. Studies exam-ining the prevalence of diabetes among patients receiving atypical antipsychotics are thoroughly discussed in Chapter 7 ("Glucose Metabolism: Effects of Atypical Antipsychotics"), this volume.

Schizophrenia

To our knowledge, three controlled studies conducted after the introduction of typical antipsychotic agents reported prevalence rates of diabetes in patients with psychotic disorders (Dynes 1969; Ryan et al. 2003; Tabata et al. 1987). Dynes

TABLE 4–1. Summary of studies linking mental illness to type 2 diabetes

Era/Population	Risk	Study types	Strengths of research/association	Limitations of research/association
Pre-1949				
Patients with psychotic and mood disorders	Two to four times healthy subjects	Predominantly case-control studies	Increased risk observed/replicated across different investigators, method of assessment of glucose dysregulation, and populations of individuals with severe mental illness Association of diabetes with severe mental illness antedates current era of pharmacotherapy Some replication of association in more rigorously conducted studies	Poorly defined mental illness diagnostic categories for study subjects Lack of control for important demographic or anthropometric factors that predispose individuals to developing diabetes Most study subjects were acutely ill Most studies did not include control subjects
Post-1949 (patients not prescribed SGAs)				
Patients with schizophrenia	Increased risk observed but magnitude undetermined	Controlled studies Large-cohort studies	The most rigorous controlled prospective study to date in medication-naive subjects showed an increased risk for diabetes Increased risk observed/replicated across different investigators, method of assessment of glucose dysregulation, and study sites	Most studies did not include data on other risk factors for diabetes or pharmacological treatment Magnitude of risk of diabetes posed by psychotic disorders alone could not be determined

TABLE 4–1.   Summary of studies linking mental illness to type 2 diabetes *(continued)*

Era/Population	Risk	Study types	Strengths of research/association	Limitations of research/association
Post-1949 (patients not prescribed SGAs) *(continued)*				
Patients with bipolar disorder	Inconclusive	Prospective cohort studies Retrospective chart review	Diagnostic category of bipolar disorder specified in studies Some prospective data with large follow-up period	Limited literature (number of patients studied) Most studies did not evaluate the impact of medications
Community samples with depressive symptoms	Increased risk up to twofold compared with nondepressed control subjects	Prospective epidemiological studies Case-control studies	Multiple community samples including ethnically and socioeconomically diverse samples Some studies control for other risk factors that increase the risk for type 2 diabetes	Heavy reliance on self-report of depressive symptoms or history of depression Failure to use clinician-administered diagnostic instruments to categorize subjects; thus studies do not distinguish depression from unipolar versus bipolar disorder

(1969) compared the prevalence of chart diagnosis of diabetes and obesity in 33 patients hospitalized with schizophrenia with 33 patients hospitalized with a variety of medical illnesses. Diabetes was significantly more prevalent in the medical group (27%) compared with the group with schizophrenia (3%). It is not surprising that the prevalence of diabetes would be higher in hospitalized patients with other medical (e.g., cardiovascular) illnesses. In contrast, the prevalence of obesity was significantly higher in patients with schizophrenia (64%) compared with the medically ill group (5%). This study is not informative regarding the prevalence of diabetes in patients with schizophrenia compared with the general population or healthy control subjects.

Tabata et al. (1987) examined the prevalence of diabetes in 248 patients with schizophrenia and 239 sedentary office workers and reported a significantly higher rate of diabetes in the schizophrenia group (9%) compared with the sedentary group (5%). Both groups might have been expected to have higher rates of diabetes compared with the general population. Unfortunately, neither the Dynes nor the Tabata et al. study included data regarding other risk factors for diabetes or examined the potential influence of antipsychotic or other pharmacological treatments.

Ryan et al. (2003) conducted the only controlled, prospective study of glucose tolerance in treatment-naïve patients with schizophrenia reported to date. In this cross-sectional study, fasting plasma concentrations of glucose, insulin, lipids, and cortisol were measured in 26 patients with DSM-IV (American Psychiatric Association 1994) schizophrenia who had never been treated with antipsychotic agents and 26 age- and sex-matched healthy control subjects. Subjects were also matched on several lifestyle variables (e.g., habitual amount of exercise and diet) and anthropometric measures. This study design thus controlled for a number of potential confounding factors that previous studies did not. The authors found that 15% of patients with schizophrenia (mean age = 34 years) met American Diabetes Association (1997) criteria for impaired fasting glucose tolerance compared with 0% in the healthy control group. Moreover, the patients with schizophrenia had significantly higher fasting glucose, insulin, and cortisol levels compared with the healthy control subjects. This important study requires replication but represents substantial evidence that factors associated with first-episode psychosis or its prodrome represent risk factors for impaired glucose tolerance in patients with schizophrenia, independent of treatment effects.

A number of surveys examined the prevalence rate of diabetes in large cohorts of patients with schizophrenia (McKee et al. 1986; Mukherjee et al. 1996; Schwarz and Munoz 1968; Thonnard-Neumann 1968). Schwarz and Munoz (1968) reported that only 0.6% of 859 patients developed new-onset diabetes following chlorpromazine initiation. Risk factors for developing diabetes were age, body weight, and ethnicity. Thonnard-Neumann (1968) compared the prevalence of diabetes in 450 female patients hospitalized in 1954 with a second group of 528 women with schizophrenia hospitalized in 1966 in order to examine the potential impact of treatment with typical antipsychotics on diabetes. The prevalence rate of diabetes increased from 4% in 1954 to 17% in 1966, and risk factors associated with diabetes in the 1966 cohort included age, obesity, and treatment with a typical antipsychotic. McKee et al. (1986) reported that 2.5% of 1,960 patients with schizophrenia had diabetes—a rate within the range of the general population in the mid-1960s, but at the upper end. Although most patients developed diabetes after treatment with typical antipsychotics, the drugs' potential role as a risk factor could not be determined without a control group. Finally, Mukherjee et al. (1996) specifically examined the role of antipsychotic treatment in the development of diabetes and found a higher prevalence of diabetes in patients not receiving treatment with typical antipsychotics compared with those who were. Age was the only risk factor identified with developing diabetes in this study. Interestingly, in a separate study, Mukherjee et al. (1989) also found an increased prevalence of T2DM in the first-degree relatives of patients with schizophrenia compared with the general population. Overall, the results of these surveys are inconclusive regarding the magnitude of risk of diabetes posed by psychotic disorders alone, apart from treatment.

Bipolar Disorder

Three studies examined the prevalence of diabetes in patients with bipolar disorder (Cassidy et al. 1999; Lilliker 1980; Musselman et al. 2003; Vestergaard and Schou 1987). Lilliker (1980) reported that 10% of 203 patients with bipolar disorder followed over 10 years developed diabetes, a rate significantly higher than that in the general population at that time. The impact of treatment was not assessed. Vestergaard and Schou (1987) followed 226 patients prospectively for an average of 2 years after initiation of lithium therapy and reported that only 0.4% developed diabetes. The possible use of adjunctive typical antipsychotics was not reported. In the most recent survey, Cassidy et al. (1999) reported that 9.9% of 357 patients with bipolar disorder had diabetes, a rate nearly triple that of the general population. The authors did not control for the possible effects of pharmacological treatment. Thus, as with surveys of the prevalence of diabetes in patients with schizophrenia, the results of these studies in patients with bipolar disorder are mixed and inconclusive.

Major Depressive Disorder

Epidemiological studies indicate that individuals with T2DM have elevated rates of depression compared with the general population and with patients with most other chronic medical illnesses (Musselman et al. 2003). In other words, individuals with T2DM are at increased risk of developing major depressive disorder. A number of studies also strongly suggest that the converse is true—namely, that patients with major depressive disorder are at increased risk for developing T2DM (Arroyo et al. 2004; L. C. Brown et al. 2005; Carnethon et al. 2003; Eaton et al. 1996; Golden et al. 2004;

Kawakami et al. 1999; Kessing et al. 2004; Palinkas et al. 2004; Saydah et al. 2003). In 1684 the British physician Thomas Willis observed that diabetes resulted from "sadness or long sorrow and other depressions and disorders" (Willis 1971). This prescient observation has been borne out in most, but not all, recent epidemiological studies.

The first modern study to suggest that depression might be a risk factor for T2DM was a community-based survey in Baltimore, Maryland (Eaton et al. 1996). Eaton et al. (1996), using the Diagnostic Interview Schedule to ascertain a diagnosis of major depression, found that lifetime diagnosis of major depressive disorder predicted a twofold increased risk of T2DM at 13-year follow-up. These observations were replicated by Kawakami et al. (1999), who, in a cohort of employed Japanese men, also found a twofold increased risk of T2DM in individuals with moderate to severe baseline depressive symptoms on the Zung Self-Rating Depression Scale after 8 years of follow-up. Carnethon et al. (2003) studied participants from the First National Health and Nutrition Examination Survey (NHANES I) who were followed as part of the NHANES I Epidemiologic Follow-Up Survey (NHEFS). The NHANES I, conducted from 1971 to 1975, was a cross-sectional survey of health conditions and health-related behaviors in a cohort of U.S. civilians aged 1–74 (Miller 1973; "Plan and Operation of the Health and Nutrition Examination Survey" 1973). After the initial evaluation, participants were contacted, and medical and healthcare records were examined in four cycles: 1982–1984, 1986, 1987–1989, and 1990–1992. The General Well-Being survey was administered as part of the NHANES I procedures and included questions about depressive symptoms rated on a Likert scale. In their analysis, Carnethon et al. (2003) examined the incidence of subsequent T2DM in individuals with high, moderate, and low depressive symptoms on the General Well-Being Depression subscale but also controlled for educational achievement, a proxy for socioeconomic status. They found that the incidence of diabetes was greatest among participants with the highest depressive symptoms but did not differ among individuals reporting moderate and low symptoms. In the subgroup of participants with less than a high school education, the risk of developing diabetes was threefold higher among those reporting high versus low depressive symptoms. These results were consistent with data from the Alameda County, California, epidemiological survey, which found that depression, obesity, and diabetes were associated with low socioeconomic status (Everson et al. 2002). Using data from the Nurses' Health Study cohort, an epidemiological follow-up study of 72,178 female nurses aged 45–72, Arroyo et al. (2004) found a modest risk ratio of 1.29 (0.96–1.72) for developing T2DM in nurses who reported depressive symptoms on the 36-item Short-Form Health Status Survey at baseline and at 4-year follow-up.

Golden et al. (2004) analyzed data on self-reported depressive symptoms (vital exhaustion questionnaire) from the Atherosclerosis Risk in Communities study, a cohort of 11,615 ethnically diverse individuals aged 45–64 who were evaluated at baseline and at 6-year follow-up. After adjustment for age, ethnicity, sex, and education, individuals in the highest quartile for baseline depressive symptoms had a 63% increased risk of developing diabetes compared with individuals in the lowest quartile (relative hazard = 1.63; 95% CI = 1.31–2.02). Palinkas et al. (2004) found that elevated scores on the Beck Depression Inventory at baseline predicted development of T2DM (odds ratio [OR] = 2.5; 95% CI = 1.29–4.87) in a cohort of 971 men and women aged 50 and older from the adult population in Rancho Bernardo, California, who were evaluated at baseline and at 8-year follow-up. The presence of T2DM was assessed using oral glucose tolerance tests. The risk of developing T2DM was independent of sex, age, exercise, and BMI when assessed by the presence of baseline depressive symptoms. Brown et al. (2005) conducted a population-based, nested case-control study using databases of Saskatchewan Health to assess the history of depression in individuals with new-onset T2DM compared with individuals without diabetes. Diagnoses of depression and diabetes were made based on diagnostic claim codes and prescription records. Individuals with new-onset diabetes were 30% more likely to have had a previous history of depression compared with individuals without diabetes. This elevated risk was limited to younger individuals aged 20–50 (adjusted OR = 1.23; 95% CI = 1.10–1.37).

In contrast to these cumulative findings suggesting a strong relationship between depressive symptoms and the development of T2DM, two studies failed to find such a link (Kessing et al. 2004; Saydah et al. 2003). Saydah et al. (2003) also utilized data from the NHEFS cohort, but they examined the relationship between scores on the Center for Epidemiologic Studies Depression Scale and subsequent development of T2DM in participants followed for an average of 9 years. After adjusting for age, sex, ethnicity, education, BMI, and physical activity, the relative hazard of diabetes among individuals with high depressive symptoms at baseline was 1.11 (95% CI = 0.79–1.56). Finally, Kessing et al. (2004) examined a national case register of all patients in Denmark from 1977 to 1997 who were discharged from a psychiatric hospital with a first-admission diagnosis of depression or bipolar disorder and compared them with a group with a first-admission diagnosis of osteoarthritis. The authors evaluated the groups for risk of being readmitted with a diagnosis of diabetes and found no significant differences in risk of subsequent readmission among the three groups. However, this study was biased toward inpatients and the development of severe and type 1 diabetes (T1DM). Interestingly, Ruzickova et al. (2003) reported that patients with bipolar disorder and diabetes had significantly higher rates of a rapid-cycling, chronic course of illness and greater rates of disability than patients with bipolar disorder without co-occurring diabetes. Similarly, several studies have suggested that patients with major depressive disorder and co-occurring diabetes have a higher recurrence rate of depression and longer duration of depressive episodes compared with patients without co-occurring diabetes (Talbot and Nouwen 2000).

Overall, these epidemiological data suggest a strong relationship between depressive symptoms and the risk for T2DM. These studies are limited by heavy reliance on self-report instruments and lack of clinician-administered diagnostic instruments. Thus, although they suggest that depressive symptoms are associated with an increased risk of developing diabetes, they do not distinguish among patients with major depressive disorder, bipolar disorder, and psychotic disorders, all of whom are likely to share a high lifetime prevalence of depressive symptoms.

Potential Mechanisms Linking Severe Mental Illness and Type 2 Diabetes

The precise mechanisms underlying the apparent increased risk of T2DM in patients with psychotic and mood disorders are unknown. There are several possible explanations for this strong association (Figure 4–1; Keck et al. 2003). First, these psychiatric disorders and diabetes might be consequences of some other process— for example, an as-yet unidentified genetic factor or a shared vulnerability to stress diathesis. Second, metabolic disturbances associated with psychotic and mood disorders may affect normal glucose regulation. Third, behavioral consequences of psychotic and mood disorders could increase the risk of T2DM. Fourth, psychotic and mood disorders may serve as an additive risk factor for T2DM and worsen glucose regulation only in combination with other risk factors in individuals at increased risk genetically for T2DM. Last, and not addressed in this chapter, treatments for psychotic and mood disorders with adverse metabolic effects could increase the risk of T2DM in patients with these illnesses.

HEREDITARY FACTORS

Genetic factors play an important role in vulnerability to psychotic and mood disorders as well as diabetes. Tentative overlap in gene regions identified with susceptibility to psychosis, mood disorders, and T2DM has been identified (Bushe and Holt 2004). Although the specific genes within these chromosomal regions have yet to be identified and the finding requires replication, this overlap could provide evidence of common linkage disequilibrium that may predispose to both mental illness and T2DM. Bushe and Holt (2004), marshaling available family studies of the prevalence of diabetes in first-degree relatives of patients with schizophrenia, observed that up to 50% of patients with schizophrenia have been reported to have positive family histories of diabetes compared with 5% of healthy control subjects. These findings suggest that genetic factors may contribute to the high prevalence rates of diabetes in patients with schizophrenia. To our knowledge, there are no published family history studies of the prevalence of diabetes in patients with bipolar disorder or major depressive disorder. Given these data, such studies are clearly needed.

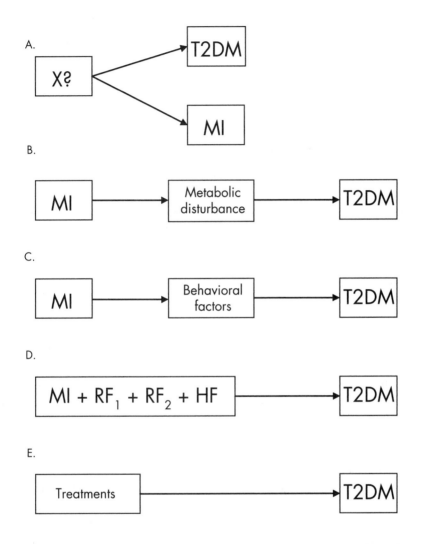

FIGURE 4–1. Five scenarios linking mental illness and type 2 diabetes mellitus (T2DM).

A. Mental illness and T2DM are the consequences of an unidentified factor.

B. Metabolic disturbances associated with mental illness cause glucose dysregulation.

C. Behavioral factors associated with mental illness may increase the risk for T2DM.

D. Mental illness in combination with other risk factors for T2DM may increase the risk of diabetes in individuals with an increased genetic risk for diabetes.

E. Treatments for mental illness increase the risk for T2DM.

HF = hereditary factor; MI = mental illness; RF = risk factor for T2DM; X? = unknown factor.

In addition to possible shared genetic linkages, it is also possible that the risk of diabetes and psychotic and mood disorders is imparted, in part, from intra-uterine disturbances during gestation. Numerous reports have linked poor fetal growth to impaired glucose tolerance (Newsome et al. 2003) and, separately, to psychotic and mood disorders (Jones 1997; Smith et al. 2001).

NEUROBIOLOGICAL FACTORS AFFECTING GLUCOSE REGULATION

Psychosis, mania, melancholic depression, and mixed states (co-occurring mania and depression) activate the sympathetic nervous system and the hypothalamic-pituitary-adrenal (HPA) stress hormone axis, producing catecholamine elevations and hypercortisolemia (Dinan 2004; Holt et al. 2004; McElroy et al. 1992; Rubin et al. 2002; Ryan and Thakore 2002; Ryan et al. 2003; Shiloah et al. 2003; Talbot and Nouwen 2000). These effects have implications on glucose metabolism that are not trivial. For example, glucocorticoids interfere with insulin function in a number of ways. Cortisol decreases glucose utilization in muscle, reduces the binding affinity of insulin receptors, and antagonizes the insulin's inhibiting effects on hepatic glucose release (Meyer and Badenhoop 2003). Hypercortisolemia also suppresses growth hormone and gonadal hormone axes (Bjorntorp and Rosmond 2000), and decreased levels of insulin-like growth factor and testosterone in men are associated with obesity and insulin resistance (Marin et al. 1993; Rosmond and Bjorntorp 1998; Seidell et al. 1990). Cortisol elevations may also be expected to interfere with leptin-mediated satiety signaling (Rosmond and Bjorntorp 1998; Zahrzewska et al. 1997). Long-term glucocorticoid therapy is associated with enduring impaired glucose metabolism in up to 25% of patients receiving such treatment (Dinan 2004). Such iatrogenic effects are analogous to the effects of repeated endogenous hypercortisolemia from recurrent and/or protracted psychotic and mood episodes. Although these physiological effects are compelling and have been established to occur during acute mood and psychotic episodes, there are no prospective studies providing long-term evidence of HPA or sympathetic nervous system overactivity in patients with these psychiatric illnesses. Despite the difficulty in conducting this type of study, given the potential confounding effects of treatment, treatment effects could nevertheless be controlled for, and correlations among symptomatic status, recovery, and biological and physiological measures of these systems could be ascertained. Such studies might ideally be conducted in patients with new-onset illness to control for the effects of illness progression and prior treatment at baseline.

BEHAVIORAL FACTORS

Individuals with psychotic and mood disorders are more likely to be single, unem-ployed, or disabled, and of lower socioeconomic status, than individuals without these illnesses (Coryell et al. 1993; Keck et al. 1998; Murray and Lopez 1996). These sociodemographic characteristics are risk factors for limited access to health-care resources and poor social support and self-care. They are also clearly consequences of psychotic and mood disorders themselves.

The lifetime prevalence rates of alcohol and substance use disorders, smoking, and obesity—all of which are risk factors for T2DM—are all significantly elevated in patients with psychotic and mood disorders (McElroy et al. 2004; Meyer and Nasrallah 2003). Binge eating disorder, a common cause of obesity, is highly comorbid with mood disorders (McElroy et al. 2005). Fagiolini et al. (2002) reported that the number of previous depressive episodes contributed to the likelihood of being overweight or obese in a cohort of 50 patients with bipolar disorder in which the overall prevalence of overweight or obesity was 68%. These provocative findings suggest that neurobiological changes (e.g., HPA overactivity) and/or behavioral changes (anergia, hyperphagia, diminished overall physical activity) associated with depressive episodes and/or negative symptoms may contribute to overweight and obesity and indirectly to the risk of T2DM. Thakore et al. (2002) found that central adiposity—strongly correlated with risk for the metabolic syndrome, of which impaired glucose tolerance is one component—was evident in drug-naïve patients with schizophrenia compared with age- and sex-matched healthy control subjects, again suggesting that risk factors for T2DM were apparent at the outset of illness and prior to treatment effects.

Poor dietary habits may also be a common behavioral pathway for patients with psychotic and mood disorders en route to developing risk for T2DM. There are few data regarding the dietary habits of individuals with mood disorders compared with the general population (Keck and McElroy 2003), although the diet of the general population in most industrialized countries falls below the World Health Organization (2003) recommendations for a healthy diet. Several studies suggest that patients with schizophrenia have worse dietary habits than the general population, including consumption of high-calorie, high-fat, low-fiber foods (S. Brown et al. 1999; McCreadie et al. 1998; World Health Organization 1979).

A number of lines of evidence from preclinical, clinical, and epidemiological data suggest that patients with psychotic and mood disorders have a high prevalence of abnormalities in phospholipid metabolism and that these abnormalities correlate with the severity and recurrence of psychotic and depressive symptoms (Horrobin and Bennett 1999; Peet 2002). Whether these abnormalities are a result of poor dietary habits, represent an important mechanism of disease, or perpetuate symptoms and are a reason for treatment refractoriness is not clear.

Conclusion

Individuals with psychotic and mood disorders appear to have an increased risk of T2DM. This increased risk may be due to neurobiological changes associated with acute psychotic and mood episodes and residual symptoms that have a systemic impact on glucose metabolism or to a genetic predisposition to insulin resistance. In addition, behavioral effects of these psychiatric illnesses, including physical inactivity and poor dietary habits, appear to play a role in this increased risk. Co-occurring psychiatric illnesses such as alcohol abuse and dependence and eating disorders may also contribute to the risk of T2DM.

KEY CLINICAL CONCEPTS

- An association between T2DM and severe mental illness, schizophrenia, bipolar disorder, and major depression has been observed for nearly a century and prior to the current era of pharmacotherapy.

- Studies conducted prior to 1949 reported rates of T2DM in patients with psychotic and mood disorders ranging from two to four times the prevailing rates of healthy subjects.

- Studies conducted after 1949 in patients with schizophrenia suggest these patients have an increased risk for T2DM. However, the magnitude of the risk from the psychotic disorder alone cannot be determined.

- The literature examining the association between bipolar disorder and T2DM is limited, and the results of these studies are inconclusive.

- Epidemiological studies suggest that individuals with depressive symptoms have an increased risk for T2DM. Thus individuals with unipolar disorder may be at increased risk, as may individuals with bipolar disorder, especially those who have recurrent depressive episodes or symptoms.

- A variety of mechanisms—including hereditary factors, neurobiological factors affecting glucose regulation, and behavioral factors—likely link severe mental illness and T2DM.

- In attempting to understand the risk for metabolic disturbances and T2DM associated with psychiatric medications, it is important to discern the risks for diabetes posed by the illnesses themselves.

References

American Diabetes Association: Report of the Expert Committee on the Diagnosis and Classification of Diabetes Mellitus. Diabetes Care 20:1183–1197, 1997

American Psychiatric Association: Diagnostic and Statistical Manual of Mental Disorders, 4th Edition. Washington, DC, American Psychiatric Association, 1994

Arroyo C, Hu FB, Ryan LM, et al: Depressive symptoms and risk of type 2 diabetes in women. Diabetes Care 27:129–133, 2004

Barrett TB, Serre P: Blood analysis and sugar tolerance in mental disease. J Nerv Ment Dis 59:561–570, 1924

Bjorntorp P, Rosmond R: Obesity and cortisol. Nutrition 16:924–936, 2000

Bowman KM, Kasanin J: The sugar content of the blood in emotional states. Arch Neurol Psychiatry 21:342–362, 1929

Braceland FJ, Meduna LJ, Vaichulis JA: Delayed action of insulin in schizophrenia. Am J Psychiatry 102:108–110, 1945

Brown LC, Majumdar SR, Newman SC, et al: History of depression increases risk of type 2 diabetes in younger adults. Diabetes Care 28:1063–1070, 2005

Brown S, Birtwistle J, Roe L, et al: The unhealthy lifestyle of people with schizophrenia. Psychol Med 29:697–701, 1999

Bushe C, Holt R: Prevalence of diabetes and impaired glucose tolerance in patients with schizophrenia. Br J Psychiatry 47(suppl):S67–S71, 2004

Cade JFJ: Lithium salts in the treatment of psychotic excitement. Med J Aust 36:349–352, 1949

Carnethon MR, Kinder LS, Fair JM, et al: Symptoms of depression as a risk factor for incident diabetes: findings from the National Health and Nutrition Examination Epidemiologic Follow-up Study. Am J Epidemiol 158:416–423, 2003

Cassidy F, Ahearn E, Carroll BJ: Elevated frequency of diabetes mellitus in hospitalized manic-depressive patients. Am J Psychiatry 156:1417–1420, 1999

Coryell W, Scheftner W, Keller M, et al: The enduring psychosocial consequences of mania and depression. Am J Psychiatry 150:720–727, 1993

Cowie DM, Parsons JP, Raphael T: Insulin and mental depression. Arch Neurol Psychiatry 12:522–533, 1924

Diethelm O: Influence of emotions on dextrose tolerance. Arch Neurol Psychiatry 36:342–360, 1936

Dinan TG: Stress and the genesis of diabetes mellitus in schizophrenia. Br J Psychiatry 47(suppl):S72–S75, 2004

Drury KK, Farron-Ridge C: Some observations of the types of blood-sugar curves found in different forms of insanity. J Ment Sci 71:8–29, 1921

Dynes JB: Diabetes in schizophrenia and diabetes in nonpsychotic medical patients. Dis Nerv Syst 30:341–344, 1969

Eaton WW, Armenian H, Gallo J, et al: Depression and risk for onset of type II diabetes: a prospective population-based study. Diabetes Care 19:1097–1102, 1996

Everson SA, Maty SC, Lynch JW, et al: Epidemiologic evidence for the relation between socioeconomic status and depression, obesity, and diabetes. J Psychosom Res 53:891–895, 2002

Fagiolini A, Frank E, Houck PR, et al: Prevalence of obesity and weight change during treatment in patients with bipolar I disorder. J Clin Psychiatry 63:528–533, 2002

Freeman H: Resistance to insulin in mentally disturbed soldiers. Arch Neurol Psychiatry 56:74–78, 1946

Glidea EF, McLean VL, Man EB: Oral and intravenous dextrose tolerance curves of patients with manic-depressive psychosis. Arch Neurol Psychiatry 49:852–859, 1943

Golden SH, Williams JE, Ford DE, et al: Depressive symptoms and the risk of type 2 diabetes: the Atherosclerosis Risk in Communities study. Diabetes Care 27:429–435, 2004

Henry GW, Mangan E: Blood in personality disorders. Arch Neurol Psychiatry 13:743–749, 1925

Holt RI, Peveler RC, Byrne CD: Schizophrenia, the metabolic syndrome and diabetes. Diabet Med 21:515–523, 2004

Horrobin DF, Bennett CN: Depression and bipolar disorder: relationships to impaired fatty acid and phospholipids metabolism and to diabetes, cardiovascular disease, immunological abnormalities, cancer, aging, and osteoporosis. Possible candidate genes. Prostaglandins Leukot Essent Fatty Acids 60:217–234, 1999

Jones P: The early origins of schizophrenia. Br Med Bull 53:135–155, 1997

Kasanin J: The blood sugar curve in mental disease. Arch Neurol Psychiatry 16:414–419,1926

Kawakami N, Takatsuka N, Shimizu H, et al: Depressive symptoms and occurrence of type 2 diabetes among Japanese men. Diabetes Care 22:1071–1076, 1999

Keck PE, McElroy SL: Bipolar disorder, obesity and pharmacotherapy-associated weight gain. J Clin Psychiatry 64:1426–1435, 2003

Keck PE Jr, McElroy SL, Strakowski SM, et al: 12-Month outcome of patients with bipolar disorder following hospitalization for a manic or mixed episode. Am J Psychiatry 155:646–652, 1998

Keck PE Jr, Buse JB, Dagogo-Jack S, et al: Managing Metabolic Concerns in Patients With Severe Mental Illness. Minneapolis, MN, Postgraduate Medicine, McGraw-Hill, 2003

Kessing LV, Nilsson FM, Siersma V, et al: Increased risk of developing diabetes in depressive and bipolar disorders? J Psychiatr Res 38:395–402, 2004

Kooy FH: Hyperglycemia in mental disorders. Brain 42:214–289, 1919

Lilliker SL: Prevalence of diabetes in a manic-depressive population. Compr Psychiatry 21:270–275, 1980

Lorenz WF: Sugar tolerance in dementia praecox and other mental disorders. Arch Neurol Psychiatry 8:184–196, 1922

Marin P, Kvist H, Lindstedt G, et al: Low concentrations of insulin-like growth factor–I in abdominal obesity. Int J Obes Relat Metab Disord 17:83–89, 1993

Maudsley H: The Pathology of the Mind: Second Part of the Physiology and Pathology of the Mind, 3rd Edition. London, Macmillan, 1879

McCowan PK, Quastel JH: Blood sugar studies in abnormal mental states. J Ment Sci 77:525–548, 1931

McCreadie R, Macdonald E, Blacklock C, et al: Dietary intake of schizophrenic patients in Nithsdale, Scotland: case-control study. BMJ 317:784–785, 1998

McElroy SL, Keck PE Jr, Pope HG Jr, et al: Clinical and research implications of the diagnosis of dysphoric or mixed mania or hypomania. Am J Psychiatry 149:1633–1644, 1992

McElroy SL, Kotwal R, Malhotra S, et al: Are mood disorders and obesity related? A review for the mental health professional. J Clin Psychiatry 65:634–651, 2004

McElroy SL, Kotwal R, Keck PE Jr, et al: Comorbidity of bipolar and eating disorders: distinct or related disorders with shared dysregulations? J Affect Disord 86:107–127, 2005

McFarland RA, Goldstein H: The biochemistry of manic-depressive psychosis. Am J Psychiatry 96:21–58, 1939

McKee HA, D'Arcy PF, Wilson PJ: Diabetes and schizophrenia: a preliminary study. J Clin Hosp Pharm 11:297–299, 1986

Meyer G, Badenhoop K: Glucocorticoid-induced insulin resistance and diabetes mellitus: receptor-, postreceptor mechanisms, local cortisol action, and new aspects of antidiabetic therapy. Med Klin 98:266–270, 2003

Meyer JM, Nasrallah HA (eds): Medical Illness and Schizophrenia. Washington, DC, American Psychiatric Publishing, 2003

Miller HW: Plan and operation of the health and nutrition examination survey. Vital Health Stat 1 1:1–46, 1973

Mukherjee S, Schnur DB, Reddy R: Family history of type 2 diabetes in schizophrenic patients (letter). Lancet 1:495, 1989

Mukherjee S, Decina P, Bocola V, et al: Diabetes mellitus in schizophrenic patients. Comp Psychiatry 37:68–73, 1996

Murray CJL, Lopez AD: The Global Burden of Disease: Summary. Cambridge, MA, Harvard School of Public Health, 1996

Musselman DL, Betan E, Larsen H, et al: Relationship of depression to diabetes types 1 and 2: epidemiology, biology, and treatment. Biol Psychiatry 54:317–329, 2003

Newcomer HS: Blood constituents and mental state. Am J Psychiatry 78:609–611, 1922

Newsome CA, Shiell AW, Fall CH, et al: Is birth weight related to later glucose and insulin metabolism? A systematic review. Diabet Med 20:339–348, 2003

Palinkas LA, Lee PP, Barrett-Connor E: A prospective study of type 2 diabetes and depressive symptoms in the elderly: the Rancho Bernardo Study. Diabet Med 21:1185–1191, 2004

Peet M: Essential fatty acids: theoretical aspects and treatment implications for schizophrenia and depression. Advances in Psychiatry Treatment 8:223–229, 2002

Plan and operation of the health and nutrition examination survey. United States: 1971–1973. Vital Health Stat 1 1:1–77, 1973

Raphael T, Parsons JP: Blood sugar studies in dementia praecox and manic-depressive insanity. Arch Neurol Psychiatry 5:681–709, 1921

Rosmond R, Bjorntorp P: The interactions between hypothalamic-pituitary-adrenal axis activity, testosterone, insulin-like growth factor I and abdominal obesity with metabolism and blood pressure in men. Int J Obes Relat Metab Disord 22:1184–1196, 1998

Rubin RR, Peyrot M: Was Willis right? Thoughts on the interaction of depression and diabetes. Diabetes Metab Res Rev 18:173–175, 2002

Ruzickova M, Slaney C, Garnham J, et al: Clinical features of bipolar disorder with and without comorbid diabetes mellitus. Can J Psychiatry 48:458–461, 2003

Ryan MC, Thakore JH: Physical consequences of schizophrenia and its treatment: the metabolic syndrome. Life Sci 71:239–257, 2002

Ryan MC, Collins P, Thakore JH: Impaired fasting glucose tolerance in first-episode, drug-naïve patients with schizophrenia. Am J Psychiatry 160:284–289, 2003

Saydah SH, Brancati FL, Golden SH, et al: Depressive symptoms and the risk of type 2 diabetes mellitus in a U.S. sample. Diabetes Metab Res Rev 19:202–208, 2003

Schwarz L, Munoz R: Blood sugar levels in patients treated with chlorpromazine. Am J Psychiatry 125:253–255, 1968

Seidell JC, Bjorntorp P, Sjostrom L, et al: Visceral fat accumulation in men is positively associated with insulin, glucose, and C-peptide levels, but negatively with testosterone levels. Metabolism 39:897–901, 1990

Shiloah E, Witz S, Abramovitch Y, et al: Effect of acute psychotic stress in nondiabetic subjects on beta-cell function and insulin sensitivity. Diabetes Care 26:1462–1467, 2003

Smith GN, Flynn SW, McCarthy N, et al: Low birthweight in schizophrenia: prematurity or poor fetal growth? Schizophr Res 47:177–184, 2001

Tabata H, Kikuoka M, Kikuoka H, et al: Characteristics of diabetes mellitus in schizo-phrenic patients. J Med Assoc Thai 70(suppl):90–93, 1987

Talbot F, Nouwen A: A review of the relationship between depression and diabetes in adults: is there a link? Diabetes Care 23:1556–1562, 2000

Thakore JH, Mann JN, Vlahos I, et al: Increased visceral fat distribution in drug-naïve and drug-free patients with schizophrenia. Int J Obes Relat Metab Disord 26:137–141, 2002

Thonnard-Neumann E: Phenothiazines and diabetes in hospitalized women. Am J Psychi-atry 124:978–982, 1968

Tod H: Studies on carbohydrate metabolism in nervous and mental disorders, I: glucose tol-erance tests in manic-depressive insanity and other depression. Edinburgh Med J 43:524–527, 1934

Tod H: Studies on carbohydrate metabolism in nervous and mental disorders, III: the dis-turbance of the glucose tolerance caused by hypnotics in clinical doses. Edinburgh Med J 44:44–46, 1937

Vestergaard P, Schou M: Does long-term lithium treatment induce diabetes mellitus? Neu-ropsychobiology 17:130–132, 1987

Whitehorn JC: The blood sugar in relation to emotional reactions. Am J Psychiatry 90:987–1005, 1934

Willis T: Diabetes: A Medical Odyssey. New York, Tuckahoe, 1971

World Health Organization: Schizophrenia: An International Follow-Up Study. New York, John Wiley, 1979

World Health Organization: Diet, Nutrition and the Prevention of Chronic Diseases. WHO Technical Report Series 916. Geneva, Switzerland, World Health Organiza-tion, 2003

Zahrzewska KE, Cusin I, Sainsbury A, et al: Glucocorticoids as counterregulatory hor-mones of leptin: toward an understanding of leptin resistance. Diabetes 46:717–719, 1997

Zimmerman U, Kraus T, Himmerich H, et al: Epidemiology, implications and mechanisms underlying drug-induced weight gain in psychiatric patients. J Psychiatr Res 37:193–220, 2003

Chapter 5

CARDIOVASCULAR DISEASE

Richard A. Bermudes, M.D.

Cardiovascular disease (CVD) is the most pressing healthcare problem and leading cause of death worldwide (Bonow et al. 2002). The World Health Organization (WHO; 2005) estimates approximately 16.7 million people around the globe die annually of CVD, particularly from heart attacks and strokes. With 80% of the burden in low- and middle-income countries, the problem has spread beyond Westernized societies. Despite the advent of coronary care units, availability of reperfusion technologies, increased public access to defibrillators, and medications such as aspirin and beta blockers, CVD accounted for 38% of all deaths in the United States in 2002 (American Heart Association 2005).

Persons with chronic and severe mental illness are at greater risk for cardiovascular morbidity and mortality compared with the general population. Patients with schizophrenia have a significantly increased burden of CVD versus the general population, and cardiovascular mortality contributes to the excess mortality associated with schizophrenia. A variety of studies of different methods and designs have confirmed this association. In a retrospective cohort study in which 3,022 individuals with schizophrenia were identified from a Canadian health database, researchers found an increased incidence of ventricular arrhythmia, heart failure, stroke, and cardiovascular mortality compared with age- and sex-matched, randomly selected, general population control subjects (Curkendall et al. 2004).

Recent data from the Clinical Antipsychotic Trials of Intervention Effectiveness (CATIE) study confirm the findings of greater risk for CVD in severely

139

mentally ill populations. Goff et al. (2005), using the Framingham CHD risk function, calculated the 10-year risk for coronary heart disease (CHD) for 689 subjects with schizophrenia at baseline. Compared with age-, race- and gender-matched control subjects, both male (9.4% vs. 7.0%) and female (6.3% vs. 4.2%) subjects had an elevated 10-year risk for CHD. Schizophrenia patients had higher rates of smoking, diabetes, and hypertension, and lower high-density lipoprotein (HDL) cholesterol values, compared with the control group. McEvoy et al. (2005) used baseline data from the CATIE study and found that males were 138% more likely to have the metabolic syndrome and females were 251% more likely, compared with a national comparison group, after controlling for age and race. Persons with the metabolic syndrome are at increased risk for CVD. These data are consistent with the excess cardiovascular mortality reported in previous studies of patients with schizophrenia (Allebeck 1989; Brown et al. 2000; Mortensen and Juel 1990; Osby et al. 2000) and in Brown's 1997 meta-analysis of mortality studies published from 1952 to 1996.

Patients with mood disorders also have increased mortality from CVD. In a systematic review of the mortality of depression, Wulsin et al. (1999) reviewed 57 studies published from 1966 through 1998. They found that although the studies linking depression to early death were poorly controlled, 29 (51%) of the 57 studies reviewed suggested depression increased the risk of death by CVD. Angst et al. (2002) prospectively followed hospitalized patients with bipolar or unipolar disorder for 22 years or more and found an elevated standardized mortality ratio (SMR) for CVD. In the subgroup analysis of unipolar and bipolar patients, unipolar patients had an SMR of 1.36 (not significant) for CVD, and bipolar patients had an SMR of 1.84 ($P<0.05$). In a population study conducted in Sweden (Osby et al. 2001), all patients with a hospital diagnosis of bipolar ($n=15,386$) or unipolar ($n=39,182$) disorder from 1973 to 1995 were identified and linked with the national cause-of-death register to determine the date and cause of death. In this sample, male or female patients with either bipolar or unipolar disorder had significantly increased SMRs for CVD compared with the general population.

Why do the mentally ill have an increased risk of mortality from CVD? First, mental illness is associated with a number of changes in an individual's health that may influence the development and course of CVD. Second, mental illness is associated with physiological changes that negatively affect the cardiovascular system. Finally, there may be an underlying factor such as stress that leads to the development of both mental illness and CVD (Figure 5–1).

This chapter addresses 1) potential relationships between mental illness and CVD, with a particular emphasis on traditional cardiac risk factor prevalence rates among the mentally ill, and 2) practical management of cardiac risk factors to assist psychiatrists in quantifying and reducing their patients' cardiac risk.

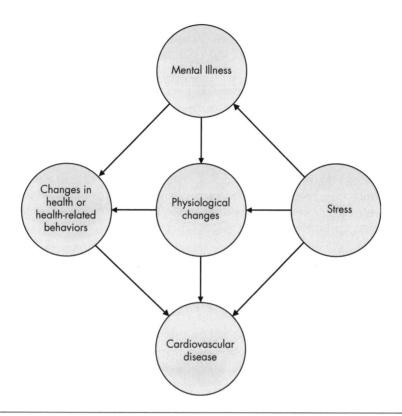

FIGURE 5–1. Plausible pathways between mental illness and cardiovascular disease.

Mental illness may be associated with mental illness via changes in physiology or changes in health or health-related behaviors. Stress may also be an underlying cause for both cardiovascular disease and mental illness.

Changes in Health

Mental illness is associated with a number of health changes that may increase the development of CVD. These health changes range from unhealthy behaviors in persons with mental illness, such as poor adherence or nonadherence, to undertreatment of the physical health of those with mental illness by the health system, to clustering of cardiovascular risk factors in persons with mental illness.

POOR ADHERENCE OR NONADHERENCE

Studies demonstrate that poor adherence to medical treatment is associated with a worse prognosis with CVD (Coronary Drug Project 1980; Gallagher et al. 1993; Horwitz et al. 1990; Irvine et al. 1999). In a group of 1,141 patients with acute myocardial infarction (MI) randomly assigned to receive amiodarone or placebo to prevent arrhythmias, poor adherence to both placebo and amiodarone was associated with an increased risk of sudden cardiac death, total cardiac mortality, and all-cause mortality (Irvine et al. 1999). In a study of adherence to lipid-lowering therapy and cardiac outcomes, patients with good adherence in both the intervention and placebo groups had lower 5-year mortality compared with patients with poor adherence (Coronary Drug Project 1980).

Although nonadherence to medical advice is common, mental illness predicts even poorer adherence and subsequent poor cardiac outcomes. For example, in a group of patients recovering from MI, those with posttraumatic stress disorder had significantly poorer adherence to aspirin and an increased likelihood of cardiovascular readmission compared with nontraumatized counterparts enrolled in the study (Shemesh et al. 2004). Carney et al. (1995) found similar results among depressed CVD patients taking aspirin therapy. Patients with depression are also less likely to adhere to cardiac rehabilitation programs after MI (Glazer et al. 2002).

The literature for psychotic disorders and adherence to medical advice for physical health conditions is less developed, although many factors that mediate adherence, such as social isolation and poor social support, are common in psychotic disorders. Furthermore, patients with schizophrenia are often nonadherent with their psychiatric medications. Rates of medication adherence among outpatients with schizophrenia approach 50% during the first year after hospital discharge (Babiker 1986; Weiden and Olfson 1995).

It is unclear whether nonadherence with specific medical treatments or nonadherence itself leads to a poor prognosis with CVD. Poor adherence may be a marker for unhealthy behaviors that lead to a poorer prognosis. Alternatively, poor adherence may be a marker for mental illness (recognized or unrecognized) that is associated with a worse prognosis in CVD.

SYSTEM NEGLECT

Individual physician attitudes and system neglect may mediate a change in health status among the mentally ill, with subsequent worsening in CVD and other physical health problems. Lawrie et al. (1996, 1998) used clinical vignettes to study attitudes of general practitioners toward individuals with mental illness. General practitioners were less happy to have patients with severe mental disorders on their lists than diabetic or healthy individuals. Similar stigma against those with mental illness has been documented in hospital settings (Aydin et al. 2003) and in nursing and medical student trainees (Llerena et al. 2002; Singh et al. 1998). System neglect also contributes to poor cardiovascular outcomes in the mentally ill. In a national cohort, Druss et al. (2000) measured the type and number of cardiovascular procedures received by post-MI patients with and without mental disorders. Individuals with mental disorders were less likely to undergo coronary revascularization procedures than those without mental disorders. In another study, those with mental illness, particularly those with comorbid substance disorders, received less preventive cardiovascular care (Druss et al. 2002).

CARDIAC RISK FACTORS

Cardiovascular risk factors consist of modifiable, nonmodifiable, and emerging risk factors (Table 5–1). Modifiable risk factors are considered targets for intervention and include elevated cholesterol, diabetes, hypertension, obesity, smoking, and sedentary lifestyle. Nonmodifiable risk factors include advancing age, family history of CVD, and gender. Our knowledge of emerging cardiovascular risk factors is evolving, but markers of inflammation, hemostasis, and immunity such as fibrinogen, C-reactive protein (CRP), and homocysteine are increasingly linked to CVD. Risk factors are additive so that the total cardiovascular risk of a person increases with each risk factor they accumulate. Modifiable risk factors are highly prevalent in persons with mental disorders, and psychiatric medications often have detrimental effects and worsen cardiovascular risk factors. Thus it is important for mental health providers to know what these risks are and to understand how cardiac risk factors contribute to increased mortality in those with mental illness.

Smoking

Tobacco smoke has deleterious effects on the cardiovascular system, increasing the risk for MI, stroke, and death. Smoking affects the cardiovascular system by 1) increasing catecholamine levels, 2) reducing HDL cholesterol levels, 3) impairing arterial vasodilation, and 4) increasing clotting (Rigotti and Pasternak 1996). These changes to the vasculature converge to cause atherosclerosis, vascular injury, and increased coagulability resulting in CHD (Villablanca et al. 2000). Compared with those who have never smoked or with former smokers, current smokers have MIs an average of 10 years earlier, even after other cardiac risk factors are controlled for (Liese et al. 2000). Smokers who stop smoking may reduce their risk for CHD by 50% (Eliasson et al. 2001). Even smokers who are elderly (>70 years) or who have suffered a cardiac event, such as an MI or bypass surgery, benefit from smoking cessation (Critchley and Capewell 2003; Hermanson et al. 1988). One review found a 36% reduction in overall mortality with smoking cessation in patients with CHD, which is a greater benefit than other secondary prevention strategies such as aspirin and beta blockers (Critchley and Capewell 2003).

Smoking is highly prevalent in the mentally ill—despite an overall reduction in smoking rates within the general population in the United States. Findings from a national sample indicate that individuals with mental illness are two times as likely to smoke as those who are not mentally ill, and may compose up to 50% of the tobacco market in the United States (Lasser et al. 2000). The rate of smoking

TABLE 5–1.   Risk factors for coronary atherosclerosis

Modifiable	Nonmodifiable	Emerging
Weight gain	Gender	Lipoprotein A
Dyslipidemia	Family history	Homocysteine
Diabetes	Age	Prothrombotic factors (fibrinogen)
Hypertension		Proinflammatory factors
Smoking		(C-reactive protein)
Sedentary lifestyle		Impaired fasting glucose
		Subclinical atherosclerosis

in schizophrenia is extremely high, and evidence suggests that persons with schizophrenia smoke a higher number of cigarettes per day. Surveys of cigarette smoking in patients with schizophrenia have found prevalence rates as high as 92% (McEvoy and Brown 1999), with the majority of studies showing rates ranging from 83% to 88% (de Leon et al. 1995; Diwan et al. 1998; Hughes et al. 1999; Masterson and O'Shea 1984; O'Farrell et al. 1983). Individuals with schizophrenia not only smoke more cigarettes (de Leon et al. 1995), but they extract more nicotine per cigarette than comparison smokers without schizophrenia (Olincy et al. 1997).

There is also a high rate of smoking among patients with major depression and bipolar disorder. Patients with major depression have a greater frequency of smoking and experience more difficulty trying to quit compared with nondepressed smokers (Fergusson et al. 2003; Glassman 1993). Smoking rates among those with bipolar disorder are high (Itkin et al. 2001; Leonard et al. 2001) and are associated with depressive and/or psychotic symptoms (Corvin et al. 2001; Glassman 1998; Glassman et al. 1992). Some studies indicate that smoking rates are higher in patients with schizophrenia compared with patients with mood disorders (de Leon et al. 2002; Diwan et al. 1998; Leonard et al. 2001). However, a recent study suggests these differences may be in part due to illness severity or functional impairment rather than diagnosis (Vanable et al. 2003).

Dyslipidemia

Numerous clinical and epidemiological studies show that an elevated blood cholesterol level is one of the major modifiable risk factors associated with CHD. Dyslipidemia is instrumental in a number of mechanisms, including vascular wall injury, impaired vascular endothelial function, and formation of atherosclerotic plaque, that ultimately lead to CVD (Levine et al. 1995). Dyslipidemia includes elevated total cholesterol (>200 mg/dL), elevated serum low-density lipoprotein (LDL) cholesterol (>130 mg/dL), elevated serum triglycerides (>150 mg/dL), and/or low serum HDL cholesterol (<40 mg/dL) (Expert Panel on Detection, Evaluation, and Treatment of High Blood Cholesterol in Adults 2001). Each of these abnormalities is linked to CHD and CVD. However, the National Cholesterol Education Program Adult Treatment Panel III (NCEP-ATP III) identified elevated LDL cholesterol as the primary target of cholesterol-lowering therapy because of the wealth of experimental animal data, epidemiological data, and treatment studies indicating elevated LDL as the major cause of CHD (Expert Panel on Detection, Evaluation, and Treatment of High Blood Cholesterol in Adults 2001).

Multiple studies demonstrate that reducing elevated LDL, increasing depressed HDL, or reducing elevated triglycerides reduces the risk of CVD, CHD, and mortality. This has been demonstrated in a variety of patient populations, including the elderly, those with previous cardiac events, persons with diabetes, persons who smoke, and in individuals with mild risk for CVD (Hanna and Wenger 2005; Safeer and Ugalat 2002). In patients with CHD, reducing LDL levels by 30%–40% reduces risk for cardiac death by 20%–40% (Long-Term Intervention With Pravastatin in Ischaemic Disease Study Group 1998; Scandinavian Simvastatin Survival Study 1994). In healthy patients (no history of CHD) with normal levels of LDL but abnormal triglycerides or HDL, risk for CHD can be reduced by as much as 32% in 5 years with statin drug treatment. Furthermore, all-cause mortality is reduced by as much as 20% over the same 5-year time period (Downs et al. 1998; Shepherd et al. 1995).

Although dyslipidemia is prevalent in persons with mental disorders, it is unclear whether these rates are elevated independent of factors that influence lipid levels in the general population. Serum lipids are influenced by a number of factors, including genetics, diet, weight, alcohol consumption, medications, and illnesses such as diabetes. Rates of dyslipidemia are high in community samples and are expected to increase with the current epidemics of obesity and diabetes. In one national survey, the third National Health and Nutrition Examination Survey (NHANES III; 1988–1994), 30% of individuals met criteria for hypertriglyceridemia, and 37% met criteria for low HDL (Ford et al. 2002). In samples of mentally ill patients, dyslipidemia ranges from 20% to 60% depending on the cholesterol parameter assessed and the profile of atypical antipsychotics prescribed in the population (Gupta et al. 2003; Meyer 2002; Saari et al. 2004).

Hypertension

The relationship between blood pressure and CVD is well known. In middle-aged white men and women, an increase of 10 mm Hg in diastolic pressure increases the risk for CVD by 37%. After adjustment for other cardiac risk factors, more than 25% of CHD events in men and women are attributable to blood pressure levels that exceed high-normal levels (≥130/85; Wilson et al. 1998). Long-term studies (follow-up over 30 years) suggest mortality from blood pressure starts at a threshold systolic pressure of approximately 140 mm Hg and a diastolic pressure of approximately 85 mm Hg. When other cardiovascular risk factors, such as smoking and/or dyslipidemia, are present, cardiovascular risk from hypertension begins at lower blood pressures (Standberg et al. 2001).

Some researchers have proposed that individuals with mental illness are at risk for hypertension, especially patients with depression and anxiety, theorizing that the autonomic hyperactivity seen in these patients and increased sympathetic tone increases their risk. Prospective studies to date have yielded conflicting results. In one group of patients followed for 4 years, no association between anxiety or depression and blood pressure was found (Shinn et al. 2001). However, in a larger national cohort followed over 20 years, symptoms of anxiety and depression at baseline predicted development of hypertension (Jonas and Lando 2000). Cross-sectional studies of the chronically mentally ill and in patients with schizophrenia have not shown elevated rates of hypertension compared with age- and gender- matched control subjects (Davidson et al. 2001).

Obesity and Diabetes

Obesity and diabetes are both established risk factors for CVD. Compared with normal-weight individuals (body mass index [BMI] 18.5–24), overweight (BMI 25–29) or obese (BMI ≥30) patients have a relative risk for CVD of 1.2 and 1.6, respectively (Wilson et al. 2002). Furthermore, the rate of weight gain and central weight distribution (truncal obesity) confer greater risk for CVD compared with weight alone (Bakx et al. 2000; Bard et al. 2001). Diabetes confers a three- to four-fold risk for CVD (Garcia et al. 1974), and current guidelines consider it a disease equivalent to having established CHD (Expert Panel on Detection, Evaluation, and Treatment of High Blood Cholesterol in Adults 2001). Even modest increases in fasting glucose can substantially increase the risk for CVD. Data from individuals followed for more than 10 years show that modest increases in fasting glucose (>110 mg/dL) can increase cardiovascular events by a third compared with individuals with lower fasting glucoses (≤80 mg/dL) (Coutinho et al. 1999; Gerstein et al. 1999).

Diabetes and obesity are prevalent in the mentally ill. The prevalence of diabetes among patients with mental illness is two times the rate in the general population, and the prevalence of obesity is 1.5–2.0 times the rate in the general population (Allison and Casey 2001; Dixon et al. 2000; Istvan et al. 1992; Zhao et al. 2006). The association of diabetes and obesity with mental illness is thoroughly reviewed in Chapter 3 ("Severe Mental Illness and Obesity") and Chapter 4 ("Severe Mental Illness and Diabetes Mellitus") in this volume.

Lifestyle Factors: Diet and Exercise

A diet rich in saturated fat and low in fiber, and a sedentary lifestyle, independently increase the risk of CHD. Certain dietary factors raise the risk of CVD, while other nutritional factors increase the risk for other metabolic problems, such as diabetes or high blood pressure, that subsequently predict poor cardiovascular outcomes. Trans fats and saturated fats increase the risk of CHD, whereas sodium increases blood pressure (Reddy and Katan 2004). A diet rich in fruits and vegetables protects against hypertension, CHD, and stroke (Appel et al. 1998; Joshipura et al. 1999; Ness and Powles 1997). Epidemiological studies examining the relationship between physical activity and CVD across different populations show that leisure time and overall physical activity are associated with a reduced risk of CHD and cardiovascular mortality (Kohl 2001; Wannamethee and Shaper 2001). Thus lifestyle habits such as dietary choices and physical activity play a large role in one's cardiovascular risk.

Several studies demonstrate that mentally ill persons have physical activity and dietary habits that may contribute to their increased cardiovascular risk. One cross-sectional survey conducted in more than 200 mentally ill outpatients showed higher levels of salt intake and lower levels of moderate exercise compared with community matched control subjects (Davidson et al. 2001). One study showed that outpatients with schizophrenia consumed less quantities of fruits and vegetables compared with healthy control subjects, even after social class was controlled for (McCreadie and Scottish Schizophrenia Lifestyle Group 2003). Brown et al. (1999) found that outpatients with schizophrenia exercised less frequently and consumed a diet high in fat and low in fiber compared with the general population. In a recent pilot study involving older adults, Anton and Miller (2005) found that high levels of depression and anger correlated positively with dietary fat intake. Studies thus have demonstrated that the dietary and exercise habits of the mentally ill place them at increased risk for CVD.

Novel Cardiovascular Risk Factors

CHD and other cardiovascular disorders occur among persons with normal lipid values and who otherwise appear to be at low clinical risk. Thirty-five percent of CVD occurs in persons without any known risk factors (Koenig 2001). The ongoing search for novel markers of cardiovascular risk is inspired by this need to better portray future cardiovascular risk as well as to improve the effectiveness of targeted interventions and to discover new targets for therapeutic and preventive interventions.

Research has focused on a number of circulating biomarkers linked to CHD and atherosclerosis. These markers include lipoprotein A (lipoprotein metabolism), homocysteine (endothelial dysfunction), fibrinogen (hemostasis), and CRP (inflammation). Available data are insufficient to support recommendations for using nonlipid markers in clinical decisions. However, studies suggest these markers add prognostic information over standard lipid measures. In a nested-control study from a prospective cohort of 14,916 physicians, CRP was the strongest nonlipid predictor for peripheral arterial disease compared with 11 other atherothrombotic biomarkers including homocysteine and fibrinogen (Ridker et al. 2001). Among 27,000 healthy American women, CRP more strongly predicted MI, ischemic stroke, coronary revascularization, and death from cardiovascular causes compared with LDL levels (Ridker et al. 2002). Even after adjustment for other traditional cardiovascular risk factors, independent effects were observed for CRP. These data suggest that novel markers such as CRP can be strong predictors of cardiovascular events and add to the prognostic information conveyed by traditional risk factors.

Depression is strongly associated with elevated levels of CRP. Kop et al. (2002) found that depression predicted elevated CRP and fibrinogen in a sample of 4,268 individuals without CVD. Data from a national cohort showed that a history of one episode of depression was strongly associated with elevated CRP in men but not women (Danner et al. 2003). Very few studies have examined this relationship outside of unipolar depression. One small pilot study found elevated CRP in acutely psychotic patients compared with control subjects; however, these levels returned to normal with resolution of the psychosis during follow-up (Ohaeri et al. 1993).

Elevated homocysteine levels have been measured in groups of depressed and psychotic patients. In 184 consecutively admitted patients with schizophrenia, Applebaum et al. (2004) found markedly increased homocysteine levels compared with control subjects. Homocysteine levels are high in depressed patients, with a significant number of patients exhibiting homocysteine levels that confer an increased risk of CVD mortality (Servus et al. 2001).

Physiological Impact of Mental Illness on Cardiovascular Disease

Mental illness may lead to physiological changes that speed the development of CVD or worsen the prognosis of patients with established CVD. These changes include activation of the hypothalamic-pituitary-adrenal (HPA) axis, cardiac rhythm disturbances, and alterations in the coagulation and inflammation pathways (Bayes et al. 1989; Fuster et al. 1992a, 1992b; Mulvihill and Foley 2002; Remme 1998). A number of these changes are associated with mental illness and poor cardiovascular health and provide a mechanistic explanation for increased CVD in persons with mental disorders.

HPA AXIS ACTIVATION

Activation of the HPA axis and the sympathoadrenal system accelerates the development of CVD. The result of HPA axis hyperactivity is increased production of cortisol from the adrenal gland. Chronic elevated levels of cortisol, whether from endogenous or exogenous sources, lead to a variety of derangements within the cardiovascular system. Cortisol promotes atherosclerosis, hypertension, vascular injury, and inhibition of normal vascular repair (Colao et al. 1999; Kemper et al. 1957; Nahas et al. 1958; Troxler et al. 1977). Chronically administered corticosteroids rapidly lead to hypercholesterolemia, hypertriglyceridemia, and hypertension in patients (Sholter and Armstrong 2000). Young and middle-aged men with elevated morning plasma cortisol have high rates of moderate to severe coronary atherosclerosis as demonstrated by coronary angiography (Troxler et al. 1977). HPA axis activation also adds to sympathoadrenal activity, resulting in elevated levels of catecholamines with subsequent vasoconstriction, platelet activation, and elevated heart rate—all of which are linked to cardiovascular system damage (Anfossi and Trovati 1996; Remme 1998).

HPA axis hyperactivity is seen in depressed patients, and recent studies show the HPA axis to be overactive in patients with bipolar disorder and in patients with schizophrenia (Gillespie and Nemeroff 2005). A variety of methods demonstrating HPA hyperactivity have been used in studies involving subjects with mental illness, including elevated corticotropin-releasing hormone in cerebrospinal fluid, decreased adrenocorticotropic hormone response to corticotropin-releasing hormone, nonsuppression of cortisol secretion in response to dexamethasone, and elevated salivary free cortisol levels in response to waking (Carroll 1982; Coryell and Tsuang 1992; Daban et al. 2005; Deshauer et al. 2003; Kathol et al. 1989; Nemeroff et al. 1984; Sharma et al. 1988; Watson et al. 2004; Yeragani 1990). In some samples of the mentally ill, evidence of HPA axis dysfunction has not been uniformly observed. For example, failure to suppress plasma levels of cortisol in response to oral dexamethasone has not been demonstrated in some studies involving patients with schizophrenia (Dewan et al. 1982; Tandon et al. 1991). However, discrepancies may be due to various methodological problems. such as sampling procedures and the use of patients taking antipsychotic medications that may suppress the HPA axis (Ryan et al. 2004). In a recent, small case-control study, first-episode drug-naïve subjects with schizophrenia were found to have higher levels of adrenocorticotropic hormone and cortisol compared with age- and sex-matched healthy control subjects (Ryan et al. 2004).

A number of studies demonstrate sympathoadrenal hyperactivity in persons with mental illness. The final end product of the sympathoadrenal system is catecholamines, and various studies show the mentally ill to have elevated catecholamine levels. Depressed patients have elevated plasma norepinephrine levels and an increased catecholamine response to orthostatic challenge (Gold et al. 2000; Maas et al. 1994). Likewise, various studies in drug-free patients with schizophrenia as well as neuroleptic-treated patients demonstrate elevated noradrenaline in cerebrospinal fluid as well as in plasma (Kemali et al. 1985, 1990; Yamamoto and Hornykiewicz 2004). Although difficult to quantify, HPA and sympathoadrenal overactivity likely play a significant role in conjunction with other factors to increase CVD in the mentally ill and worsen the prognosis for patients with underlying CVD.

CARDIAC ARRHYTHMIAS

Certain cardiac rhythm disturbances predict a poorer prognosis for patients with CVD. Decreased heart rate variability (HRV) and ventricular arrhythmias are both risk factors for sudden cardiac death in patients with CVD (Curtis and O'Keefe 2002). HRV, a measure of the average fluctuation in heart rate, is a sensitive marker of autonomic dysfunction and reflects the interplay between sympathetic and parasympathetic input to the heart's pacemaker (Low and Pfeifer 1997). In one group of patients with CVD, those with low HRV were 5.3 times as likely to die within 31 months of follow-up compared with those with normal HRV (Kleiger et al. 1987). Patients with mental illness have high rates of these same rhythm disturbances, which may place them at a higher risk for sudden cardiac death. In an unmedicated group of patients with schizophrenia, Bär et al. (2005) assessed HRV and found that, compared with matched control subjects, those with schizophrenia had significantly decreased parasympathetic responses during tilt maneuvers and a deep breathing test. In another study, first-episode drug-naïve patients with psychosis displayed less short-term heart rate reactivity and HRV under conditions of different mental loads compared with healthy control subjects, which suggests dysfunction in the autonomic nervous system (Valkonen-Korhonen et al. 2003). Patients with CHD and depression are more likely to have episodes of ventricular tachycardia and decreased HRV compared with control subjects (Carney et al. 1993, 2001). Other electrocardiographic abnormalities found in depressed patients include reduced baroreflex sensitivity, higher QT variability, and increased QT dispersion (Nahshoni et al. 2000; Watkins and Grossman 1999; Yeragani et al. 2000). Based on this evidence, mental illness may impact prognosis in CVD through mechanisms involving decreased parasympathetic tone, with subsequent disturbances in HRV, resting heart rate, and QT interval.

ALTERATIONS IN COAGULATION AND INFLAMMATION

Mental illness may worsen the course of CVD by leading to alterations in coagulation and inflammation. Changes in proinflammatory cytokines and hemostasis (blood coagulation, anticoagulation, fibrinolysis, and platelet activity) are instrumental in the development and prognosis of CVD (Fuster et al. 1992a, 1992b; Koenig 2001). Indicators of platelet activity and inflammation are higher among depressed individuals and patients with schizophrenia with and without CVD (Kop et al. 2002; Nemeroff and Musselman 2000; Rothermundt et al. 2001; Walsh et al. 2002). Platelet reactivity in depressed patients is 40% higher compared with control subjects, and functional changes in platelet surface receptors (implicated in changes in hemostasis) have been found in drug-naïve patients with first-episode schizophrenia (Musselman et al. 1996; Walsh et al. 2002).

In summary, a variety of mechanisms link mental illness and CVD. It is unlikely that one pathway explains the high prevalence of CVD among the mentally ill. Abnormalities evident within the HPA axis, autonomic system, and inflammation and coagulation pathways provide a physiological basis for the negative impact of mental illness on the cardiovascular system.

Stress as a Common Underlying Cause for Cardiovascular Disease and Mental Illness

There are a variety of definitions for *stress* used in the literature, and most epidemiological studies use self-report measures to evaluate the effects of stress. Thus there is some difficulty in characterizing stress. Nonetheless, it is implicated in the development and prognosis of CVD and mental illness. A national (N>74,000) prospective study conducted in Japan found stress to predict MI and coronary artery disease in women but not in men (Iso et al. 2002). Individuals who perceive they lack control on the job and report high levels of job strain are at increased risk for progression of atherosclerosis and CHD (Bosma et al. 1997; Everson et al. 1997). Stress complicates MI and affects prognosis and the risk for reinfarction (Rosengren et al. 1991), but results are not consistent across studies (Jenkinson et al. 1993; Welin et al. 2000). In community and clinical samples, stressful life experiences correlate with the onset and course of depressive disorders (Monroe et al. 2001). A longitudinal study of 680 twin pairs studying genetic, life event, and temperament factors found a stressful event in the preceding year was the most powerful predictor for depression (Kendler et al. 1993). Likewise, psychosocial stress is included in most etiological models of schizophrenia, frequently as a precipitating factor for psychosis in vulnerable individuals (Corcoran et al. 2003).

How does stress influence the pathogenesis of both CVD and mental disorders as well as a host of other disease conditions? This question still challenges investigators. Adaptation in response to stressful events involves activation of a number of systems and includes neural, neuroendocrine, and immunological mechanisms and is referred to as *allostasis* (Sterling and Eyer 1988). Through allostasis, the autonomic nervous system, HPA axis, and the cardiovascular, metabolic, and immune systems protect the body by responding to stress, whether external or internal (McEwen 1998a). When these adaptive systems are activated chronically, overstimulated, or are performing maladaptively, "allostatic load" ensues and subsequently leads to disease states (McEwen and Stellar 1993). The HPA axis and the sympathetic nervous system are the most common allostatic responses. When these systems are activated, catecholamines are released from nerves and the adrenal medulla, which leads to the release of corticotropin from the pituitary gland. Corticotropin initiates the release of cortisol from the adrenal cortex. With the increase in catecholamines and cortisol, adaptive processes in a variety of cells and tissues are initiated. When the threat is gone, the infection is resolved, or the environment is improved, the body returns to basal levels of cortisol and catecholamines. However, if inactivation does not occur or if there is hyperactivity of allostasis, exposure to stress hormones occurs over months or years, with subsequent development of allostatic load and disease states (McEwen 1998a, 1998b). Thus when individuals sustain long periods of stress or have maladaptive changes in their stress response system, they may be at risk for adverse cardiovascular and mental health outcomes. CVD and mental disorders may be two outcomes of the same causative factor.

Clinical Recommendations and Conclusions

Two published studies have addressed whether treating patients with mental disorders affects CVD outcome. Both trials attempted to treat patients with major depression in order to reduce the cardiac-event rate. The Sertraline Antidepressant Heart Attack Randomized Trial tested the selective serotonin reuptake inhibitor (SSRI) sertraline against placebo in a double-blind, multicenter trial in hospitalized patients with unstable angina or MI (Glassman et al. 2002). After a 2-week single-blind placebo run-in, patients were randomly assigned to receive sertraline in flexible dosages of 50–200 mg/day ($n=186$) or placebo ($n=183$) for 24 weeks. The primary outcome measure was change from baseline in left ventricular ejection fraction; secondary measures included surrogate cardiac measures and cardiovascular adverse events as well as scores on the Hamilton Rating Scale for Depression and the Clinical Global Impression—Improvement scale. Sertraline had no significant effect on mean left ventricular ejection fraction, treatment-emergent increase in ventricular premature complex runs, or other cardiac measures. In the total randomized sample, the Clinical Global Impression—Improvement scale ($P=0.049$), but not the Hamilton Rating Scale for Depression ($P=0.14$), favored sertraline. Although these results suggest sertraline is a safe treatment for depression in patients with recent MI or unstable angina, its efficacy for reducing depression and improving cardiac outcomes in this population was not significant (Sheps et al. 2003).

The Enhancing Recovery in Coronary Disease Patients Randomized Trial determined whether treatment of depression and low perceived social support (LPSS), using cognitive-behavioral therapy (CBT; augmented with an SSRI when indicated), reduced mortality and recurrent infarction in patients within 28 days after MI (Berkman et al. 2003). In this multicenter study, patients were randomly assigned to receive usual medical care or a CBT-based psychosocial intervention consisting of 11 individual sessions throughout 6 months plus group therapy when feasible. Patients in the intervention with a poor response also received SSRIs. The primary endpoint was death or recurrent MI; secondary outcomes included change in ratings for depression or LPSS at 6 months. Although improvement in psychosocial outcomes (depression and LPSS) at 6 months favored treatment, after an average follow-up of 29 months there was no significant difference in event-free survival between usual care (75.9%) and the psychosocial intervention (75.8%).

It is unclear whether the interventions in these two trials failed to affect cardiac prognosis because of a less than robust effect on depression measures or because they failed to correct the dysregulated physiology that might explain the increased morbidity and mortality seen when these two conditions occur together. Furthermore, there are a number of methodological complexities associated with research regarding mental illness and CVD, including difficulties in the definition and measurement of mental illness or symptoms of mental illness, complexities in the conduct of large-scale trials with behavioral interventions such as CBT, ethical considerations surrounding the use of placebo, and interpretation of trial results. Although there is currently no evidence from clinical trials suggesting that we can change cardiac outcomes by treating mental illness such as depression, evidence from post hoc analysis from both these trials supports additional research in this area (Carney et al. 2004; Serebruany et al. 2003; Taylor et al. 2005).

Thus primary prevention of CVD in the mentally ill focuses on risk factor identification and treatment (risk factor modification). The goal of risk factor modification is to slow the progression of atherosclerotic disease, which is the cause of the majority of cardiovascular morbidity. Persons with more risk factors (e.g., hypertension, hyperlipidemia, smoking) are at increased risk for CVD; as one accumulates risk factors, the risk for a morbid cardiovascular event increases (Expert Panel on Detection, Evaluation, and Treatment of High Blood Cholesterol in Adults 2001). However, risk factors may be viewed as markers rather than direct evidence for atherosclerotic disease. Some individuals who harbor risk factors are free from disease, whereas others without risk factors have atherosclerotic disease (Magliano et al. 2003).

The NCEP has provided regular guidelines for heart disease prevention and other CVD-related conditions since 1988 (Expert Panel on Detection, Evaluation, and Treatment of High Blood Cholesterol in Adults 1988). The ATP III, the most recent meeting of this panel, issued an evidence-based set of guidelines on heart disease risk factor modification and cholesterol management in 2001 (Expert Panel on Detection, Evaluation, and Treatment of High Blood Cholesterol in Adults 2001). More recently, a NCEP report was issued with modified recommendations from ATP III incorporating outcomes from five major clinical trials of statin therapy published since 2001 (Grundy et al. 2004).

Risk categorization in patients without CHD or other forms of CVD is determined by a two-step process. First, the number of risk factors is counted. Table 5–2 lists the major cardiac risk factors according to ATP III (Expert Panel on Detection, Evaluation, and Treatment of High Blood Cholesterol in Adults

TABLE 5–2. Adult Treatment Panel III coronary heart disease (CHD) major risk factors that modify low-density lipoprotein goals

- Cigarette smoking
- Hypertension (blood pressure ≥ 140/90 or on a antihypertensive medication)
- Low HDL cholesterol (<40 mg/dL)[a]
- Family history of premature CHD (CHD in male first-degree relative <55 years; CHD in female first-degree relative <65 years)
- Age (men ≥ 45 years; women ≥ 55 years)

Note. Low-density lipoprotein (LDL) is excluded because these risk factors modify LDL treatment goals. Diabetes is regarded as a CHD risk equivalent. HDL=high-density lipoprotein.
[a]HDL cholesterol ≥ 60 mg/dL counts as a "negative" risk factor; its presence removes one risk factor from the total count.
Source. Reprinted from Expert Panel on Detection, Evaluation, and Treatment of High Blood Cholesterol in Adults 2001.

2001). For example, a 45-year-old woman who smokes, is not hypertensive, whose mother died from CHD at age 60, and who has an HDL level of 55 mg/dL has two major risk factors (smoking and family history) for CHD. As patients accumulate major risk factors, their categorical risk increases as well (Table 5–3). Second, for patients with more than one risk factor, the Framingham scoring method is carried out to better identify individuals whose 10-year risk warrants intensive management. An individual with one major risk factor would be categorized as being at low risk, whereas an individual with two risk factors, depending on other risk factors, may be categorized as being at moderate risk, moderate-high risk, or high risk (see Chapter 9, "Translating What We Have Learned Into Practice," this volume, for Framingham scoring method). Although the Framingham system may be time consuming and tedious, this step is warranted because it allows better targeting of intensive management to patients who will most likely benefit. From this risk assessment, the ATP III established LDL cholesterol goals in order to improve primary prevention of CHD—that is, as patients accumulate risk factors and their risk categorization increases, LDL therapeutic goals and interventions are lowered and intensified.

Patients with two or more risk factors should have their 10-year cardiovascular risk calculated or be referred to a primary care doctor for further risk categorization and comanagement. Diet and lifestyle modification, with a focus on weight reduction, exercise training, and smoking cessation, should be readily available to those with mental illness because these interventions are the foundation of cardiac risk reduction. Although integrated medical and psychiatric care is not com-

TABLE 5–3. Adult Treatment Panel III coronary heart disease (CHD) risk classification for adults and low-density lipoprotein (LDL) goals

Number of cardiac risk factors[a]	Risk category	LDL goal (mg/dL)
0–1	Low risk	< 160
2+ (10-year Framingham risk 10%–20%)	Moderate risk	< 130
CHD or CHD-equivalent condition (10-year Framingham risk >20%)	High risk	< 100

[a]Risk factors are listed in Table 5–2.

Source. Reprinted from Expert Panel on Detection, Evaluation, and Treatment of High Blood Cholesterol in Adults 2001.

mon, efforts to augment the number of specialists (e.g., dieticians, recreational therapists, primary care physicians, nurse practitioners) who deliver these treatments should be increased within publicly funded mental healthcare systems. Although it is often presumed that patients with severe and debilitating mental illness will not respond to such behavioral and lifestyle interventions, preliminary evidence from studies does not support this notion (Littrell et al. 2003; Menza et al. 2004). Finally, psychiatrists can change medications to improve patients' cardiovascular risk profile (Casey et al. 2003; Weiden et al. 2003). In Phase 2T of the CATIE study (the "tolerability pathway"), among the 61 patients who gained more than 7% of their body weight in Phase 1, 42% of those assigned to ziprasidone lost more than 7% of their body weight. For patients in this group assigned to risperidone, 20% lost more than 7% of their body weight. Furthermore, patients switched to ziprasidone and risperidone had significant reductions in triglycerides and cholesterol (Stroup et al. 2006). Even minor reductions in triglycerides, LDL, weight, and waist circumference can lead to significant reductions in cardiovascular risk.

Improving cardiovascular risk and overall health begins with clinicians acknowledging the vulnerability of patients with mental disorders to CVD. Furthermore, clinicians cannot lose sight of the impact of medical problems on mental health outcomes. Given the high risk for CVDs in the mentally ill, cardiac risk factor assessment should be performed in mental health treatment settings. Cardiac risk factor modification has led to dramatic reductions in CHD morbidity and mortality in the non–mentally ill, and these interventions should be available to those with mental illness given their high risk for CVD.

KEY CLINICAL CONCEPTS

- Individuals with mental illness are at greater risk for cardiovascular morbidity and mortality compared with the general population.
- Mental illness and CVD may be related through a variety of mechanisms, including changes in health status, physiological changes that may influence the development of CVD, and underlying factors that lead to the development of both mental illness and CVD.
- Modifiable cardiovascular risk factors are highly prevalent in persons with mental illness, and psychiatric medications often have detrimental effects on cardiovascular risk. Thus it is important for mental health providers to understand cardiovascular risk classification and modification strategies.
- Patients with two or more cardiovascular risk factors should have their 10-year cardiovascular risk estimated and be referred to a primary care center for further risk reduction.

References

Allebeck P: Schizophrenia: a life shortening disease. Schizophr Bull 15:81–89, 1989

Allison DB, Casey DE: Antipsychotic-induced weight gain: a review of the literature. J Clin Psychiatry 62 (suppl 7):22–31, 2001

American Heart Association: Heart disease and stroke statistics: 2005 update. Dallas, TX, American Heart Association, 2005

Anfossi G, Trovati M: Role of catecholamines in platelet function: pathophysiological and clinical significance. Eur J Clin Invest 26:353–370, 1996

Angst F, Stassen H, Clayton P, et al: Mortality of patients with mood disorders: follow-up over 34–38 years. J Affect Disord 68:167–181, 2002

Anton SD, Miller PM: Do negative emotions predict alcohol consumption, saturated fat intake, and physical activity in older adults? Behav Modif 29:677–688, 2005

Appel LJ, Moore TJ, Obarzanek E, et al: A clinical trial of the effects of dietary patterns on blood pressure. N Engl J Med 336:1117–1124, 1998

Applebaum J, Shimon H, Sela BA, et al: Homocysteine levels in newly admitted schizophrenic patients. J Psychiatr Res 38:413–416, 2004

Aydin N, Yigit A, Inandi T, et al: Attitudes of hospital staff toward mentally ill patients in a teaching hospital, Turkey. Int J Soc Psychiatry 49:17–26, 2003

Babiker I: Noncompliance in schizophrenia. Psychiatr Dev 4:329–337, 1986

Bakx JC, van den Hoogen HJ, Deurenberg P, et al: Changes in serum total cholesterol levels over 18 years in a cohort of men and women: the Nijmegen cohort study. Prev Med 30:138–145, 2000

Bär KJ, Letzsch A, Jochum G, et al: Loss of efferent vagal activity in acute schizophrenia. J Psychiatr Res 39:519–527, 2005

Bard JM, Charles MA, Juhan-Vague I, et al: Accumulation of triglyceride-rich lipoprotein in subjects with abdominal obesity: the Biguanides and Prevention of the Risk of Obesity (BIGPRO) 1 study. Arterioscler Thromb Vasc Biol 21:407–414, 2001

Bayes DL, Coumel P, Leclercq JF: Ambulatory sudden cardiac death: mechanisms of production of fatal arrhythmia on the basis of data from 157 cases. Am Heart J 117:151–159, 1989

Berkman LF, Blumenthal J, Burg M, et al: Effects of treating depression and low perceived social support on clinical events after myocardial infarction: the Enhancing Recovery in Coronary Heart Disease Patients (ENRICHD) Randomized Trial. JAMA 289:3106–3116, 2003

Bonow RO, Smaha LA, Smith SC, et al: The international burden of cardiovascular disease: responding to the emerging global epidemic. Circulation 106:1602–1605, 2002

Bosma H, Marmot MG, Hemingway H, et al: Low job control and risk of coronary heart disease: Whitehall II (prospective cohort) study. BMJ 314:558–565, 1997

Brown S: Excess mortality of schizophrenia: a meta-analysis. Br J Psychiatry 171:502–508, 1997

Brown S, Inskip H, Barraclouch B: Causes of excess mortality of schizophrenia. Br J Psychiatry 177:212–217, 2000

Brown S, Birtwistle J, Roe L, et al: The unhealthy lifestyle of people with schizophrenia. Psychol Med 29:697–701, 1999

Carney RM, Feedland KE, Rich MW, et al: Ventricular tachycardia and psychiatric depression in patients with coronary artery disease. Am J Med 95:23–28, 1993

Carney RM, Freedland KE, Eisen SA, et al: Major depression and medication adherence in elderly patients with coronary artery disease. Health Psychol 14:88–90, 1995

Carney RM, Blumenthal JA, Stein PK, et al: Depression, heart rate variability, and acute myocardial infarction. Circulation 104:2024–2028, 2001

Carney RM, Blumenthal JA, Freedland KE, et al: Depression and late mortality after myocardial infarction in the Enhancing Recovery in Coronary Heart Disease (ENRICHD) study. Psychosom Med 66:466–474, 2004

Carroll BJ: Use of the dexamethasone test in depression. J Clin Psychiatry 43:44–50, 1982

Casey DE, Carson WH, Saha AR, et al: Switching patients to aripiprazole from other antipsychotic agents: a multicenter randomized study. Psychopharmacology (Berl) 166:391–399, 2003

Colao A, Pivonello R, Spieza S, et al: Persistence of increased cardiovascular risk in patients with Cushing's disease after five years of successful cure. J Clin Endocrinol Metab 84:2664–2672, 1999

Corcoran C, Walker E, Huot R, et al: The stress cascade and schizophrenia: etiology and onset. Schizophr Bull 29:671–692, 2003

Coronary Drug Project: Influence of adherence to treatment and response of cholesterol on mortality in the coronary drug project. N Engl J Med 303:1038–1041, 1980

Corvin A, O'Mahony E, O'Reagan M, et al: Cigarette smoking and psychotic symptoms in bipolar disorder. Br J Psychiatry 179:35–38, 2001

Coryell W, Tsuang D: Hypothalamic-pituitary-adrenal axis hyperactivity and psychosis: recovery during an 8-year follow-up. Am J Psychiatry 149:1033–1039, 1992

Coutinho M, Gerstein HC, Wang Y, et al: The relationship between glucose and incident cardiovascular events: a metaregression analysis of published data from 20 studies of 95,783 individuals followed for 12.4 years. Diabetes Care 22:233–240, 1999

Critchley JA, Capewell S: Mortality risk reduction associated with smoking cessation in patients with coronary heart disease: a systematic review. JAMA 290:86–97, 2003

Curkendall S, Mo J, Glasser D, et al: Cardiovascular disease in patients with schizophrenia in Saskatchewan, Canada. J Clin Psychiatry 65:715–720, 2004

Curtis BM, O'Keefe JH Jr: Autonomic tone as a cardiovascular risk factor: the dangers of chronic fight or flight. Mayo Clin Proc 77:45–54, 2002

Daban C, Vieta E, Mackin P, et al: Hypothalamic-pituitary-adrenal axis and bipolar disorder. Psychiatr Clin North Am 28:469–480, 2005

Danner M, Kasl SV, Abramson JL, et al: Association between depression and C-reactive protein. Psychosom Med 65:347–356, 2003

Davidson S, Judd F, Jolley D, et al: Cardiovascular risk factors for people with mental illness. Aust N Z J Psychiatry 35:196–202, 2001

de Leon J, Dadvand M, Canuso C, et al: Schizophrenia and smoking: an epidemiological survey in a state hospital. Am J Psychiatry 152:453–455, 1995

de Leon J, Diaz FJ, Rogers T, et al: Initiation of daily smoking and nicotine dependence in schizophrenia and mood disorders. Schizophr Res 56:47–54, 2002

Deshauer D, Duffy A, Alda M, et al: The cortisol awaking response in bipolar disorder: a pilot study. Can J Psychiatry 48:462–466, 2003

Dewan MJ, Pandurangi AK, Boucher ML, et al: Abnormal dexamethasone suppression test results in chronic schizophrenic patients. Am J Psychiatry 139:1501–1503, 1982

Diwan A, Castine M, Pomerleau CS, et al: Differential prevalence of cigarette smoking in patients with schizophrenic vs mood disorders. Schizophr Res 33:113–118, 1998

Dixon L, Weiden P, Delahanty J, et al: Prevalence and correlates of diabetes in national schizophrenia samples. Schizophr Bull 26:903–912, 2000

Downs JR, Clearfield M, Weis S, et al: Primary prevention of acute coronary events with lovastatin in men and women with average cholesterol levels: results of the Air Force/Texas Coronary Atherosclerosis Prevention Study. JAMA 279:1615–1622, 1998

Druss BG, Bradford DW, Rosenheck RA, et al: Mental disorders and use of cardiovascular procedures after myocardial infarction. JAMA 283:506–511, 2000

Druss BG, Rosenheck RA, Desai MM, et al: Quality of preventive medical care for patients with mental disorders. Med Care 40:129–136, 2002

Eliasson B, Hjalmarson A, Kruse E, et al: Effect of smoking reduction and cessation on cardiovascular risk factors. Nicotine Tob Res 3:249–255, 2001

Everson SA, Lynch JW, Chesney MA, et al: Interaction of workplace demands and cardiovascular reactivity in progression of carotid atherosclerosis: population based study. BMJ 314:553–558, 1997

Expert Panel on Detection, Evaluation, and Treatment of High Blood Cholesterol in Adults: Report of the National Cholesterol Education Program Expert Panel on Detection, Evaluation and Treatment of High Blood Cholesterol in Adults. Arch Intern Med 148:36–69, 1988

Expert Panel on Detection, Evaluation, and Treatment of High Blood Cholesterol in Adults: Executive Summary of the Third Report of the National Cholesterol Education Program (NCEP) Expert Panel on Detection, Evaluation, and Treatment of High Blood Cholesterol in Adults (Adult Treatment Panel III). JAMA 285:2486–2497, 2001

Ford ES, Giles WH, Dietz WH: Prevalence of the metabolic syndrome among U.S. adults: findings from the Third National Health and Nutrition Examination Survey. JAMA 287:356–359, 2002

Fergusson DM, Goodwin RD, Horwood LJ: Major depression and cigarette smoking: results of a 21-year longitudinal study. Psychol Med 33:1357–1367, 2003

Fuster V, Badimon L, Badimon JJ, et al: The pathogenesis of coronary artery disease and the acute coronary syndromes, part 1. N Engl J Med 326:242–250, 1992a

Fuster V, Badimon L, Badimon JJ, et al: The pathogenesis of coronary artery disease and the acute coronary syndromes, part 2. N Engl J Med 326:310–318, 1992b

Gallagher E, Viscoli C, Horwitz R: The relationship of treatment adherence to the risk for death after myocardial infarction in women. JAMA 270:742–744, 1993

Garcia MJ, McNamara PM, Gordon T, et al: Morbidity and mortality in diabetes in the Framingham population: sixteen year follow-up study. Diabetes 23:105–111, 1974

Gerstein HC, Pais P, Pogue J, et al: Relationship of glucose and insulin levels to the risk of myocardial infarction: a case control study. J Am Coll Cardiol 33:612–619, 1999

Gillespie CF, Nemeroff CB: Hypercortisolemia and depression. Psychosom Med 67(suppl):S26–S28, 2005

Glassman AH: Cigarette smoking: implications for psychiatric illness. Am J Psychiatry 150:546–553, 1993

Glassman AH: Psychiatry and cigarettes. Arch Gen Psychiatry 55:692–693, 1998

Glassman AH, Covey LS, Dalack GW, et al: Cigarette smoking, major depression and schizophrenia. Clin Neuropharmacol 15(suppl):560A–561A, 1992

Glassman AH, O'Connor CM, Califf RM, et al: Sertraline treatment of major depression in patients with acute MI or unstable angina. JAMA 288:701–709, 2002

Glazer K, Emery C, Frid D, et al: Psychological predictors of adherence and outcomes among patients in cardiac rehabilitation. J Cardiopulm Rehabil 22:40–46, 2002

Goff DC, Sullivan LM, McEvoy JP, et al: A comparison of ten-year cardiac risk estimates in schizophrenia patients from the CATIE study and matched controls. Schizophr Res 80:45–53, 2005

Gold PW, Gabry KE, Yasuda MR, et al: Divergent endocrine abnormalities in melancholic and atypical depression: clinical and pathophysiologic implications. Endocrinol Metab Clin North Am 31:37–62, 2000

Gupta S, Steinmeyer C, Frank B, et al: Hyperglycemia and hypertriglyceridemia in real world patients on antipsychotic therapy. Am J Ther 10:348–355, 2003

Grundy SM, Cleeman JI, Merz CN, et al: Implications of recent clinical trials for the National Cholesterol Education Program Adult Treatment Panel III guidelines. Circulation 110:227–239, 2004

Hanna IR, Wenger NK: Secondary prevention of coronary heart disease in elderly patients. Am Fam Physician 71:2289–2296, 2005

Hermanson B, Omenn GS, Kronmal RA, et al: Beneficial six-year outcome of smoking cessation in older men and women with coronary artery disease: results from the CASS registry. N Engl J Med 319:1365–1369, 1988

Horwitz R, Viscoli C, Berkman L, et al: Treatment adherence and risk of death after myocardial infarction. Lancet 336:542–545, 1990

Hughes JR, Goldstein MG, Hurt RD, et al: Recent advances in the pharmacotherapy of smoking. JAMA 281:72–76, 1999

Irvine J, Baker B, Smith J, et al: Poor adherence to placebo or amiodarone therapy predicts mortality: results from the CAMIAT study. Psychosom Med 61:566–575, 1999

Iso H, Date C, Yamamoto A, et al: Perceived mental stress and mortality from cardiovascular disease among Japanese men and women: The Japan Collaborative Cohort Study for Evaluation of Cancer Risk Sponsored by Monbusho (JACC Study). Circulation 106:1229–1236, 2002

Istvan J, Zavela K, Weidner G: Body weight and psychological distress in NHANES I. Int J Obes Relat Metab Disord 16:999–1003, 1992

Itkin O, Nemetes B, Einat H: Smoking habits in bipolar and schizophrenic outpatients in southern Israel. J Clin Psychiatry 62:269–272, 2001

Jenkinson CM, Madeley RJ, Mitchell JR, et al: The influence of psychosocial factors on survival after myocardial infarction. Public Health 107:305–317, 1993

Jonas BS, Lando JF: Negative affect as a prospective risk factor for hypertension. Psychosom Med 62:188–196, 2000

Joshipura KJ, Ascherio A, Manson JF, et al: Fruit and vegetable intake in relation to risk of ischemic stroke. JAMA 282:1233–1239, 1999

Kathol RG, Jaeckle RS, Lopez JF, et al: Consistent reduction of ACTH responses to stimulation with CRH, vasopressin, and hypoglycaemia in patients with major depression. Br J Psychiatry 155:468–478, 1989

Kemali D, Maj M, Iorio G, et al: Relationship between CSF noradrenaline levels, C-EEG indicators of activation and psychosis ratings in drug-free schizophrenic patients. Acta Psychiatr Scand 71:19–24, 1985

Kemali D, Maj M, Galderisi S, et al: Factors associated with increased noradrenaline levels in schizophrenic patients. Prog Neuropsychopharmacol Biol Psychiatry 14:49–59, 1990

Kemper JW, Baggenstoss AH, Slocumb CH: The relationship of therapy with cortisone to the incidence of vascular lesions in rheumatoid arthritis. Ann Intern Med 6:831–851, 1957

Kendler KS, Kessler RC, Neale MC, et al: The prediction of major depression in women: toward an integrated etiologic model. Am J Psychiatry 150:1139–1148, 1993

Kleiger RE, Miller JP, Bigger JT, et al: Decreased heart rate variability and its association with increased mortality after acute myocardial infarction. Am J Cardiol 59:256–262, 1987

Koenig W: Inflammation and coronary heart disease: an overview. Cardiol Rev 9:31–35, 2001

Kohl HW III: Physical activity and cardiovascular disease: evidence for a dose response. Med Sci Sports Exerc 33(suppl):S472–S483, 2001

Kop WJ, Gottdiener JS, Tangen CM, et al: Inflammation and coagulation factors in persons >65 years of age with symptoms of depression but without evidence of myocardial ischemia. Am J Cardiol 89:419–424, 2002

Lasser K, Boyd JW, Wollhandler S, et al: Smoking and mental illness: a population-based prevalence study. JAMA 284:2606–2610, 2000

Lawrie S, Parsons C, Patrick J, et al: A controlled trial of general practitioners' attitudes to patients with schizophrenia. Health Bull 54:201–203, 1996

Lawrie S, Martin K, McNeill G, et al: General practitioners' attitudes to psychiatric and medical illness. Psychol Med 28:1463–1467, 1998

Leonard S, Adler LE, Benhammou K, et al: Smoking and mental illness. Pharmacol Biochem Behav 70:561–570, 2001

Levine GN, Keaney JF, Vita JA: Cholesterol reduction in cardiovascular disease: clinical benefits and possible mechanisms. N Engl J Med 332:512–521, 1995

Liese AD, Hense HW, Brenner H, et al: Assessing the impact of classical risk factors on myocardial infarction by rate advancement periods. Am J Epidemiol 52:884–888, 2000

Littrell KH, Hilligoss NM, Kirshner CD, et al: The effects of an educational intervention on antipsychotic-induced weight gain. J Nurs Scholarsh 35:237–241, 2003

Llerena A, Caceres M, Penas L, et al: Schizophrenia stigma among medical and nursing school undergraduates. Eur Psychiatry 17:298–299, 2002

Long-Term Intervention With Pravastatin in Ischaemic Disease Study Group: Prevention of cardiovascular events and death with pravastatin patients with coronary heart disease and a broad range of initial cholesterol levels: the Long-Term Intervention With Pravastatin in Ischaemic Disease Study Group. N Engl J Med 339:1349–1357, 1998

Low PA, Pfeifer MA: Standardization of autonomic function, in Clinical Autonomic Disorders. Edited by Low PA. New York, Little, Brown, 1997, pp 287–295

Maas JW, Katz MM, Koslow SH, et al: Adrenomedullary function in depressed patients. J Psychiatr Res 28:357–367, 1994

Magliano DJ, Liew D, Ashton EL, et al: Novel biomedical risk markers for cardiovascular disease. J Cardiovasc Risk 10:21–55, 2003

Masterson E, O'Shea B: Smoking and malignancy in schizophrenia. Br J Psychiatry 145:429–432, 1984

McCreadie RG, Scottish Schizophrenia Lifestyle Group: Diet, smoking and cardiovascular risk in people with schizophrenia: descriptive study. Br J Psychiatry 183:534–539, 2003

McEvoy JP, Brown S: Smoking in first-episode patients with schizophrenia. Am J Psychiatry 156:1120–1121, 1999

McEvoy JP, Meyer JM, Goff DC, et al: Prevalence of the metabolic syndrome in patients with schizophrenia: baseline results from the Clinical Antipsychotic Trials of Intervention Effectiveness (CATIE) schizophrenia trial and comparison with national estimates from NHANES III. Schizophr Res 80:19–32, 2005

McEwen B: Protective and damaging effects of stress mediators. N Engl J Med 338:171–179, 1998a

McEwen BS: Stress, adaptation, and diseases: allostasis and allostatic load. Ann NY Acad Sci 840:33–44, 1998b

McEwen B, Stellar E: Stress and the individual: mechanisms leading to disease. Arch Intern Med 153:2093–2101, 1993

Menza M, Vreeland B, Minsky S, et al: Managing atypical antipsychotic-associated weight gain: 12-month data on a multimodal weight control program. J Clin Psychiatry 65:471–477, 2004

Meyer JM: A retrospective comparison of weight, lipid, and glucose changes at one year between risperidone- and olanzapine-treated inpatients: metabolic outcomes after 1 year. J Clin Psychiatry 63:425–433, 2002

Monroe SM, Harkness K, Simons AD, et al: Life stress and the symptoms of major depression. J Nerv Ment Dis 189:168–175, 2001

Mortensen P, Juel K: Mortality and causes of death in schizophrenic patients in Denmark. Acta Psychiatr Scand 81:372–377, 1990

Mulvihill NT, Foley JB: Inflammation in acute coronary syndromes. Heart 87:210–204, 2002

Musselman DL, Tomer A, Manatunga AK, et al: Exaggerated platelet reactivity in major depression. Am J Psychiatry 153:1313–1317, 1996

Nahas CG, Brunson JG, King WM, et al: Functional and morphologic changes in heart lung preparations following administration of adrenal hormones. Am J Pathol 34: 717–729, 1958

Nahshoni E, Aizenberg D, Strasberg B, et al: QT dispersion in the surface electrocardiogram in elderly patients with major depression. J Affect Disord 60:197–200, 2000

Nemeroff CB, Musselman DL: Are platelets the link between depression and ischemic heart disease? Am Heart J 140(suppl):S57–S62, 2000

Nemeroff CB, Widerlov E, Bissette G, et al: Elevated concentrations of CSF corticotropin-releasing factor-like immunoreactivity in depressed patients. Science 226:1342–1344, 1984

Ness AR, Powles JW: Fruit and vegetables, and cardiovascular disease: a review. Int J Epidemiol 26:1–13, 1997

O'Farrell TJ, Connors GJ, Upper D: Addictive behaviors among hospitalized psychiatric patients. Addict Behav 8:329–333, 1983

Ohaeri JU, Heo CC, Lagundoye OO: The profile of C-reactive proteins in functional psychotic states in a cohort in Nigeria. Acta Psychiatr Scand 88:252–255, 1993

Olincy A, Young DA, Freedman R: Increased levels of the nicotine metabolite cotinine in schizophrenic smokers compared to other smokers. Biol Psychiatry 42:1–5, 1997

Osby U, Correia N, Brandt L, et al: Time trends in schizophrenia mortality in Stockholm County, Sweden: cohort study. BMJ 321:483–484, 2000

Osby U, Brandt L, Correia N, et al: Excess mortality in bipolar and unipolar disorder in Sweden. Arch Gen Psychiatry 58:844–850, 2001

Reddy KS, Katan MB: Diet, nutrition and the prevention of hypertension and cardiovascular diseases. Public Health Nutr 7:167–186, 2004

Remme WJ: The sympathetic nervous system and ischemic heart disease. Eur Heart J 19(suppl):F62–F71, 1998

Ridker PM, Stampfer MJ, Rifai N: Novel risk factors for systemic atherosclerosis: a comparison of C-reactive protein, fibrinogen, homocysteine, lipoprotein (a), and standard cholesterol screening as predictors of peripheral arterial disease. JAMA 285:2481–2485, 2001

Ridker PM, Rifai N, Rose L, et al: Comparison of C-reactive protein and low-density lipoprotein cholesterol levels in the prediction of first cardiovascular events. N Engl J Med 347:1557–1565, 2002

Rigotti NA, Pasternak RC: Cigarette smoking and coronary heart disease: risks and management. Cardiol Clin 14:51–68, 1996

Rosengren A, Tibblin G, Wilhelmsen L: Self-perceived psychological stress and incidence of coronary artery disease in middle-aged men. Am J Cardiol 68:1171–1175, 1991

Rothermundt M, Arolt V, Bayer TA: Review of immunological and immunopathological findings in schizophrenia. Brain Behav Immun 15:319–339, 2001

Ryan M, Sharifi N, Condren R, et al: Evidence of basal pituitary-adrenal overactivity in first episode, drug naïve patients with schizophrenia. Psychoneuroendocrinology 29: 1065–1070, 2004

Saari K, Koponen H, Laitinen J, et al: Hyperlipidemia in persons using antipsychotic medication: a general population-based birth cohort study. J Clin Psychiatry 65:547–550, 2004

Safeer RS, Ugalat PS: Cholesterol treatment guidelines update. Am Fam Physician 65:871–880, 2002

Scandinavian Simvastatin Survival Study: Randomised trial of cholesterol lowering in 4444 patients with coronary heart disease: the Scandinavian Simvastatin Survival Study (4S). Lancet 344:1383–1389, 1994

Serebruany VL, Glassman AH, Malinin AI, et al: Platelet/endothelial biomarkers in depressed patients treated with the selective serotonin reuptake inhibitor sertraline after acute coronary events: the Sertraline AntiDepressant Heart Attack Randomized Trial (SADHART) Platelet Substudy. Circulation 108:939–944, 2003

Servus WE, Littman AB, Stoll AL: Omega-3 fatty acids, homocysteine, and the increased risk of cardiovascular mortality in major depressive disorder. Harv Rev Psychiatry 9:280–293, 2001

Sharma RP, Pandey GN, Janicak PG, et al: The effect of diagnosis and age on the DST: a metaanalytic approach. Biol Psychiatry 5:555–568, 1988

Shemesh E, Yehuda R, Milo O, et al: Posttraumatic stress, non-adherence, and adverse outcome in survivors of myocardial infarction. Psychosom Med 66:521–526, 2004

Shepherd J, Cobbe SM, Ford I, et al: Prevention of coronary heart disease with pravastatin in men with hypercholesterolemia: West of Scotland Coronary Prevention Study Group. N Engl J Med 333:1301–1307, 1995

Sheps DS, Freedland KE, Golden RN, et al: ENRICHD and SADHART: implications for future biobehavioral intervention efforts. Psychosom Med 65:1–2, 2003

Shinn EH, Poston WS, Kimball KT, et al: Blood pressure and symptoms of depression and anxiety: a prospective study. Am J Hypertens 14:660–664, 2001

Sholter DE, Armstrong PW: Adverse effects of corticosteroids on the cardiovascular system. Can J Cardiol 16:505–511, 2000

Singh S, Baxter H, Standen P, et al: Changing the attitudes of "tomorrow's doctors" towards mental illness and psychiatry: a comparison of two teaching models. Med Educ 32:115–120, 1998

Standberg TE, Salomaa VV, Vanhanen HT, et al: Blood pressure and mortality during an up to 32-year follow-up. J Hypertens 19:35–39, 2001

Sterling P, Eyer J: Allostasis: a new paradigm to explain arousal pathology, in Handbook of Life Stress, Cognition, and Health. Edited by Fisher S, Reason J. New York, Wiley, 1988, pp 629–649

Stroup TS, Lieberman JA, McEvoy JP, at al: Effectiveness of olanzapine, quetiapine, risperidone, and ziprasidone in patients with chronic schizophrenia following discontinuation of a previous atypical antipsychotic. Am J Psychiatry 163:611–622, 2006

Tandon R, Mazzara C, De Quardo J, et al: Dexamethasone suppression test in schizophrenia: relationship to symptomatology ventricular enlargement, and outcome. Biol Psychiatr 29:953–964, 1991

Taylor CB, Youngblood ME, Catellier D, et al: Effects of antidepressant medication on morbidity and mortality in depressed patients after myocardial infarction. Arch Gen Psychiatry 62:792–798, 2005

Troxler RG, Sprague EA, Albanese RA, et al: The association of elevated plasma cortisol and early atherosclerosis as demonstrated by coronary angiography. Atherosclerosis 26: 151–162, 1977

Valkonen-Korhonen M, Tarvainen MP, Ranta-Aho P, et al: Heart rate variability in acute psychosis. Psychophysiology 40:716–726, 2003

Vanable PA, Carey MP, Carey KB, et al: Smoking among psychiatric outpatients: relationship to substance use, diagnosis, and illness severity. Psychol Addict Behav 4:259–265, 2003

Villablanca AC, McDonald JM, Rutledge JC: Smoking and cardiovascular disease. Clin Chest Med 21:159–172, 2000

Viscoli C, Horwitz R, Singer B: Beta-blockers after myocardial infarction: influence of first-year clinical course on long-term effectiveness. Ann Intern Med 118:99–105, 1993

Walsh MT, Ryan M, Hillmann A, et al: Elevated expression of integrin alpha(IIb) beta(IIIa) in drug-naive, first-episode schizophrenic patients. Biol Psychiatry 52:874–879, 2002

Wannamethee SG, Shaper AG: Physical activity in the prevention of cardiovascular disease: an epidemiological perspective. Sports Med 31:101–114, 2001

Watkins LL, Grossman P: Association of depressive symptoms with reduced baroreflex cardiac control in coronary artery disease. Am Heart J 137:452–457, 1999

Watson S, Gallagher P, Ritchie JC, et al: Hypothalamic-pituitary-adrenal axis function in patients with bipolar disorder. Br J Psychiatry 184:496–502, 2004

Weiden P, Olfson M: Cost of relapse in schizophrenia. Schizophr Bull 21:419–429, 1995

Weiden PJ, Daniel DG, Simpson G, et al: Improvement in indices of health status in outpatients with schizophrenia switched to ziprasidone. J Clin Psychopharmacol 23:595–600, 2003

Welin C, Lapppas G, Wilhelmsen L: Independent importance of psychosocial factors for prognosis after myocardial infarction. J Intern Med 247:629–639, 2000

Wilson PW, D'Agostino RB, Levy D, et al: Prediction of coronary heart disease using risk factor categories. Circulation 97:1837–1847, 1998

Wilson PW, D'Agostino, RB, Sullivan L, et al: Overweight and obesity as determinants of cardiovascular risk: the Framingham experience. Arch Intern Med 162:1867–1872, 2002

World Health Organization: WHO publishes definitive atlas on global heart disease and stroke epidemic (news release). Available online at http://www.who.int/mediacentre/news/releases/2004/pr68/en/index.html. Accessed August 27, 2005

Wulsin L, Vaillant G, Wells V. A systematic review of the mortality of depression. Psychosom Med 61:6–17, 1999

Yamamoto K, Hornykiewicz O: Proposal for a noradrenaline hypothesis of schizophrenia. Prog Neuropsychopharmacol Biol Psychiatry 28:913–22, 2004

Yeragani VK: The incidence of abnormal dexamethasone suppression in schizophrenia: a review and a meta-analytic comparison with the incidence in normal controls. Can J Psychiatry 35:128-132, 1990

Yeragani VK, Pohl R, Jampala VC, et al: Increased QT variability in patients with panic disorder and depression. Psychiatry Res 93:225–235, 2000

Zhao W, Chen Y, Lin M, et al: Association between diabetes and depression: sex and age differences. Public Health 120:696–704, 2006

Chapter 6

ANTIPSYCHOTIC-ASSOCIATED WEIGHT GAIN

A Synthesis and Clinical Recommendations

Roger S. McIntyre, M.D., F.R.C.P.C.
Joanna K. Soczynska, B.Sc.
Kamran Bordbar, M.D.
Jakub Z. Konarski, M.Sc.

Antipsychotics, both first and second generation, are broad-spectrum neurotherapeutic agents capable of attenuating myriad psychopathological symptoms. As a class of agents, the second-generation antipsychotics are promoted as offering several therapeutic advantages when compared with the older first-generation agents (e.g., enhanced efficacy for neurocognitive deficits, reduced propensity for neurological adverse events). Nevertheless, significant weight gain associated with many of the available second-generation drugs detracts from their therapeutic potential and patient acceptance.

In this chapter, we aim to provide the practicing clinician with a synthesis of the extant literature reporting on the association between antipsychotic usage and weight gain. The chapter is organized into three areas of focus: 1) the liability and correlates of antipsychotic-associated weight gain (AAWG); 2) the putative mechanisms of AAWG; 3) and the strategies preliminarily evaluated as management approaches for AAWG.

We conducted a Medline search of all English-language articles from 1966 to 2005, using the following keywords: overweight, obesity, body mass index (BMI), weight gain, schizophrenia, psychosis, psychotic disorders, bipolar disorder, major depressive disorder, conventional antipsychotics, atypical antipsychotics, clozapine, olanzapine, risperidone, quetiapine, ziprasidone, aripiprazole, genetics, peptides, leptin, weight loss, bariatric, topiramate, sibutramine, orlistat, behavioral therapy, Weight Watchers, and antidepressants. The search was supplemented with a manual review of summary articles and references germane to this topic. Throughout the chapter, the use of the word *significant* denotes statistical significance of $P < 0.05$.

Antipsychotic-Associated Weight Gain: Liability and Correlates

The synthesis and interpretation of investigations reporting AAWG requires familiarity with the methodological limitations of the data. For example, most studies do not sufficiently adjust for sociodemographics, dietary habits, comorbidity (e.g., binge eating disorder, hypothyroidism), patient behavior (e.g., inactivity, smoking), family history, premorbid weight status, illness-associated weight change, body composition, and concomitant treatment effects.

Moreover, reports do not differentiate a patient's weight prior to the onset of his or her psychiatric illness from the effects of the illness itself or from the treatment provided. Importantly, most studies report weight gain with the last observation carried forward (LOCF) imputation method. This method often underestimates the weight gain propensity associated with treatment (i.e., patients who gain significant weight are less likely to complete the full duration of the study). Nevertheless, results from extant studies describing weight gain correlates are presented in Figure 6–1 and Table 6–1.

STUDIES OF DIFFERENTIAL LIABILITY AMONG ANTIPSYCHOTICS

Weight gain associated with first-generation antipsychotics was reported soon after their introduction (McIntyre et al. 2001b). The short-term (i.e., 10-week) weight gain liability of both first- and second-generation agents was estimated in a meta-analysis of 81 studies primarily evaluating patients with schizophrenia (Figure 6–1; Allison et al. 1999). A weight gain liability spectrum was reported in which clozapine (4.0 kg) represented the high end, followed by olanzapine (3.5 kg), thioridazine (3.5 kg), sertindole (2.9 kg), chlorpromazine (2.1 kg), risperidone (2.0 kg), and ziprasidone (0.04 kg). Other reports have estimated the weight gain liability of quetiapine and aripiprazole to be similar to that of risperidone and ziprasidone, respectively (Borison et al. 1996; Peuskens and Link 1997).

Weight gain reported categorically as a change in basal weight (i.e., ≥7%) further illustrates the differential liability for weight gain among antipsychotics. Relative to placebo, aripiprazole, ziprasidone, and risperidone are associated with

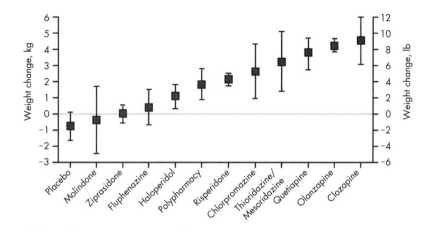

FIGURE 6–1. Weight gain liability of antipsychotics with short-term (10-week) treatment.

Source. Reprinted from Allison DB, Mentore JL, Heo M, et al.: "Antipsychotic-Induced Weight Gain: A Comprehensive Research Synthesis." *American Journal of Psychiatry* 156:1686–1696, 1999. Copyright 1999, American Psychiatric Association. Used with permission.

approximately 2 times, quetiapine 4 times, and olanzapine 10 times the placebo incidence (Casey et al. 2004).

There are relatively few multiyear studies reporting AAWG. As with most adverse events, patients tolerating medications (i.e., minimal weight gain) are more likely to remain in a lengthier study. Hence interpretative caution is required when evaluating AAWG in studies employing the LOCF imputation method. Nevertheless, differential weight gain trajectory curves are reported among the available agents.

For most second-generation antipsychotics, the rate of weight gain increase is highest within the initial 2–3 months of treatment, although a longer hazard period has been reported with olanzapine (6–9 months) and clozapine (>1 year). It is important to emphasize that these estimates are extrapolated from populations of heterogeneous patients. Within these studies, individual patients exhibit significant interindividual variation, with some patients manifesting a slow yet inexorable increase in body weight over several years (Casey et al. 2004).

BODY COMPOSITION STUDIES

Eder et al. (2001) evaluated anthropometrics and body composition in olanzapine-treated patients ($n = 10$) versus a healthy comparison group ($n = 10$). Body composition was determined every 4 weeks by impedance analysis. The patient group exhibited significant weight gain (mean = 3.3 kg), most of which represented an increase

TABLE 6–1. Antipsychotic-associated weight gain: correlates

Variable	Findings	Study
Age	Younger more at risk	Kelly et al. 1998; Kinon et al. 1998; Lane et al. 2003; Wetterling and Mussigbrodt 1999
Sex	Females more than males	Gopalaswamy and Morgan 1985
	Males more than females	Kinon et al. 1998
	No difference in males and females	Lane et al. 2003
Ethnicity	Nonwhites gained more weight than whites	Basson et al. 2001; Lane et al. 2003
Environment	More weight gain in inpatients	Lane et al. 2003
Cigarette smoking	No association	Ellingrod et al. 2002
Appetite increase	Positive association	Brady 1989; Kinon et al. 1998
Baseline weights	Normal or underweight at pretreatment baseline at higher risk	Kinon et al. 1998; Lane et al. 2003
Previous treatment exposure	Antipsychotic naïve at higher risk	Wetterling and Mussigbrodt 1999
	Number or duration of prior hospitalizations: no association	Lane et al. 2003
Dose	Positive association	Lane et al. 2003; Nemeroff 1997
	No association	Ganguli 1999; Johnson and Breen 1979

TABLE 6–1. Antipsychotic-associated weight gain: correlates *(continued)*

Variable	Findings	Study
Duration	Risperidone weight gain 3.3 kg after 1 year	Amery et al. 1997
	Risperidone (mean modal daily dosage=4.9 mg) weight gain 2.3 kg after 2 years	Csernansky et al. 1999
	Olanzapine (mean daily dosage=15 mg; SD 2.5) weight gain 11.8 kg after 1 year	Beasley et al. 1997
	Olanzapine weight gain tapers between weeks 30 and 40	Eli Lilly (unpublished data); Nemeroff 1997
	Clozapine weight gain greatest during first year but continued up to 36 months and then plateaued	Umbricht et al. 1994
	Plateaued at 20 weeks with olanzapine and clozapine versus 10 weeks with risperidone	Wirshing et al. 1999
Formulation	Oral and depot equally likely	Gaulin et al. 1999; Johnson and Breen 1979
Plasma level	Threshold dose-weighted plasma concentration of 20.6 ng/mL associated with increased likelihood of weight gain during olanzapine treatment	Perry et al. 2005

TABLE 6–1. Antipsychotic-associated weight gain: correlates *(continued)*

Variable	Findings	Study
Clinical response	Positive relation	Bustillo et al. 2003; Dobmeier et al. 2000; Gupta et al. 1999; Jalenques et al. 1996; Kinon et al. 1998; Kryspin-Exner 1996; Lane et al. 2003; Leadbetter et al. 1992; Planansky and Heilizer 1959
	No relation	Lamberti et al. 1992; Umbricht et al. 1994
	Positive relationship with olanzapine and clozapine, no relationship with risperidone and haloperidol	Czobor et al. 2002
	Negative relationship with clozapine	Zhang et al. 2003
Antipsychotic class	Atypical more than conventional	Allison et al. 1999; Wetterling and Mussigbrodt 1999

Source. Reprinted from Keck PE, Buse JB, Dagogo-Jack S, et al.: "Metabolic Disease and Severe Mental Illness," in *Managing Metabolic Concerns in Patients With Severe Mental Illness*. Minneapolis, MN, Postgraduate Medicine, McGraw-Hill, 2003. Copyright 2003, Vendome Group LLC. Used with permission.

in body fat (2.2 kg). A separate investigation of first-episode schizophrenic patients treated with chlorpromazine, risperidone, and quetiapine also reported a significant increase in subcutaneous and intraabdominal adipose tissue depots. An increase in adiposity in these patients was associated with a significant increase in leptin concentration, dysglycemia, and dyslipidemia (Zhang et al. 2004).

Ryan et al. (2004) evaluated and compared body composition (with computed tomography) in first-episode medication-naïve schizophrenic patients ($n=$ 19) relative to a matched control group. Prior to therapy with a second-generation antipsychotic (risperidone or olanzapine), the patient group exhibited a relatively higher mean percentage of intraabdominal fat and plasma cortisol level. Both risperidone and olanzapine were associated with significant weight gain, with no significant increase in intraabdominal fat. The dissociation between use of second-generation antipsychotics and intraabdominal fat is surprising, potentially explained by the small sample size and the possibility of type II error.

The findings above, when taken together, indicate there is a continuum of weight gain liability among the antipsychotics. As a class, the second-generation agents impart more weight gain than the first, with the highest weight gain liability reported with olanzapine, clozapine, and the low-potency first-generation antipsychotics. The increase in weight associated with the use of antipsychotics represents an increase in adiposity.

The extent and significance of AAWG invites the need to refine baseline variates that may be predictive of weight gain (see Table 6–1). Most variates examined to date have weak or equivocal associations with AAWG, with some exceptions. For example, significant associations between AAWG and age, basal BMI, and improvement in psychopathology have been reported (Keck et al. 2003a). These observations have led to hypotheses regarding putative mechanisms of AAWG and have drawn attention to potential high-risk patients (e.g., pediatric patients).

As an illustration, orexins (hypocretins) are peptides that are only expressed in the lateral hypothalamus and perifornical area. Orexins stimulate feeding behavior and increase regional dopamine concentration. Olanzapine is associated with an increase in c-fos protein expression in orexin-containing neurons. These data suggest that olanzapine may simultaneously engage neurological systems that subserve feeding behaviors and psychopathological symptoms (Fadel et al. 2002; Nakamura et al. 2000; Sakurai et al. 1998; Uramura et al. 2001).

Medication-Associated Weight Gain: Mechanisms

The balance between energy intake and expenditure ostensibly determines net body weight (Tappy et al. 2003). Energy expenditure can be further partitioned into resting energy expenditure and activity-related expenditure (Speakman and Selman 2003). Weight gain is a highly complex multifactorial phenotype with a heritable liability of approximately 70% (Hebebrand et al. 2001). Energy intake and expenditure are tightly regulated by a panoply of central and peripheral energy homeostasis mechanisms. It is likely that AAWG is subserved by several mechanisms, with an increase in appetite, via affinity for central appetite-stimulating systems, occupying a central role (Gale et al. 2004).

REGULATION OF ENERGY EXPENDITURE AND INTAKE

Monoamines

Compelling evidence indicates that the catecholamines are salient to appetite, feeding behavior, and body weight regulation. For example, an absolute or relative decrease in the hypothalamic availability of dopamine is associated with an increase in feeding behavior in animal models. Preliminary evidence also suggests that obese patients may have a decreased availability (i.e., downregulation) of striatal dopamine D_2 receptors (G.J. Wang et al. 2001). These observations have provided the impetus for the development of monoamine-based anorexiants (e.g., amphetamine) and further suggest a mechanistic model for AAWG (Parada et al. 1989, 1991).

Serotonin is the most scrutinized monoamine in the research and treatment of obesity (Wirtshafter 2001). Serotonin is a satiety factor that also influences food preferences (i.e., inhibiting the ingestion of carbohydrate and promoting consumption of protein or fat) (De Vry and Schreiber 2000; Harvey and Bouwer 2000; Meguid et al. 2000). Preclinical studies of serotonin 5-HT_{2C} knockout mice are frequently cited as a proof of principle that serotonin and its receptors are relevant to feeding behavior and metabolism.

For example, Tecott et al. (1995) bred a 5-HT_{2C} knockout mouse that became obese later in life and developed what was described, based on laboratory evidence, as an obesity syndrome (i.e., increased insulin and leptin) and a propensity for seizures. Several investigations have also reported significant associations between psychotropic medication in vitro affinity for the 5-HT_{2C} receptor and propensity for AAWG (Goodall et al. 1988; Tecott et al. 1995; Vickers et al. 2000).

Histamine

Histamine and its receptors (H_1, H_2, and H_3) are integral to the regulation of body weight, drinking, and feeding behavior (Eder et al. 2001). Histamine receptor H_1 knockout mice are desensitized to the anorectic effects of leptin, which may presage their propensity to increases in feeding behavior and obesity (Masaki et al. 2001). Several investigations have reported on the association between in vitro histamine receptor affinity and a propensity to AAWG (Wirshing et al. 1999).

For example, Kroeze et al. (2003) reported an association between AAWG ($n = 17$ antipsychotics) and in vitro affinity for 12 neurotransmitter receptors. In vitro affinity for the H_1 histamine receptor had the highest correlation with short-term AAWG for both the first- and second-generation antipsychotics. Weight gain was also correlated with in vitro affinity for the α_{1A}, 5-HT$_{2C}$, and 5-HT$_6$ receptors, whereas affinities for eight other receptors (D$_2$, α_{2A}, α_{2B}, α_{2C}, 5-HT$_{1A}$, 5-HT$_{2A}$, 5-HT$_7$, and M$_3$) were not associated with short-term weight gain (Table 6–2).

Muscarinic Cholinergic Receptors

In vitro affinity for muscarinic cholinergic receptors (MCR) has not been consistently reported to correlate with AAWG. Nevertheless, neurotherapeutic agents associated with weight gain (e.g., low-potency first-generation antipsychotics, tricyclic antidepressants, and paroxetine) all exhibit relatively high in vitro affinity for MCR. Moreover, Yamada et al. (2001) reported that MCR (i.e., M$_3$ receptor) knockout mice exhibited a decrease in feeding behavior with resultant reductions in weight, peripheral fat, leptin, and insulin.

Amino Acid Neurotransmitters

Glutamate and γ-aminobutyric acid (GABA) have reciprocal interactions with each other and have been shown to modulate appetite and feeding behavior. GABAergic medications promote weight gain, and agonists at the glutamate *N*-methyl-D-aspartate (NMDA) receptor (e.g., glycine) stimulate feeding behavior. Although antipsychotics modulate both glutamate and GABAergic systems, the association with AAWG has not been parsed out (Baptista et al. 2000; Gordon and Price 1999; Ketter et al. 1999; Picard et al. 2000; Stanley et al. 1997).

Reproductive Hormones

Associations between AAWG and reproductive hormones (e.g., estrogen, prolactin) have been preliminarily examined. Excess weight and obesity is associated with androgenization in human females and hypogonadism in males. It is reported that antipsychotic treatment is associated with a decrease in plasma estradiol levels in female treated rats. Baptista et al. (1997) hypothesized that the plasma estradiol:testosterone ratio may affect the responsivity of "satiety" neurons in the lateral hypothalamus (Parada et al. 1989).

Sustained hyperprolactinemia is associated with repeated administration of first- and some second-generation antipsychotics (e.g., risperidone). Prolactin stimulates food intake, fat deposition, and lipolysis and decreases insulin binding and glucose uptake in adipocytes isolated from pregnant women (Flint et al. 2003). It has been conjectured that sustained hyperprolactinemia may be an effect mediator of AAWG (Baptista 1999; Baptista et al. 1997). If elevation of prolactin level is a relevant mechanism, it is not likely primary, because the antipsychotics with the highest weight gain propensity (e.g., clozapine, olanzapine) are not associated with sustained hyperprolactinemia.

TABLE 6–2. Correlation between propensity of 17 drugs to induce weight gain and affinity (log K_i) for 12 receptors

Receptor	Spearman correlation	
	ρ	P
D_2	0.361	NS
H_1	−0.723	< 0.01
α_{1A}	−0.537	< 0.05
α_{2A}	−0.370	NS
α_{2B}	−0.361	NS
α_{2C}	−0.323	NS
5-HT_{1A}	−0.208	NS
5-HT_{2A}	−0.373	NS
5-HT_{2C}	−0.493	< 0.05
5-HT_6	−0.521	< 0.05
5-HT_7	0.113	NS
M_3	−0.408	NS

Source. Adapted by permisison from Macmillan Publishers Ltd. from Kroeze WK, Hufeisen SJ, Popadak BA, et al.: "H_1-Histamine Receptor Affinity Predicts Short-Term Weight Gain for Typical and Atypical Antipsychotic Drugs." *Neuropsychopharmacology* 28:519–526, 2003. Copyright Macmillan Publishers Ltd. Used with permission.

Cytokines

Proinflammatory cytokines (e.g., interleukins, tumor necrosis factor–α, interferon) mediate sickness and appetitive behaviors and metabolic and immune functioning (Musselman et al. 2003). Cytokines are also reported to mediate glucose, protein, and lipid metabolism (Stumvoll et al. 2005). Administration of several psychotropic agents (e.g., antidepressants, antipsychotics) has been reported to alter plasma concentrations of several proinflammatory cytokines and their respective soluble receptors. For example, chronic clozapine administration is associated with an increase in plasma tumor necrosis factor–α, interleukin-2, and leptin concentration (Argiles et al. 1997; Auwerx and Staels 1998; Bromel et al. 1998; Dandona et al. 1998; Haack et al. 1999; Hauner et al. 1998; Hinze-Selch et al. 2000; Kraus et al. 2002; Old 1985; Uysal et al. 1997; K.Y. Wang et al. 2000). A very promising research vista for the future is to characterize the role of cytokines in the pathophysiology of mental disorders (e.g., mood disorders) and their relevance to medication-associated adverse events.

Leptin

Leptin is an adipocyte-derived peptide that regulates energy intake, energy expenditure, the neuroendocrine axis, and possibly the size of the peripheral adipose tissue depot (Yanovski and Yanovski 1999). The association between changes in plasma leptin concentrations and AAWG has been comprehensively reviewed elsewhere (Baptista et al. 2004). The findings, when taken together, indicate that leptin may not be a primary mechanism of AAWG, but an important secondary role has been suggested (Hagg et al. 2001; McIntyre et al. 2003; Melkersson and Hulting 2001). For example, Haupt et al. (2005) reported on the relationship between adiposity and plasma leptin concentration in schizophrenic patients ($n=72$) receiving antipsychotic therapy. This group was compared with a contemporaneously examined group of healthy adult control subjects ($n=124$). The investigators reported that adiposity-related elevation in plasma leptin concentration in antipsychotic-treated patients with schizophrenia was highly comparable with that observed in the control group. These effects remained significant after adjustment for adiposity and gender.

Ghrelin

Ghrelin is a 28-amino acid orexigenic peptide. The concentration of ghrelin is inversely associated with energy balance (i.e., increased in states of negative energy balance). In rodents, circulating total and active ghrelin levels are reduced in the ob/ob and db/db mice (Ariyasu et al. 2002). Ghrelin is isolated from the human stomach and is believed to act at the level of the hypothalamus via neuropeptide Y and agouti-related protein (Shintani et al. 2001). Ghrelin and leptin appear to exert opposing effects on appetite and feeding behavior.

Murashita et al. (2005) examined the effect of olanzapine on plasma ghrelin, leptin, and other metabolic parameters in olanzapine-treated schizophrenia patients ($n=7$). Most patients reported a significant increase in appetite, mean body weight, and mean body fat percentage. Plasma leptin, plasma total ghrelin (which includes inactive des-acyl ghrelin), and active ghrelin also increased significantly. The predicted decrease in leptin levels, associated with a high circulating ghrelin concentration, was not observed.

Energy Expenditure

Antipsychotic effects on energy expenditure have been preliminarily examined. Graham et al. (2005) evaluated changes in body weight, body composition, and energy expenditure in first-episode psychotic patients ($n=9$) treated with olanzapine. Body composition was assessed using dual energy x-ray absorptiometry at the first and last visit. Substrate utilization (respiratory quotient) and resting energy expenditure were determined by indirect calorimetry.

The median increase in body weight was 4.7 kg, or 7.3% of baseline weight. Measures of body fat percentage and absolute fat mass increase with olanzapine

(3.8% and 4.3 kg, respectively) indicated that the increase in body fat accounted for 74% of total weight gain. There was no evidence of lower baseline energy expenditure in subjects who gained the most weight, although the respiratory quotient increased significantly with olanzapine treatment (median change 0.12, a 14% increase). There was also a significant positive correlation between change in respiratory quotient and change in weight. These data indicate that a decrease in resting energy expenditure does not mediate olanzapine-associated weight gain; instead, it may be mediated by a decreased fatty acid oxidation (Heilbronn et al. 2004).

Gothelf et al. (2002) examined caloric intake and energy expenditure as mediators of olanzapine-associated weight gain in male adolescent schizophrenic inpatients. Subjects were treated with olanzapine ($n=10$) or haloperidol ($n=10$) and evaluated at baseline and after 4 weeks of treatment. Parameters of interest were anthropometry, caloric intake, and energy expenditure. Resting energy expenditure was measured by indirect calorimetry after an overnight fast with a metabolic monitor. Activity-related expenditure was measured by means of an accelerometer positioned above the right hip and a heart rate monitor.

The mean BMI was reported to significantly increase over the subsequent 4 weeks (baseline 24.5 kg/m^2; week 4, 25.8 kg/m^2). The caloric intake for the olanzapine-treated group increased by 589 kcal/day (27%). There were no changes in diet composition, although a significant increase in abdominal circumference was noted. It was also reported that there were no significant differences in resting energy expenditure noted in olanzapine-treated patients. The small sample and low baseline activity level may obfuscate an effect of olanzapine on energy expenditure. Nevertheless, olanzapine-associated weight gain may be parsimoniously explained by an increase in energy intake.

Food Preference and Satiety Signaling

Patients receiving antipsychotic medications frequently report a change in the subjective feeling of fullness and satiety, food preferences, hyperphagia, and in some cases, de novo binge eating (Theisen et al. 2003). Hartfield et al. (2003) reported results from a preclinical study indicating that clozapine and olanzapine are associated with an increase in fat intake (versus a decrease with haloperidol). The increased energy intake associated with the use of antipsychotics suggests dysregulation of central mechanisms (e.g., hypothalamic) that subserve energy homeostasis. From a clinical perspective, patients should be encouraged to consume a balanced diet and not rely on a subjective sense of satiety as a surrogate marker of adequate food consumption.

Uncoupling Proteins

Uncoupling proteins (UCPs) occupy a pivotal role in regulating energy expenditure through peripheral mechanisms. The UCP 1, 2, and 3 isoforms exhibit tissue selectivity, with UCP 1 located in brown adipose tissue, UCP 2 ubiquitous in its distribution (with a preponderance in white adipose tissue), and UCP 3 located in skeletal muscle (Hesselink et al. 2003). An increased expression of UCPs would be predictive of weight loss via increased heat dissipation. Several appetite suppressants and neurotherapeutic agents (e.g., topiramate) modulate UCP transcription (Berraondo et al. 2000; Nagase et al. 2001; Tai et al. 1996). These molecular effects would suggest that a significant change in body weight could occur in a eucaloric patient via an increase in heat loss mechanisms. It remains a testable hypothesis that AAWG may be associated with a functional or quantitative decrease in heat dissipation protein activity.

Peroxisome Proliferator-Activated Receptor

As reported earlier in this chapter, AAWG represents a significant increase in body adiposity. Peroxisome proliferator-activated receptors are cell surface receptors that promote the conversion of non–lipid-storing pre-adipocytes to mature adipocytes. It is not known if the increase in total body fat associated with the use of antipsychotics represents adipocyte cell proliferation and/or hypertrophy (Yanovski and Yanovski 1999).

PHARMACOGENETICS

Differences among individuals in their predisposition to AAWG indicate that common variations of the DNA sequence (i.e., polymorphisms) may account for the observed weight gain (see Table 6–3). Alternatively, polymorphisms may be in linkage disequilibrium with other more salient gene(s). For example, genes that are responsible for AAWG may be more prevalent than expected by random assortment due to their co-inheritance with other, more salient genes. Polymorphisms encode for proteins that differ in activity and/or conformation (Basile et al. 2001). These changes may portend differential patterns of response and adverse events among the available antipsychotics. Pharmacogenetic investigations have attempted to identify associations between AAWG and disparate polymorphisms. Polymorphisms that encode proteins involved in medication pharmacodynamics and pharmacokinetics have been an area of most inquiry.

The 5-HT$_{2C}$ receptor gene (*5HT2C*) is located on the X chromosome at q24 and has a promoter polymorphism consisting of a *C* to *T* transversion at position −759 in the 5′-flanking region (Niswender et al. 1998; Pooley et al. 2004). In human subjects, polymorphism of the *5HT2C* may be associated with the development of obesity and insulin resistance in normal subjects. The variant *T* allele may offer a protective effect against weight gain perhaps related to higher transcriptional level of this gene affecting appetite regulation and resistance to obesity (Yuan et al. 2000). These findings have provided the impetus to examine the role of *5HT2C* polymorphisms in AAWG (Buckland et al. 2005).

TABLE 6–3. Pharmacogenetic studies

Study	Treatment	Sample size (N)	Diagnosis	Ethnicity	Period of weight assessment	Polymorphisms	Results
Rietschel et al. 1996	Clozapine	149	Schizophrenia/ Schizoaffective disorder (DSM-IV)	German	$\geq$28 days	Four in *DRD4* (48-bp repeat in exon 3, 12-bp repeat in exon 1, 13-bp deletion in exon 1, Gly11Arg substitution)	Nonsignificant
Rietschel et al. 1997	Clozapine	152	Schizophrenia/ Schizoaffective disorder (DSM-IV)	German	$\geq$28 days	One in the 5-HT$_{2C}$ receptor (Cys23Ser)	Nonsignificant
Hong et al. 2001	Clozapine	93	Schizophrenia (DSM-IV)	Chinese	Monthly for 4 months	Four in the serotonergic system: 5-HTT (short/ long allele), 5-HT$_{2A}$ (102T/C), 5-HT$_{2C}$ (Cys23Ser), 5-HT$_6$ (267C/T)	Nonsignificant

TABLE 6–3. Pharmacogenetic studies *(continued)*

Study	Treatment	Sample size (N)	Diagnosis	Ethnicity	Period of weight assessment	Polymorphisms	Results
Basile et al. 2001	Clozapine	80	Schizophrenia (DSM-III-R)	Caucasian (58) African American (22)	6 weeks	Four in serotonergic receptors: 5-HT$_{1A}$ (CA-repeat), 5-HT$_{2A}$ (102T/C), 5-HT$_{2A}$ (His452/Tyr), 5-HT$_{2C}$ (Cys23Ser); two in histamine H$_1$ (promoter) and H$_2$ (G-1018A) receptors; one in *CYP1A2* (C → A in the first intron); two adrenergic receptors ADRα1 (Arg347Cys), ADRβ3 (Trp64Arg); one in the TNF-α gene (G-308A)	Nonsignificant (trends for 5-HT$_{2C}$, ADRα1, ADRβ3, and TNF-α)
Ellingrod et al. 2002	Olanzapine	11	Schizophrenia (DSM-III-R and DSM-IV)	Caucasian	Weekly, up to 47 weeks	Two in *CYPD26* (allele 1* represents the wild type whereas alleles 3* and 4* represent two distinct polymorphisms)	Heterozygous (1*/3*, 1*/4*) gained more weight ($P = 0.0097$)

TABLE 6–3. Pharmacogenetic studies *(continued)*

Study	Treatment	Sample size (N)	Diagnosis	Ethnicity	Period of weight assessment	Polymorphisms	Results
Hong et al. 2002	Clozapine	88	Schizophrenia (DSM-IV)	Han Chinese	4 months	Two in the H_1 receptor (Glu349Asp, Leu449Ser)	Nonsignificant for Glu349Asp; all patients were homozygotes for Leu449
Reynolds et al. 2002	Chlorpromazine (69) Risperidone (46) Clozapine (4) Fluphenazine (3) Sulpiride (1)	123	Schizophrenia (DSM-IV)	Han Chinese	Weekly, up to 10 weeks	One in the $5\text{-}HT_{2C}$ gene (−759C/T)	Less weight gain with −759T allele ($P=0.003$)
Basile et al. 2002	Clozapine	80	Schizophrenia (DSM-III-R)	Caucasian (58) African American (22)	6 weeks	One in the $5\text{-}HT_{2C}$ gene (−759C/T)	Hemizygous men with T allele gained more weight ($P=0.047$)
Tsai et al. 2002	Clozapine	80	Schizophrenia/ Schizoaffective disorder	Han Chinese	4 months	One in the $5\text{-}HT_{2C}$ gene (−759C/T)	Nonsignificant

TABLE 6–3. Pharmacogenetic studies *(continued)*

Study	Treatment	Sample size (N)	Diagnosis	Ethnicity	Period of weight assessment	Polymorphisms	Results
Hong et al. 2002	Clozapine	88	Schizophrenia (DSM-IV)	Han Chinese from Taiwan	4 months	Histamine H_1 receptor (Glu349Asp)	Nonsignificant
Reynolds et al. 2003	Clozapine	32	First-episode schizophrenia	Han Chinese	6 weeks	One in the 5-HT_{2C} gene (−759C/T)	Less weight gain with −759T variant allele; effect strongest in the male patients
Zhang et al. 2003	Antipsychotics	117	First-episode schizophrenia	Han Chinese	10 weeks	*Taq*I A polymorphism of dopamine D_2 receptor gene (*DRD2*)	Nonsignificant
Pooley et al. 2004	Psychological	120	Obese	Female	12 months	Prevalence of 5-HT_{2C} gene (−759C/T)	C allele more common (*P*=0.008); heterozygotes lost less weight than homozygotes after 6 months (*P*=0.006) and 12 months (*P*=0.009)

TABLE 6–3. Pharmacogenetic studies *(continued)*

Study	Treatment	Sample size (N)	Diagnosis	Ethnicity	Period of weight assessment	Polymorphisms	Results
Theisen et al. 2004	Clozapine	97	Schizophrenia spectrum disorder (ICD-10)	German Caucasian	12 weeks	One in the 5-HT$_{2C}$ gene (−759C/T)	Nonsignificant
Templeman et al. 2005	Risperidone (26) Olanzapine (19) Haloperidol (10) Quetiapine (11) Ziprasidone (6) Amisulpride (1)	73	First-episode psychosis	Spanish Caucasian	6 weeks, 3 months, 9 months	5-HT$_{2C}$ gene (−759C/T) and leptin (−2548A/G)	Less weight gain with −759T variant allele; significant association between −2548 leptin polymorphism and antipsychotic-induced weight gain at 9 months but not 6 weeks or 3 months
Miller et al. 2005	Clozapine	41	Treatment-refractory schizophrenia (DSM-IV)	Caucasian (35) African American (5) Hispanic (1)	6 months	One in the 5-HT$_{2C}$ gene (−759C/T)	Less weight gain with −759T variant allele; stronger trend in males

TABLE 6–3. Pharmacogenetic studies *(continued)*

Study	Treatment	Sample size (*N*)	Diagnosis	Ethnicity	Period of weight assessment	Polymorphisms	Results
Muller et al. 2005	Olanzapine (21) Risperidone (13) Haloperidol (13) Clozapine (12)	59	Chronic schizophrenia/ schizoaffective (DSM-IV)	African American (33) Caucasian (15) Hispanic (8) Asian Pacific (2) American Indian (1)	14 weeks	SNAP-25 gene (sites *Dde*I, *Mnl*I and *Taq*I)	*Mnl*I and *Taq*I associated with both clinical response (*P*=0.01 and *P*=0.03) and weight gain (*P*=0.01 and *P*=0.04) but not *Dde*I; significant association with more weight gain in the T/T genotype of *Mnl*I (cf. T/G or G/G) and C/C genotype of *Taq*I (cf. T/C or T/T)

Note. DRD4=dopamine D_4 receptor gene; 5-HT=serotonin; ICD-10=*International Classification of Diseases*, 10th Revision; SNAP-25=synaptosomal-associated protein of 25 kDa; TNF-α=tumor necrosis factor–α.

Source. Adapted from Muller DJ, Muglia P, Fortune T et al.: "Pharmacogenetics of Antipsychotic-Induced Weight Gain." *Pharmacological Research* 49:309–329, 2004. Copyright 2004, Elsevier Health Sciences. Used with permission.

Clozapine exhibits a pleiotropic receptor profile, including a high affinity for the D_4 receptor. Rietschel et al. (1996) did not find a significant association among four polymorphisms for the D_4 gene (*DRD4*) and clozapine-induced weight gain in a cohort ($N=149$) of schizophrenic and schizoaffective patients. Zhang et al. (2003) also did not find an association between antipsychotic-induced weight gain and the *Taq1* A polymorphism of the dopamine D_2 receptor gene (*DRD2*).

Polymorphisms for the histamine receptors have also been scrutinized. Hong et al. (2002) failed to find an association between clozapine-associated weight gain in schizophrenia patients and two polymorphisms for the histamine H_1 receptor. Basile et al. (2001) also reported a nonsignificant association between clozapine-associated weight gain and a single nucleotide polymorphism for the histamine H_1 receptor gene or the G-1018A polymorphism of the histamine H_2 receptor gene.

Reynolds et al. (2002) reported that Han Chinese patients with first-episode schizophrenia ($N=123$) were significantly less likely to exhibit AAWG if they had the −759C/T polymorphism in the promoter region of *5HT2C*. It was also reported in this population that the −759C/T polymorphism accounted for up to 18% (32% in males) of variance in weight gain attributable to clozapine use (Reynolds et al. 2003).

Templeman et al. (2005) reported on the associations between the *5HT2C* −759C/T and leptin −254A/G polymorphisms and AAWG in patients with first-episode psychosis. The prescribed antipsychotics were risperidone ($n=26$), olanzapine ($n=19$), haloperidol ($n=10$), quetiapine ($n=11$), ziprasidone ($n=6$), and amisulpride ($n=1$). Patients with the variant T/TC genotype gained significantly less weight after 6 weeks, 3 months, and 9 months of antipsychotic treatment. This association was reported in patient groups with a "very low" (<18) and "very high" (>28) initial BMI.

No significant association between the leptin genotype and baseline BMI or change in BMI at 6 weeks or 6 months was noted. After 9 months of treatment, patients with the GG genotype trended toward a greater BMI increase than those with AA or AG genotypes (GG=5.8; AG=3.6; AA=3.4). Subjects with the A allele (AA/AG) had a significant increase in BMI (AA/AG=3.58 vs. GG=5.81). These data extend previous findings indicating that the −759 genotype may offer long-term protection against AAWG. The −2548A/G leptin polymorphism was associated with long-term weight increases in patients while receiving antipsychotic medication.

Miller et al. (2005) reported that the −759T allele may be protective against AAWG. The −759T allele frequency was lower in subjects exhibiting an increase of 7% or more from their basal BMI. Subjects without a −759T allele were also at a significantly higher risk for AAWG and an increase in BMI relative to those without this polymorphism.

The synaptosomal-associated protein of 25 kDa (SNAP-25) is a presynaptic plasma protein involved in vesicle docking and fusion machinery mediating secretion of neurotransmitters. SNAP-25 is regionally distributed and is involved in cellular plasticity and synaptogenesis. Postmortem studies have reported lower SNAP-25 immunoreactivity in cortical and subcortical (hippocampus and cerebellum) brain regions. SNAP-25 may affect insulin release from pancreatic cells and may also be relevant to insulin receptor function (Ma et al. 2005). Muller et al. (2005) scrutinized polymorphisms of SNAP-25 gene (sites *Dde*I, *Mnl*I and *Tai*I) and their association with antipsychotic drug response and weight gain.

It was reported that the *Mnl*I and the *Tai*I polymorphisms, but not the *Dde*I polymorphism, were associated with clinical response and weight gain. The T/T genotype of the *Mnl*I polymorphism was significantly associated with greater weight gain than the T/G genotype or the G/G genotype. Similar results were reported for the *Tai*I polymorphism, where carriers of the C/C genotype gained significantly more weight than carriers of the T/C and T/T genotypes (Muller et al. 2005).

Studies scrutinizing associations between AAWG and polymorphisms have also tested for associations with drug-metabolizing proteins. For example, olanzapine is metabolized by several cytochrome (CYP) isoenzymes (Prior and Baker 2003). Ellingrod et al. (2002) reported a positive association between variants of the *CYP2D6* genotype and olanzapine-associated weight gain. These results cohere with other data suggesting that an increase in olanzapine plasma concentration may predispose to and portend weight gain (Perry et al. 2005).

Taken together, AAWG is likely subserved by several disparate neurobiological mechanisms. Appetite stimulation via interaction with central receptors at the level of the hypothalamus is likely a predominant mechanism. Disturbances in a variety of immune/inflammatory markers are putative mechanisms that have only been preliminarily articulated. A coherent and comprehensive model of AAWG mechanisms is not currently available. Persons with major depressive disorder, bipolar disorder, and schizophrenia comprise an at-risk group for obesity and associated metabolic disturbances (McIntyre and Konarski 2005). It is conjectured that mechanisms for AAWG may overlap with the neurobiological substrates of some psychiatric symptoms (McIntyre et al. 2001a).

Prevention and Treatment of Medication-Associated Weight Gain

GENERAL MANAGEMENT

The National Institutes of Health has called for the implementation of weight-loss strategies for all overweight persons with two or more risk factors for obesity-associated diseases (see Table 6–4 and Figure 6–2). The edifice of any successful weight

TABLE 6–4. Antipsychotic use and management of induced weight gain: initial assessment

History	Risk factors (age, sex)
	Previous antipsychotic use
	Previous weight gain with antipsychotics
	Current/past history of metabolic disorders (obesity, diabetes mellitus, dyslipidemia, gestational diabetes)
	Eating disorder (bulimia nervosa, binge eating)
	Activity and exercise pattern
	Diet (caloric intake, diet composition [carbohydrates, fat, protein])
	Smoking
	Family history of overweight
Physical examination	Weight
	Height
	Body mass index
	Waist-to-hip ratio
	Waist circumference
Laboratory results	Fasting blood sugar
	Fasting lipid profile

loss program is a healthy, balanced diet along with an increase in physical activity. Bariatric pharmacotherapy is recommended for adults who manifest a BMI of 27 or more plus obesity-related medical conditions or a BMI of 30 or more in the absence of any conditions (National Institutes of Health 1998).

Some patients are at risk of rapid weight gain with atypical antipsychotic administration. For example, up to 15% of patients receiving olanzapine are at risk of rapid weight gain (defined as $\geq$7% of their baseline weight within 6 weeks of therapy) (Kinon et al. 2005). These data suggest that weight gain treatment interventions should be offered prior to the initiation of antipsychotic therapy (i.e., primary prevention).

Weight gain associated with antipsychotic use, if not adequately addressed, would be predicted to have serious health consequences (Fontaine et al. 2001). Relatively modest reductions in weight are associated with clinically significant health benefits. Psychiatric populations are complex and require a careful individualization of the treatment plan. For example, unique to the psychiatric population are cognitive impairment, comorbidity (e.g., binge eating disorder, alcohol abuse), adverse health behaviors (e.g., smoking), disability, low socioeconomic status, sedentary lifestyle, consumption of high-liquid carbohydrate diet, and insufficient access to primary and preventative healthcare.

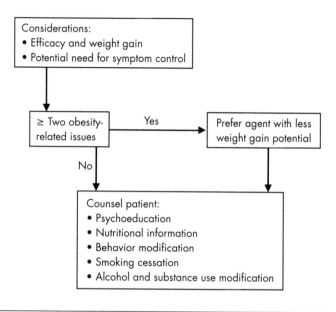

FIGURE 6–2. Choice of antipsychotic.

An intervention algorithm is presented in Figure 6–3.

The provision of basic education about weight management and healthy dietary choices is an inexpensive, effective, and paradigmatic intervention. It is inexorably true that most obese individuals do not routinely receive weight loss advice from their primary healthcare provider (Druss et al. 2001; Evans and Charney 2003). Patient dietary habits, eating behaviors, concomitant drug and alcohol use, and opportunistic screening for obesity-associated morbidity and family medical history are integral components of patient evaluation and monitoring (McIntyre et al. 2004).

Patients should be informed of the differences in caloric density among commonly consumed foods and beverages (Schulze et al. 2004) and counseled on smoking cessation and reasonable alcohol consumption. The physical and mental health benefits of weight loss need to be clearly presented along with practical resources for exercise that are accessible and affordable (Avenell et al. 2004; Fontaine et al. 2004; Keck et al. 2003b). Patient body weight, BMI, and waist-to-hip ratio should be measured and monitored on a routine basis.

Straker et al. (2005) evaluated the clinical utility and cost-effectiveness of screening for metabolic syndrome in a heterogeneous group of psychiatric patients receiving antipsychotic therapy. The overall prevalence of the metabolic syndrome was estimated at approximately 29%. Abdominal obesity and elevated fasting blood glucose (>110 mg/dL) identified 100% of the patients with the

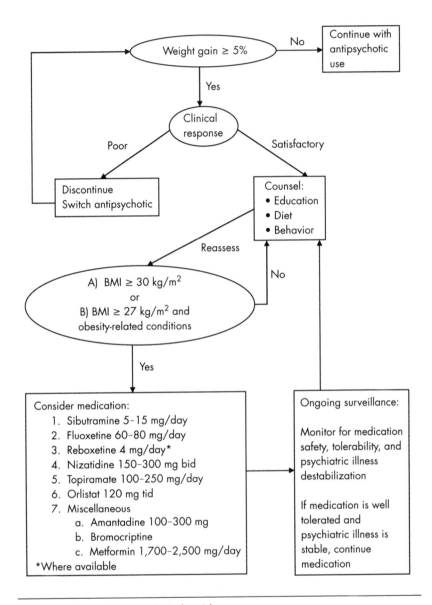

FIGURE 6–3.   Intervention algorithm.

metabolic syndrome. These data indicate that combining measurements of waist circumference and fasting blood glucose is a reasonable and cost-effective proxy of the metabolic syndrome in these patients.

Treatment of AAWG, much as in the management of weight gain in general, should emphasize primary prevention. Most studies reporting on the effectiveness of treatment interventions for AAWG have attempted to reverse weight gain already accrued (i.e., secondary prevention). Vreeland et al. (2003) examined the effectiveness of a multimodal weight management program in schizophrenic patients ($N=31$). All patients were receiving a second-generation antipsychotic for a minimum of 3 months and had a BMI of 26 or more, or they had experienced a weight gain of 2.3 kg or more within 2 months of initiating the index medication. The educational programs emphasized nutritional counseling, exercise, behavior interventions, and healthy weight management techniques.

At the completion of the study period, patients assigned to the intervention group lost significantly more weight (mean = 2.7 kg, or 2.7% of body weight), than patients assigned to the control group (mean gain = 2.9 kg, or 3.1% of body weight). The corresponding mean change in BMI was a drop from 34.32 to 33.34 (0.98 points, or 2.85%) in the intervention group and an increase from 33.4 to 34.6 (1.2 points, or 3.6%) in the control group (Vreeland et al. 2003).

Ball et al. (2001) combined an exercise regimen with the Weight Watchers program for schizophrenic patients ($N=21$) who gained significant weight after olanzapine treatment was initiated. This investigation failed to find a significant effect on BMI, with the exception of a small group of male patients. The negative findings of this study may reflect insufficient power and type II error.

Menza et al. (2004) evaluated the effect of a comprehensive, multimodal, 12-month weight management "healthy living" program in overweight patients with schizophrenia ($N=31$) receiving antipsychotic treatment. The intervention group exhibited a significant decrease in weight (i.e., −3.0 kg [6.6 lb]) and BMI (i.e., −1.74, or 5.1%). The intervention group also exhibited improvement in systolic and diastolic blood pressure, waist-to-hip ratio, exercise participation, and hemoglobin A_{1c} levels.

In summary, preliminary studies evaluating behavioral interventions as a strategy to manage AAWG appear effective and acceptable to patients. A consistent feature of these programs is their comprehensiveness, self-management, education focus, and longitudinal administration. Mental healthcare providers in many regions may find that the comprehensiveness of these programs is not feasible. Cost-effectiveness studies and partnerships with obesity clinics (and their resources) is warranted.

PHARMACOLOGICAL STRATEGIES

As previously mentioned, bariatric pharmacotherapy for obesity is recommended for use in adults who have a BMI of 27 or more plus obesity-related medical conditions or a BMI of 30 or more in the absence of such conditions ((National Institutes of Health 1998; Yanovski and Yanovski 2002). There is no pharmacological treatment for AAWG that has been proved to be reliably efficacious and safe. Nevertheless, several medication approaches are under active investigation (Khan et al. 1987; Raison and Klein 1997).

Appetite-Suppressant Medications

Several small studies have reported on the safety and efficacy of conventional appetite suppressants in schizophrenic populations (e.g., *d*-fenfluramine, fenfluramine, bromocriptine, and phenylpropanolamine). The efficacy results of these agents have largely been underwhelming, and importantly, their use is associated with many hazards (e.g., exacerbation of psychoses) (Baptista 1999).

Sibutramine hydrochloride is a bariatric treatment that engages both serotonin and norepinephrine and is effective for obesity and binge eating disorder (James et al. 2000; Wirth and Krause 2001). Henderson et al. (2005) conducted a 12-week, double-blind, placebo-controlled trial with adjunctive sibutramine (10–15 mg) in olanzapine-treated schizophrenic and schizoaffective patients ($N=37$). All patients previously stabilized with olanzapine reported a history of weight gain and had a BMI greater than 30 kg/m^2 or a BMI of 27 kg/m^2 plus another cardiovascular risk factor. In addition, all patients were offered group support and behavioral interventions. At the completion of the study, the sibutramine-treated patients exhibited a significant reduction in weight relative to the placebo group (8.3 lb vs. 1.8 lb). A small increase in systolic blood pressure was reported along with common sibutramine-associated adverse events (e.g., dry mouth, constipation, blurred vision). Caution is warranted when prescribing sibutramine because of reports of hypomanic induction and toxic interactions with serotonergic antidepressants (Benazzi 2002; Giese and Neborsky 2001).

Topiramate has been proved to favorably influence abnormal and chaotic eating behavior, weight, and associated psychopathology in patients with bulimia nervosa, binge eating disorder, and obesity (Bray et al. 2003; Hedges et al. 2003; Hoopes et al. 2003; McElroy et al. 2003). McElroy et al. (2003) reported a net loss of 6 kg and a mean decrease in BMI of 6% from baseline in bipolar patients ($N=37$) receiving adjunctive topiramate (mean dose=420 mg) for up to 1 year. Nickel et al. (2005) compared the efficacy of topiramate (250 mg/day) in a 10-week, randomized, double-blind, placebo-controlled study in women ($N=43$) who had gained weight with olanzapine. The topiramate-treated patients exhibited significant weight loss (5.6 kg). Topiramate has few pharmacokinetic drug interactions but is associated with cognitive slowing, which may further burden patients experiencing sedation or somnolence with antipsychotics.

Amantadine is indicated for the prevention and treatment of influenza and improves symptoms of Parkinson's disease, likely through enhancing dopamine neurotransmission. Several open studies have reported positive results with the use of amantadine for AAWG (Floris et al. 2001). Amantadine also has few pharmacokinetic interactions; however, it may increase propensity for anticholinergic adverse events in patients concomitantly receiving some antipsychotics (e.g., clozapine, chlorpromazine).

Conflicting results describing the efficacy of the histamine antagonist nizatidine have been reported. Cavazzoni et al. (2003) evaluated nizatidine as an antidote for olanzapine-associated weight gain in patients with schizophrenia ($N=175$). Eligible patients were randomly assigned to receive olanzapine (5–20 mg/day) in combination with nizatidine (150 mg bid, 300 mg bid, or placebo) for 16 weeks. The nizatidine groups did not differ significantly compared with the placebo group, although the higher-dosage nizatidine group had numerically less weight gain. In other studies, nizatidine (150 mg bid) was demonstrated to be superior to placebo for olanzapine-associated weight gain but not beneficial for quetiapine-associated weight gain (Atmaca et al. 2003).

The efficacy of the insulin-sensitizing agent metformin (500 mg tid) for AAWG (olanzapine, risperidone, and quetiapine) or valproic-associated weight gain was evaluated in a small, 12-week investigation of a pediatric sample. Patients ($N=19$; mean age = 14.1 ± 2.5 years) exhibiting 10% or more weight gain with index therapy were eligible. Metformin was associated with a significant reduction in BMI (2.22 kg/m^2) and weight (2.93 kg) (Baptista et al. 2001).

Fluoxetine (20–60 mg/day) treatment for AAWG has been examined in two randomized, double-blind, placebo-controlled trials, both of which failed to demonstrate the superiority of fluoxetine to placebo (Bustillo et al. 2003; Poyurovsky et al. 2002).

Reboxetine is a selective norepinephrine reuptake inhibitor approved for the symptomatic treatment of depression in several European countries. Poyurovsky et al. (2003) evaluated the efficacy of reboxetine (4 mg/day) in patients ($N=26$) hospitalized with schizophrenia. All patients experiencing a first episode of the illness were assigned to either reboxetine ($n=13$) or placebo ($n=13$) as an adjunctive treatment to olanzapine (10 mg/day). Patients in both groups gained weight at the end of the study, with completers in the olanzapine/reboxetine group gaining significantly less weight (2.5 kg ± 2.7) than the olanzapine/placebo group (5.5 ± 3.1 kg). Smaller changes in BMI were also noted in the combination group (0.86 ± 0.88 kg/m^2) compared with the olanzapine monotherapy group (1.84 ± 0.99 kg/m^2).

Nutrient Absorption Reducers

Orlistat is currently approved by the U.S. Food and Drug Administration as a weight-loss agent. Orlistat is an ex vivo agent with minimal systemic absorption and central nervous system effects (Heck et al. 2000). There are no currently available randomized, controlled trials evaluating the efficacy of orlistat for AAWG. The results of small open studies have suggested that orlistat may be an antidote for psychotropic medication–associated weight gain (Hilger et al. 2002).

Conclusion

To recapitulate, AAWG is a serious adverse event associated with many of the first- and second-generation antipsychotics. Antipsychotic-associated weight gain mostly reflects an increase in adiposity and thus may presage obesity-related morbidity. Young age is the best established correlate of weight gain, implying that pediatric patients receiving antipsychotics are most at risk. A variety of mechanisms likely subserve AAWG, with an increase in appetite via engagement of central neurotransmitters occupying a pivotal role.

Treatment options for AAWG emphasize prevention, education, diet, and behavior modification. Several medications are effective for AAWG; the most rigorous data support the use of topiramate and sibutramine. Taken together, however, the efficacy and safety of bariatric treatments are not well established for AAWG. Clinical research will need to determine which multicomponent treatment strategy is most cost-effective, pragmatic, effective, and safe for AAWG.

KEY CLINICAL CONCEPTS

- Clinically significant AAWG is defined by the U.S. Food and Drug Administration as 7% or more of baseline weight.

- As a class, second-generation antipsychotics, versus first-generation antipsychotics, are associated with more weight gain. Relative to placebo, aripiprazole, ziprasidone, and risperidone are associated with approximately 2 times ($\geq 7\%$ from baseline), quetiapine 4 times, and olanzapine 10 times the placebo incidence of categorically significant weight gain.

- AAWG correlates may include younger age, nonwhite ethnicity, appetite increase, normal or underweight status at pretreatment, and positive clinical response.

- Appetite stimulation with increased food intake via interactions with central receptors at the level of the hypothalamus is likely the predominant mechanism of AAWG. This correlation to date is most predicted by H_1 affinity, followed by α_{1A}, 5-HT_{2C}, and 5-HT_6 receptor affinity.

- Other mechanisms involved with AAWG may include increased food intake via dysregulation of neuropeptides (i.e., leptin), cytokines, and UCPs that have roles in appetite, satiety, food preferences, and energy expenditure.

- Polymorphisms that encode for proteins important in the regulation of weight or the metabolism of medication may be responsible for the differential weight effects of atypical antipsychotics.

- Treatment of AAWG should begin with primary prevention, although specific primary prevention strategies or programs have yet to be defined by the literature.

- Behavioral interventions with assessment of weight gain–associated medical conditions are first-line treatment for individuals with AAWG. Some patients may benefit from bariatric pharmacotherapy.

References

Allison DB, Mentore JL, Heo M, et al: Antipsychotic-induced weight gain: a comprehensive research synthesis. Am J Psychiatry 156:1686–1696, 1999

Amery W, Zuiderwijk P, Lemmens P: Safety profile of risperidone. Presented at the 10th European College of Neuropsychopharmacology Congress, Vienna, September 1997

Argiles JM, Lopez-Soriano J, Busquets S, et al: Journey from cachexia to obesity by TNF. FASEB J 11:743–751, 1997

Ariyasu H, Takaya K, Hosoda H, et al: Delayed short-term secretory regulation of ghrelin in obese animals: evidenced by a specific RIA for the active form of ghrelin. Endocrinology 143:3341–3350, 2002

Atmaca M, Kuloglu M, Tezcan E, et al: Nizatidine treatment and its relationship with leptin levels in patients with olanzapine-induced weight gain. Hum Psychopharmacol 18:457–461, 2003

Auwerx J, Staels B: Leptin. Lancet 351:737–742, 1998

Avenell A, Broom J, Brown TJ, et al: Systematic review of the long-term effects and economic consequences of treatments for obesity and implications for health improvement. Health Technol Assess 8:182, 2004

Ball MP, Coons VB, Buchanan RW: A program for treating olanzapine-related weight gain. Psychiatr Serv 52:967–969, 2001

Baptista T: Body weight gain induced by antipsychotic drugs: mechanisms and management. Acta Psychiatr Scand 100:3–16, 1999

Baptista T, Molina MG, Martinez JL, et al: Effects of the antipsychotic drug sulpiride on reproductive hormones in healthy premenopausal women: relationship with body weight regulation. Pharmacopsychiatry 30:256–262, 1997

Baptista T, Lacruz A, de Mendoza S, et al: Body weight gain after administration of antipsychotic drugs: correlation with leptin, insulin and reproductive hormones. Pharmacopsychiatry 33:81–88, 2000

Baptista T, Hernandez L, Prieto LA, et al: Metformin in obesity associated with antipsychotic drug administration: a pilot study. J Clin Psychiatry 62:653–655, 2001

Baptista T, Zarate J, Joober R, et al: Drug induced weight gain, an impediment to successful pharmacotherapy: focus on antipsychotics. Curr Drug Targets 5:279–299, 2004

Basile VS, Masellis M, McIntyre RS, et al: Genetic dissection of atypical antipsychotic induced weight gain: novel preliminary data on the pharmacogenetic puzzle. J Clin Psychiatry 62(suppl):45–66, 2001

Basile VS, Masellis M, De Luca V, et al: 759C/T genetic variation of 5-HT$_{2C}$ receptor and clozapine-induced weight gain. Lancet 360(9347):1790–1791, 2002

Basson BR, Kinon BJ, Taylor CC, et al: Factors influencing acute weight change in patients with schizophrenia treated with olanzapine, haloperidol, or risperidone. J Clin Psychiatry 62:231–238, 2001

Beasley CM Jr, Tollefson GD, Tran PV: Safety of olanzapine. J Clin Psychiatry 58(suppl): 13–17, 1997

Benazzi F: Organic hypomania secondary to sibutramine-citalopram interaction. J Clin Psychiatry 63:165, 2002

Berraondo B, Marti A, Duncan JS, et al: Up-regulation of muscle UCP2 gene expression by a new beta3-adrenoceptor agonist, trecadrine, in obese (cafeteria) rodents, but down-regulation in lean animals. Int J Obes Relat Metab Disord 24:156–163, 2000

Borison RL, Arvanitis LA, Miller BG: ICI 204,636, an atypical antipsychotic: efficacy and safety in a multicenter, placebo-controlled trial in patients with schizophrenia. U.S. SEROQUEL Study Group. J Clin Psychopharmacol 16:158–169, 1996

Brady KT: Weight gain associated with psychotropic drugs. South Med J 82:611–617, 1989

Bray GA, Hollander P, Klein S, et al: A 6-month randomized, placebo-controlled, dose-ranging trial of topiramate for weight loss in obesity. Obes Res 11:722–733, 2003

Bromel T, Blum WF, Ziegler A, et al: Serum leptin levels increase rapidly after initiation of clozapine therapy. Mol Psychiatry 3:76–80, 1998

Buckland PR, Hoogendoorn B, Guy CA, et al: Low gene expression conferred by association of an allele of the 5-HT2C receptor gene with antipsychotic-induced weight gain. Am J Psychiatry 162:613–615, 2005

Bustillo JR, Lauriello J, Parker K, et al: Treatment of weight gain with fluoxetine in olanzapine-treated schizophrenic outpatients. Neuropsychopharmacology 28:527–529, 2003

Casey DE, Haupt DW, Newcomer JW, et al: Antipsychotic-induced weight gain and metabolic abnormalities: implications for increased mortality in patients with schizophrenia. J Clin Psychiatry 65(suppl):4–18, 2004

Cavazzoni P, Tanaka Y, Roychowdhury SM, et al: Nizatidine for prevention of weight gain with olanzapine: a double-blind placebo-controlled trial. Eur Neuropsychopharmacol 13:81–85, 2003

Csernansky J, Okamato A, Brecher M: Risperidone versus haloperidol for prevention of relapse in schizophrenia and schizoaffective disorders. Biol Psychiatry 45(suppl):1–7, 1999

Czobor P, Volavka J, Sheitman B, et al: Antipsychotic-induced weight gain and therapeutic response: a differential association. J Clin Psychopharmacol 22:244–251, 2002

Dandona P, Weinstock R, Thusu K, et al: Tumor necrosis factor-alpha in sera of obese patients: fall with weight loss. J Clin Endocrinol Metab 83:2907–2910, 1998

De Vry J, Schreiber R: Effects of selected serotonin 5-HT(1) and 5-HT(2) receptor agonists on feeding behavior: possible mechanisms of action. Neurosci Biobehav Rev 24:341–353, 2000

Dobmeier M, Haen E, Mueller J: Therapeutic drug monitoring of olanzapine. Presented at the 153rd Annual Meeting of the American Psychiatric Association, Chicago, IL, 2000

Druss BG, Bradford WD, Rosenheck RA, et al: Quality of medical care and excess mortality in older patients with mental disorders. Arch Gen Psychiatry 58:565–572, 2001

Eder U, Mangweth B, Ebenbichler C, et al: Association of olanzapine-induced weight gain with an increase in body fat. Am J Psychiatry 158:1719–1722, 2001

Ellingrod VL, Miller D, Schultz SK, et al: CYP2D6 polymorphisms and atypical antipsychotic weight gain. Psychiatr Genet 12:55–58, 2002

Evans DL, Charney DS: Mood disorders and medical illness: a major public health problem. Biol Psychiatry 54:177–180, 2003

Fadel J, Bubser M, Deutch AY: Differential activation of orexin neurons by antipsychotic drugs associated with weight gain. J Neurosci 22:6742–6746, 2002

Flint DJ, Binart N, Kopchick J, et al: Effects of growth hormone and prolactin on adipose tissue development and function. Pituitary 6:97–102, 2003

Floris M, Lejeune J, Deberdt W: Effect of amantadine on weight gain during olanzapine treatment. Eur Neuropsychopharmacol 11:181–182, 2001

Fontaine KR, Heo M, Harrigan EP, et al: Estimating the consequences of antipsychotic-induced weight gain on health and mortality rate. Psychiatry Res 101:277–288, 2001

Fontaine KR, Barofsky I, Bartlett SJ, et al: Weight loss and health-related quality of life: results at 1-year follow-up. Eat Behav 5:85–88, 2004

Gale SM, Castracane VD, Mantzoros CS: Energy homeostasis, obesity and eating disorders: recent advances in endocrinology. J Nutr 134:295–298, 2004

Ganguli R: Weight gain associated with antipsychotic drugs. J Clin Psychiatry 60(suppl): 20–24, 1999

Gaulin BD, Markowitz JS, Caley CF, et al: Clozapine-associated elevation in serum triglycerides. Am J Psychiatry 156:1270–1272, 1999

Giese SY, Neborsky R: Serotonin syndrome: potential consequences of Meridia combined with demerol or fentanyl. Plast Reconstr Surg 107:293–294, 2001

Goodall E, Oxtoby C, Richards R, et al: A clinical trial of the efficacy and acceptability of D-fenfluramine in the treatment of neuroleptic-induced obesity. Br J Psychiatry 153: 208–213, 1988

Gopalaswamy AK, Morgan R: Too many chronic mentally disabled patients are too fat. Acta Psychiatr Scand 72:254–258, 1985

Gordon A, Price LH: Mood stabilization and weight loss with topiramate. Am J Psychiatry 156:968–969, 1999

Gothelf D, Falk B, Singer P, et al: Weight gain associated with increased food intake and low habitual activity levels in male adolescent schizophrenic inpatients treated with olanzapine. Am J Psychiatry 159:1055–1057, 2002

Graham KA, Perkins DO, Edwards LJ, et al: Effect of olanzapine on body composition and energy expenditure in adults with first-episode psychosis. Am J Psychiatry 162:118–123, 2005

Gupta S, Droney T, Al Samarrai S, et al: Olanzapine: weight gain and therapeutic efficacy. J Clin Psychopharmacol 19:273–275, 1999

Haack M, Hinze-Selch D, Fenzel T, et al: Plasma levels of cytokines and soluble cytokine receptors in psychiatric patients upon hospital admission: effects of confounding factors and diagnosis. J Psychiatr Res 33:407–418, 1999

Hagg S, Soderberg S, Ahren B, et al: Leptin concentrations are increased in subjects treated with clozapine or conventional antipsychotics. J Clin Psychiatry 62:843–848, 2001

Hartfield AW, Moore NA, Clifton PG: Effects of clozapine, olanzapine and haloperidol on the microstructure of ingestive behaviour in the rat. Psychopharmacol (Berl) 167:115–122, 2003

Harvey BH, Bouwer CD: Neuropharmacology of paradoxic weight gain with selective serotonin reuptake inhibitors. Clin Neuropharmacol 23:90–97, 2000

Hauner H, Bender M, Haastert B, et al: Plasma concentrations of soluble TNF-alpha receptors in obese subjects. Int J Obes Relat Metab Disord 22:1239–1243, 1998

Haupt DW, Luber A, Maeda J, et al: Plasma leptin and adiposity during antipsychotic treatment of schizophrenia. Neuropsychopharmacology 30:184–191, 2005

Hebebrand J, Sommerlad C, Geller F, et al: The genetics of obesity: practical implications. Int J Obes Relat Metab Disord 25(suppl):10–18, 2001

Heck AM, Yanovski JA, Calis KA: Orlistat, a new lipase inhibitor for the management of obesity. Pharmacotherapy 20:270–279, 2000

Hedges DW, Reimherr FW, Hoopes SP, et al: Treatment of bulimia nervosa with topiramate in a randomized, double-blind, placebo-controlled trial, part 2: improvement in psychiatric measures. J Clin Psychiatry 64:1449–1454, 2003

Heilbronn L, Smith SR, Ravussin E: Failure of fat cell proliferation, mitochondrial function and fat oxidation results in ectopic fat storage, insulin resistance and type II diabetes mellitus. Int J Obes Relat Metab Disord 28(suppl):12–21, 2004

Henderson DC, Copeland PM, Daley TB, et al: A double-blind, placebo-controlled trial of sibutramine for olanzapine-associated weight gain. Am J Psychiatry 162:954–962, 2005

Hesselink MK, Mensink M, Schrauwen P: Human uncoupling protein-3 and obesity: an update. Obes Res 11:1429–1443, 2003

Hilger E, Quiner S, Ginzel I, et al: The effect of orlistat on plasma levels of psychotropic drugs in patients with long-term psychopharmacotherapy. J Clin Psychopharmacol 22:68–70, 2002

Hinze-Selch D, Schuld A, Kraus T, et al: Effects of antidepressants on weight and on the plasma levels of leptin, TNF-alpha and soluble TNF receptors: a longitudinal study in patients treated with amitriptyline or paroxetine. Neuropsychopharmacology 23:13–19, 2000

Hong CJ, Lin CH, Yu YW, et al: Genetic variants of the serotonin system and weight change during clozpine treatment. Pharmacogenetics 11:265–268, 2001

Hong CJ, Lin CH, Yu YW, et al: Genetic variant of the histamine-1 receptor (Glu349asp) and body weight change during clozapine treatment. Psychiatr Genet 12:169–171, 2002

Hoopes SP, Reimherr FW, Hedges DW, et al: Treatment of bulimia nervosa with topiramate in a randomized, double-blind, placebo-controlled trial, part 1: improvement in binge and purge measures. J Clin Psychiatry 64:1335–1341, 2003

Jalenques I, Tauveron I, Albuisson E, et al: Weight gain and clozapine. Encephale 22:77–79, 1996

James WP, Astrup A, Finer N, et al: Effect of sibutramine on weight maintenance after weight loss: a randomised trial. STORM Study Group. Sibutramine Trial of Obesity Reduction and Maintenance. Lancet 356:2119–2125, 2000

Johnson DAW, Breen M: Weight changes with depot neuroleptic maintenance therapy. Acta Psychiatr Scand 59:525–528, 1979

Keck PE, Buse JB, Dagogo-Jack S, et al: Managing metabolic concerns in patients with severe mental illness. Postgraduate Medicine Special Report. Minneapolis, MN, McGraw-Hill, 2003a

Keck PE Jr, Buse JB, Dagogo-Jack S, et al: Metabolic disease and severe mental illness, in Managing Metabolic Concerns in Patients With Severe Mental Illness. Minneapolis, MN, Postgraduate Medicine, McGraw-Hill, 2003b

Kelly DL, Conley RR, Love RC, et al: Weight gain in adolescents treated with risperidone and conventional antipsychotics over six months. J Child Adolesc Psychopharmacol 18:151–159, 1998

Ketter TA, Post RM, Theodore WH: Positive and negative psychiatric effects of antiepileptic drugs in patients with seizure disorders. Neurology 53:53–67, 1999

Khan SA, Spiegel DA, Jobe PC: Psychotomimetic effects of anorectic drugs. Am Fam Physician 36:107–112, 1987

Kinon BJ, Basson B, Szynanski KA, et al: Factors associated with weight gain during olanzapine treatment. Poster Session No. 10, presented at the 38th Annual Meeting for New Clinical Drug Evaluation Unit Program, Boca Raton, FL, June 1998

Kinon BJ, Kaiser CJ, Ahmed S, et al: Association between early and rapid weight gain and change in weight over one year of olanzapine therapy in patients with schizophrenia and related disorders. J Clin Psychopharmacol 25:255–258, 2005

Kraus T, Haack M, Schuld A, et al: Body weight, the tumor necrosis factor system, and leptin production during treatment with mirtazapine or venlafaxine. Pharmacopsychiatry 35:220–225, 2002

Kroeze WK, Hufeisen SJ, Popadak BA, et al: H1-histamine receptor affinity predicts short-term weight gain for typical and atypical antipsychotic drugs. Neuropsychopharmacology 28:519–526, 2003

Kryspin-Exner W: Beitrage zum verlauf des korpergewichtes bei psychosen. Wien Klin Wochenschr 1947:68–72, 1996

Lamberti JS, Bellnier T, Schwarzkopf SB: Weight gain among schizophrenic patients treated with clozapine. Am J Psychiatry 149:689–690, 1992

Lane HY, Chang YC, Cheng YC, et al: Effects of patient demographics, risperidone dosage, and clinical outcome on body weight in acutely exacerbated schizophrenia. J Clin Psychiatry 64:316–320, 2003

Leadbetter R, Shutty M, Pavalonis D, et al: Clozapine-induced weight gain: prevalence and clinical relevance. Am J Psychiatry 149:68–72, 1992

Ma Z, Portwood N, Foss A, et al: Evidence that insulin secretion influences SNAP-25 through proteasomal activation. Biochem Biophys Res Common 329:1118–1126, 2005

Masaki T, Yoshimatsu H, Chiba S, et al: Central infusion of histamine reduces fat accumulation and upregulates UCP family in leptin-resistant obese mice. Diabetes 50:376–384, 2001

McElroy SL, Arnold LM, Shapira NA, et al: Topiramate in the treatment of binge eating disorder associated with obesity: a randomized, placebo-controlled trial. Am J Psychiatry 160:255–261, 2003

McIntyre RS, Konarski JZ: Tolerability profiles of atypical antipsychotics in the treatment of bipolar disorder. J Clin Psychiatry 66(suppl):28–36, 2005

McIntyre RS, Mancini DA, Basile VS: Mechanisms of antipsychotic-induced weight gain. J Clin Psychiatry 62(suppl):23–29, 2001a

McIntyre RS, McCann SM, Kennedy SH: Antipsychotic metabolic effects: weight gain, diabetes mellitus, and lipid abnormalities. Can J Psychiatry 46:273–281, 2001b

McIntyre RS, Mancini DA, Basile VS, et al: Antipsychotic-induced weight gain: bipolar disorder and leptin. J Clin Psychopharmacol 23:323–327, 2003

McIntyre RS, Konarski JZ, Yatham LN: Comorbidity in bipolar disorder: a framework for rational treatment selection. Hum Psychopharmacol 19:369–386, 2004

Meguid MM, Fetissov SO, Varma M, et al: Hypothalamic dopamine and serotonin in the regulation of food intake. Nutrition 16:843–857, 2000

Melkersson KI, Hulting AL: Insulin and leptin levels in patients with schizophrenia or related psychoses: a comparison between different antipsychotic agents. Psychopharmacol (Berl) 154:205–212, 2001

Menza M, Vreeland B, Minsky S, et al: Managing atypical antipsychotic-associated weight gain: 12-month data on a multimodal weight control program. J Clin Psychiatry 65:471–477, 2004

Miller DD, Ellingrod VL, Holman TL, et al: Clozapine-induced weight gain associated with the $5HT_{2C}$ receptor −759C/T polymorphism. Am J Med Genet B Neuropsychiatr Genet 133:97–100, 2005

Muller DJ, Muglia P, Fortune T et al: Pharmacogenetics of antipsychotic-induced weight gain. Pharmacol Res 49:309–329, 2004

Muller DJ, Klempan TA, De Luca V, et al: The SNAP-25 gene may be associated with clinical response and weight gain in antipsychotic treatment of schizophrenia. Neurosci Lett 379:81–89, 2005

Murashita M, Kusumi I, Inoue T, et al: Olanzapine increases plasma ghrelin level in patients with schizophrenia. Psychoneuroendocrinology 30:106–110, 2005

Musselman DL, Betan E, Larsen H, et al: Relationship of depression to diabetes types 1 and 2: epidemiology, biology, and treatment. Biol Psychiatry 54:317–329, 2003

Nagase I, Yoshida T, Saito M: Up-regulation of uncoupling proteins by beta-adrenergic stimulation in L6 myotubes. FEBS Lett 494:175–180, 2001

Nakamura T, Uramura K, Nambu T, et al: Orexin-induced hyperlocomotion and stereotypy are mediated by the dopaminergic system. Brain Res 873:181–187, 2000

National Institutes of Health: Clinical guidelines on the identification, evaluation, treatment of overweight and obesity in adults: the evidence report. Obes Res 6:51S–209S, 1998

Nemeroff CB: Dosing the antipsychotic medication olanzapine. J Clin Psychiatry 58(suppl):45–49, 1997

Nickel MK, Nickel C, Muehlbacher M, et al: Influence of topiramate on olanzapine-related adiposity in women: a random, double-blind, placebo-controlled study. J Clin Psychopharmacol 25:211–217, 2005

Niswender CM, Sanders-Bush E, Emeson RB: Identification and characterization of RNA editing events within the 5-HT2C receptor. Ann N Y Acad Sci 861:38–48, 1998

Old LJ: Tumor necrosis factor (TNF). Science 230:630–632, 1985

Parada MA, Hernandez L, Paez X, et al: Mechanism of the body weight increase induced by systematic sulpiride. Pharmacol Biochem Behav 33:45–50, 1989

Parada MA, Puig DP, Hernandez L, et al: Ventromedial hypothalamus vs. lateral hypothalamic D2 satiety receptors in the body weight increase induced by systematic sulpiride. Physiol Behav 50:1161–1165, 1991

Perry PJ, Argo TR, Carnahan RM, et al: The association of weight gain and olanzapine plasma concentrations. J Clin Psychopharmacol 25:250–254, 2005

Peuskens J, Link CG: A comparison of quetiapine and chlorpromazine in the treatment of schizophrenia. Acta Psychiatr Scand 96:265–273, 1997

Picard F, Deshaies Y, Lalonde J, et al: Topiramate reduces energy and fat gains in lean (Fa/?) and obese (fa/fa) zucker rats. Obes Res 8:656–663, 2000

Planansky K, Heilizer F: Weight changes in relation to the characteristics of patients on chlorpromazine. J Clin Exp Psychopathol 20:53–57, 1959

Pooley EC, Fairburn CG, Cooper Z, et al: A 5-HT$_{2C}$ receptor promoter polymorphism Am J Med Genet 126B:124–127, 2004

Poyurovsky M, Pashinian A, Gil-Ad I, et al: Olanzapine-induced weight gain in patients with first-episode schizophrenia: a double-blind, placebo-controlled study of fluoxetine addition. Am J Psychiatry 159:1058–1060, 2002

Poyurovsky M, Isaacs I, Fuchs C, et al: Attenuation of olanzapine-induced weight gain with reboxetine in patients with schizophrenia: a double-blind, placebo-controlled study. Am J Psychiatry 160:297–302, 2003

Prior TI, Baker GB: Interactions between the cytochrome P450 system and the second-generation antipsychotics. J Psychiatry Neurosci 28:99–112, 2003

Raison CL, Klein HM: Psychotic mania associated with fenfluramine and phentermine use. Am J Psychiatry 154:711, 1997

Reynolds GP, Zhang ZJ, Zhang XB: Association of antipsychotic drug-induced weight gain with a 5-HT$_{2C}$ receptor gene polymorphism. Lancet 359:2086–2087, 2002

Reynolds GP, Zhang Z, Zhang X: Polymorphism of the promoter region of the serotonin 5-HT(2C) receptor gene and clozapine-induced weight gain. Am J Psychiatry 160:677–679, 2003

Rietschel M, Naber D, Oberlander H, et al: Efficacy and side-effects of clozapine: testing for association with allelic variation in the dopamine D4 receptor gene. Neuropsychopharmacology 15:491–496, 1996

Rietschel M, Naber D, Fimmers R, et al: Efficacy and side-effects of clozapine not associated with variation in the 5-HT$_{2C}$ receptor. Neuroreport 8(8):1999–2003, 1997

Ryan MC, Flanagan S, Kinsella U, et al: The effects of atypical antipsychotics on visceral fat distribution in first episode, drug-naïve patients with schizophrenia. Life Sci 74:1999–2008, 2004

Sakurai T, Amemiya A, Ishii M, et al: Orexins and orexin receptors: a family of hypothalamic neuropeptides and G protein-coupled receptors that regulate feeding behavior. Cell 92:573–585, 1998

Schulze MB, Manson JE, Ludwig DS, et al: Sugar-sweetened beverages, weight gain, and incidence of type 2 diabetes in young and middle-aged women. JAMA 292:927–934, 2004

Shintani M, Ogawa Y, Ebihara K, et al: Ghrelin, an endogenous growth hormone secretagogue, is a novel orexigenic peptide that antagonizes leptin action through the activation of hypothalamic neuropeptide Y/Y1 receptor pathway. Diabetes 50:227–232, 2001

Speakman JR, Selman C: Physical activity and resting metabolic rate. Proc Nutr Soc 62:621–634, 2003

Stanley BG, Butterfield BS, Grewal RS: NMDA receptor coagonist glycine site: evidence for a role in lateral hypothalamic stimulation of feeding. Am J Physiol 273:790–796, 1997

Straker D, Correll CU, Kramer-Ginsberg E, et al: Cost-effective screening for the metabolic syndrome in patients treated with second-generation antipsychotic medications. Am J Psychiatry 162:1217–1221, 2005

Stumvoll M, Goldstein BJ, van Haeften TW: Type 2 diabetes: principles of pathogenesis and therapy. Lancet 365:1333–1346, 2005

Tai TA, Jennermann C, Brown KK, et al: Activation of the nuclear receptor peroxisome proliferator-activated receptor gamma promotes brown adipocyte differentiation. J Biol Chem 271:29909–29914, 1996

Tappy L, Binnert C, Schneiter P: Energy expenditure, physical activity and body-weight control. Proc Nutr Soc 62:663–666, 2003

Tecott LH, Sun LM, Akana SF, et al: Eating disorder and epilepsy in mice lacking 5-HT2c serotonin receptors. Nature 374:542–546, 1995

Templeman LA, Reynolds GP, Arranz B, et al: Polymorphisms of the 5-HT$_{2C}$ receptor and leptin genes are associated with antipsychotic drug-induced weight gain in Caucasian subjects with a first-episode psychosis. Pharmacogenet Genomics 15:195–200, 2005

Theisen FM, Linden A, Konig IR, et al: Spectrum of binge eating symptomatology in patients treated with clozapine and olanzapine. J Neural Transm 110:111–121, 2003

Tsai SJ, Hong CJ, Yu YW, et al: −759C/T genetic variation of 5-HT$_{2C}$ receptor and clozapine-induced weight gain. Lancet 360(9347):1790, 2002

Theisen FM, Hinney A, Bromel T, et al: Lack of association between the −759C/T polymorphism of the 5-HT$_{2C}$ receptor gene and clozapine-induced weight gain among German schizophrenic individuals. Psychiatr Genet 14(3):139–142, 2004

Umbricht DS, Pollack S, Kane JM: Clozapine and weight gain. J Clin Psychiatry 55(suppl):157–160, 1994

Uramura K, Funahashi H, Muroya S, et al: Orexin-a activates phospholipase C- and protein kinase C-mediated Ca^{2+} signaling in dopamine neurons of the ventral tegmental area. Neuroreport 12:1885–1889, 2001

Uysal KT, Wiesbrock SM, Marino MW, et al: Protection from obesity-induced insulin resistance in mice lacking TNF-alpha function. Nature 389:610–614, 1997

Vickers SP, Benwell KR, Porter RH, et al: Comparative effects of continuous infusion of MCPP, Ro 60–0175 and d-fenfluramine on food intake, water intake, body weight and locomotor activity in rats. Br J Pharmacol 130:1305–1314, 2000

Vreeland B, Minsky S, Menza M, et al: A program for managing weight gain associated with atypical antipsychotics. Psychiatr Serv 54:1155–1157, 2003

Wang GJ, Volkow ND, Logan J, et al: Brain dopamine and obesity. Lancet 357:354–357, 2001

Wang KY, Arima N, Higuchi S, et al: Switch of histamine receptor expression from H2 to H1 during differentiation of monocytes into macrophages. FEBS Lett 473:345–348, 2000

Wetterling T, Mussigbrodt HE: Weight gain: side effect of atypical neuroleptics? J Clin Psychopharmacol 19:316–321, 1999

Wirshing DA, Wirshing WC, Kysar L, et al: Novel antipsychotics: comparison of weight gain liabilities. J Clin Psychiatry 60:358–363, 1999

Wirth A, Krause J: Long-term weight loss with sibutramine: a randomized controlled trial. JAMA 286:1331–1339, 2001

Wirtshafter D: The control of ingestive behavior by the median raphe nucleus. Appetite 36:99–105, 2001

Yamada M, Miyakawa T, Duttaroy A, et al: Mice lacking the M3 muscarinic acetylcholine receptor are hypophagic and lean. Nature 410:207–212, 2001

Yanovski JA, Yanovksi SZ: Recent advances in basic obesity research. JAMA 282:1504–1506, 1999

Yanovski SZ, Yanovski JA: Obesity. N Engl J Med 346:591–602, 2002

Yuan X, Yamada K, Ishiyama-Shigemoto, et al: Identification of polymorphic loci in the promoter region of the serotonin 5-HT2C receptor gene and their association with obesity and type II diabetes. Diabetologia 43:373–376, 2000

Zhang ZJ, Yao ZJ, Zhang XB, et al: No association of antipsychotic agent-induced weight gain with a DA receptor gene polymorphism and therapeutic response. Acta Pharmacol Sin 24:235–240, 2003

Zhang ZJ, Yao ZJ, Liu W, et al: Effects of antipsychotics on fat deposition and changes in leptin and insulin levels: magnetic resonance imaging study of previously untreated people with schizophrenia. Br J Psychiatry 184:58–62, 2004

Chapter 7

GLUCOSE METABOLISM

Effects of Atypical Antipsychotics

John W. Newcomer, M.D.

A range of evidence suggests that treatment with some antipsychotic medications is associated with an increased risk for insulin resistance, hyperglycemia, and dyslipidemia compared with no treatment or treatment with alternative antipsychotics (Newcomer 2005). Evidence for drug effects on these risk factors for type 2 diabetes mellitus (T2DM), along with the results of population-based analyses of diabetes incidence during antipsychotic treatment, suggests that these same antipsychotics do increase risk for T2DM (Newcomer 2005). Interpretation of the literature has been complicated by a small number of reports suggesting that patients with mental disorders such as schizophrenia have an increased prevalence of abnormalities in weight regulation and glucose metabolism (e.g., insulin resistance) prior to initiation of antipsychotic therapy (Kasanin 1926). However, these studies have produced inconsistent results that are difficult to interpret (Reynolds 2006; Ryan et al. 2003; Thakore 2005; Zhang et al. 2004). For example, one study found evidence of impaired fasting glucose in acutely hospitalized, unmedicated patients with elevated plasma cortisol levels, in whom hypercortisolemia may contribute to an increase in plasma glucose (Ryan et al. 2003). Hypercortisolemia, however, is not typically observed in chronically ill outpatients with schizophrenia or in antipsychotic-treated patients (Newcomer et al. 2002), so this study may overestimate the degree of hyperglycemia that could persist past an acute episode, hospitalization, and/or the agitated state. Further complicating this literature, early studies in this area (see Haupt and Newcomer 2001a, 2002) did not control for age, body weight, adiposity, ethnicity, and/or diet and activity levels, suggesting that differences in key factors such as diet and activity level between patients and control subjects may contribute to some or all of the observed abnormalities. In contrast to the limited conclusions that can be drawn from the small literature on unmedicated patients, there is a large literature concerning medication effects that indicate a consistent effect of certain medications on risk for abnormalities in glucose metabolism.

This chapter examines the evidence for an association between dysregulation of glucose and lipid metabolism and the related risk of T2DM during treatment with any of the six second-generation antipsychotics currently available in the United States: clozapine, risperidone, olanzapine, quetiapine, ziprasidone, and aripiprazole. Literature references were identified primarily via Medline searches. In addition to the Medline searches, abstracts presented at selected scientific meetings were searched. Finally, published reports of key pivotal studies examining the safety and efficacy of the different second-generation antipsychotics in patients with schizophrenia were reviewed for glucose and lipid data. The reports identified in this review can be broadly divided into three categories (Table 7–1): 1) case reports, chart reviews, U.S. Food and Drug Administration (FDA) Med-Watch–based reports, and other uncontrolled observational studies; 2) large, controlled, observational database analyses using prescription, administrative, or (less commonly) population-based databases; and 3) controlled experimental studies, including randomized clinical trials, although not all categories of study are available for each antipsychotic agent. These three categories of reports provide different levels of evidence to assess the impact of antipsychotic agents on the different metabolic parameters.

Case reports, chart reviews, and open observational studies all provide uncontrolled, largely anecdotal evidence and are generally useful for hypothesis generation only. Relevant controlled observational database analyses, a few using population-based data, can provide higher or lower levels of evidence depending on the methodology and the study endpoints used. Finally, controlled experimental studies, including prospective, randomized, controlled clinical trials, are designed to address specific questions and can be useful for "hypothesis testing."

Level 1 Evidence: Case Reports and Other Uncontrolled Observational Studies

FIRST-GENERATION ANTIPSYCHOTICS

Early reports of abnormal glucose regulation occurred following the introduction of chlorpromazine and other low-potency phenothiazines. Cases of new-onset T2DM and exacerbation of existing diabetes were associated with phenothiazine treatment (see Haupt and Newcomer 2001a); in one report, the prevalence of di-

TABLE 7–1. Types of studies relating antipsychotics to dysregulation of glucose and lipid metabolism in patients with mental illness

Level of evidence	Types of studies	Study strengths	Study limitations
1	Case reports, chart reviews, U.S. Food and Drug Administration MedWatch reports	Allows for early documentation of anecdotal evidence for an association, useful for hypothesis generation only	Does not show causality, does not control for other factors or conditions that may appear to strengthen (or weaken) the association with the outcome
2	Observational database studies	Generally takes advantage of existing databases, allows review of a large number of prescriptions	Lack of verification of diagnosis, high rates of polypharmacy, lack of verification medication was received, no knowledge of pretreatment conditions, and no direct measures of metabolism
3	Controlled experimental studies, randomized clinical trials (primary and secondary outcome data)	Useful for hypothesis testing	Time-intensive and challenging to conduct, fund, and administer

abetes increased from 4.2% to 17.2% following the introduction of chlorpromazine therapy (Thonnard-Neumann 1968). In addition, phenothiazine treatment
has been associated with adverse changes in plasma lipid levels and increases in
body weight (Amdisen 1964; Clark et al. 1970). However, not all first-generation
antipsychotic agents appear to show the same propensity for adverse effects on glucose regulation as phenothiazines. Reports of diabetes associated with the use of
high-potency first-generation agents such as haloperidol have been limited, suggesting potential variability among medications in their effects on glucose metabolism. Koller et al. (2003) identified 20 reports of hyperglycemia with haloperidol
treatment from the FDA MedWatch drug surveillance system and published reports from an estimated 6.5 million years of patient exposure.

SECOND-GENERATION ANTIPSYCHOTICS

Review of the greater number of cases of new-onset T2DM associated with clozapine (Koller et al. 2001), olanzapine (Koller and Doraiswamy 2002), and risperidone (Koller et al. 2003) in the FDA MedWatch database, as well as in published
reports and meetings abstracts, provides a number of interesting observations in
addition to raw counts of adverse events. These cases emerged from estimated
years of patient exposure (based on numbers of U.S. prescriptions and mean duration of therapy through February 2002) that ranged from 679,000 years for clozapine to 2.1 million years for olanzapine to 3.1 million years for risperidone
(Koller et al. 2003). These case reports suggest that whereas the majority of new-
onset T2DM cases were associated with substantial weight gain or obesity, approximately 25% of the cases were not. These analyses also have suggested that most
new-onset cases of T2DM occurred within the first 6 months after initiation of
treatment. Cases were typically (i.e., approximately 75% of the time) associated
with substantial weight gain or obesity, and as many as half of them involved individuals with no family history of diabetes. In some of the cases, there was a close
temporal relationship between initiation and discontinuation of treatment and development or resolution of the hyperglycemia-related adverse event. These cases
formed the basis for early hypotheses concerning weight gain–related and weight
gain–independent effects of antipsychotic medications on the risk for T2DM.

Clozapine

A case series for clozapine that included data from the FDA MedWatch Drug Surveillance System (January 1990 to February 2001; Koller et al. 2001) identified a
total of 384 cases: 323 were new-onset hyperglycemia, 54 represented patients
with exacerbation of preexisting diabetes, and 7 involved patients with unclear diabetes history. Among patients with definitive new-onset diabetes (i.e., blood glucose or hemoglobin A_{1c} [HbA_{1c}] diagnosis), more than 75% were age 50 years
or younger, suggesting that many were below the typical age at onset for T2DM.

Diabetes occurred within 1 month of starting clozapine therapy for 27% of patients and within 3 months for 54% of patients. Exacerbation of preexisting diabetes also occurred rapidly after clozapine initiation—within 1 month for 38% of patients and within 3 months for 64% of individuals. For the majority of patients, glycemic control improved following withdrawal of clozapine treatment. Follow-up data, available for 54 of the 110 patients who had their clozapine therapy withdrawn, showed that 42 patients (78%) experienced improvement. The severity of hyperglycemia associated with clozapine therapy ranged from mild glucose intolerance to ketoacidosis and hyperosmolar coma. Fifty-one patients (45 with new-onset diabetes) experienced blood glucose levels of 700 mg/dL or higher. Metabolic acidosis or ketosis accompanied hyperglycemia in 80 cases, most of which ($n=73$) involved new-onset diabetes. There were 25 deaths during hyperglycemic episodes; acidosis or ketosis was reported in 16 of these. Body weight data, available for 146 patients, showed obesity or substantial weight gain in most but no evidence of obesity or substantial weight gain in 38 individuals (26%). Other early case reports concerning clozapine treatment have been analyzed elsewhere (Ananth et al. 2002).

The occurrence of diabetes in patients with psychotic disorders who are treated with clozapine has also been examined in observational clinical series and reviews of patient records. A 5-year naturalistic study (Henderson et al. 2000) examined the incidence of treatment-emergent diabetes in patients with schizophrenia or schizoaffective disorder treated with clozapine. A total of 82 patients who had received clozapine therapy for at least 1 year were included in the study. Patients were treated at an outpatient clinic, and demographic and laboratory data (including fasting blood glucose [FBG] and lipid levels) were available at treatment initiation and at 6-month intervals thereafter. Patients had a mean age of 36.4 years, and only 4 were more than 50 years old. In all, 25 patients (30.5%) were diagnosed with T2DM by primary care physicians after initiation of clozapine therapy. Fourteen patients were treated with oral hypoglycemic agents and four with insulin. One of the insulin-treated patients experienced two episodes of diabetic ketoacidosis within 6 months of starting treatment, although the authors reported that this may be unrelated to clozapine and may represent a case of type 1 diabetes. An additional 5 patients who experienced elevated FBG values during the 5-year study period were subsequently diagnosed and treated for diabetes. In total, 36.6% of the patients in the study sample were diagnosed with diabetes within 5 years of initiating clozapine therapy. Body weight increased significantly during the study, although some patients did not gain weight and still developed diabetes.

Some studies have used patient records to retrospectively assess the prevalence of hyperglycemia among patients with schizophrenia or other psychotic illness treated with clozapine. One study identified 28 patients with hyperglycemia (fasting plasma glucose [FPG] ≥110 mg/dL), 6 of whom were diagnosed with diabetes on the basis of American Diabetic Association criteria (FPG≥126 mg/dL), among 121 patients diagnosed with schizophrenia from October 1999 through September 2000 (Sernyak et al. 2003). Patients identified with diabetes had a significantly greater body mass index (BMI; 33.1 kg/m^2) than those in the normal (<110 mg/dL) or impaired FPG (≥110 to <126 mg/dL) groups (28.8 kg/m^2 and 27.3 kg/m^2, respectively; P=0.041).

A small number of observational studies have measured plasma insulin levels in patients treated with clozapine. These studies can provide evidence of either decreased insulin secretion or increased secretion, suggesting decreased tissue insulin sensitivity. Melkersson and Hulting (2001) reported elevated fasting insulin levels in 7 of 14 patients receiving clozapine therapy, although median insulin levels remained within normal limits. Similarly, increases in mean insulin and glucose levels were observed in six patients with schizophrenia treated with clozapine (Yazici et al. 1998). Two studies have reported a positive correlation between insulin levels and clozapine serum concentration (Melkersson and Dahl 2003; Melkersson et al. 1999).

Olanzapine

A case series for olanzapine that included data from MedWatch (January 1994 to mid-May 2001), published reports (Medline, to mid-May 2001), and meeting abstracts over a similar period identified a total of 237 cases of diabetes or hyperglycemia in association with olanzapine therapy (Koller and Doraiswamy 2002). These reports included 188 cases (79%) of newly diagnosed hyperglycemia and 44 cases (19%) of exacerbation of preexisting diabetes, with 5 cases involving patients with an uncertain history. For 73% of patients, onset occurred within 6 months of starting olanzapine. For patients with definitive, new-diagnosed diabetes, 47% of cases occurred within 3 months and 70% within 6 months of starting therapy. For those patients with exacerbation of disease, 84% of events occurred within 3 months of starting olanzapine therapy. Limited data were available regarding withdrawal and rechallenge with olanzapine. Of 76 case patients evaluated, improvement was reported for 60 patients (79%) after the withdrawal of olanzapine. Among 10 patients rechallenged with olanzapine therapy, 8 experienced worsening glycemic control. For 4 patients, this occurred within 8 days of the resumption of olanzapine therapy.

The severity of hyperglycemia ranged from mild glucose intolerance to diabetic ketoacidosis and hyperosmolar coma. In 69 cases (64 involving new-onset diabetes), blood glucose levels of 700 mg/dL or more were recorded; in 41 patients (38 involving new-onset diabetes), blood glucose values exceeded 1,000 mg/dL. Changes in mental state (confusion or obtundation) accompanied hyperglycemia in 43 patients, whereas for 17 patients pancreatitis or hyperamylasemia was associated with hyperglycemia. Diabetic ketoacidosis was a frequent occurrence in the reported cases of diabetes or hyperglycemia associated with olanzapine therapy. Metabolic acidosis or ketosis was reported in 80 of the 237 cases (33.8%). The majority of these 80 cases ($n = 74$; 93%) involved new-onset diabetes. In addition, the proportion of fatalities among the cases of diabetic ketoacidosis was high (11.3%) relative to the optimal outcomes generally reported in nonpsychiatric samples (e.g., 3%–5%), with acidosis or ketosis reported in 9 of the 15 deaths observed in the olanzapine cases. In an addendum to the paper, the authors reported on an additional 52 cases of hyperglycemia (newly diagnosed, $n = 35$; exacerbation, $n = 12$) that were identified when the FDA MedWatch search was extended to February 2002 (Koller and Doraiswamy 2002). Again the incidence of diabetic ketoacidosis was relatively high, with 20 reports of ketosis or acidosis associated with hyperglycemia (38.5%). There were also 5 reports of pancreatitis among the cases. In all, 10 deaths occurred among these 52 patients.

A number of case reports concerning hyperglycemia and olanzapine have been published (Azriel Mira 2002; Bechara and Goldman-Levine 2001; Beliard et al. 2003; Bettinger et al. 2000; Bonanno et al. 2001; Chang et al. 2003; Dewan 2003; Domon and Webber 2001; Fertig et al. 1998; Gatta et al. 1999; Goldstein et al. 1999; Kozian 2002; Kropp et al. 2001; Lindenmayer and Patel 1999; Malyuk et al. 2002; Meatherall and Younes 2002; Melkersson and Hulting 2002; Muench and Carey 2001; Ober et al. 1999; Opp and Hildebrandt 2002; Ragucci and Wells 2001; Ramankutty 2002; Riccitelli and Baker 2002; Rigalleau et al. 2000; Roefaro and Mukherjee 2001; Rojas et al. 2001; Seaburg et al. 2001; Selva and Scott 2001; Straker et al. 2002; Tavakoli and Arguisola 2003; Torrey and Swalwell 2003; Von Hayek et al. 1999; Wirshing et al. 1998). Details from these case reports are consistent with cases reviewed by Ananth et al. (2002). A substantial proportion of reports involve diabetic ketoacidosis, and many patients are younger than is typical for the development of T2DM in the general population. Diabetes or ketoacidosis can occur shortly after the initiation of olanzapine therapy and in the absence of weight gain, although cases also occur after prolonged olanzapine therapy. One relatively high-profile case of diabetic ketoacidosis, which resulted in death, was reported with olanzapine therapy in a 12-week, double-blind study comparing olanzapine and divalproex sodium for the treatment of acute mania in patients with bipolar disorder (Zajecka et al. 2002). The 53-year-old patient had no prior history or family history of diabetes and had a normal blood glucose level at baseline (86 mg/dL).

Risperidone

Data from MedWatch (1993 to February 2002), published reports (Medline, to February 2002), and selected abstracts from national psychiatric meetings were previously used to identify a total of 131 cases of diabetes or hyperglycemia associated with risperidone therapy (Koller et al. 2003). Of these reports, 78 cases (60%) involved newly diagnosed hyperglycemia, and 46 cases (35%) involved exacerbation of preexisting diabetes; in the remaining 7 cases, this distinction could not clearly be made. Of the 78 patients with new-onset hyperglycemia, 55 met diagnostic criteria for diabetes and 10 were receiving antidiabetic medication and/or were acidotic or ketotic at the time of hyperglycemia. In addition, there were a further six reports of acidosis with risperidone treatment that were not associated with hyperglycemia.

For risperidone-treated patients with newly diagnosed hyperglycemia, the mean age at onset was 34.8 ($\pm$15.7) years. These patients were significantly younger than risperidone-treated patients with exacerbation of existing diabetes (mean age= 48.8$\pm$17.5 years; $P<0.001$). Time from the start of risperidone therapy to the onset of hyperglycemia ranged from 1 day to 48 months among the 96 patients with available data, and for 65 of these patients (68%) onset occurred within 6 months of starting treatment. Risperidone therapy was withdrawn in 47 patients and reduced in 5 patients. Outcome data for these patients were limited, although improved glycemic control was reported for 12 of these patients.

The severity of hyperglycemia associated with risperidone treatment ranged from mild glucose intolerance to diabetic ketoacidosis and hyperosmolar coma. Thirty-one patients (24 with new-onset diabetes) experienced blood glucose levels of 500 mg/dL or above. Metabolic acidosis or ketosis was reported for 26 patients treated with risperidone, the majority of whom ($n=22$) experienced new-onset diabetes. There were four deaths among patients receiving risperidone monotherapy; 3 of these patients had had acidosis or ketosis. Limited body weight data, available for 37 patients, suggested that approximately 20% of patients were not substantially overweight or had not had significant weight gain.

In contrast to the large number of published case reports of diabetes or diabetic ketoacidosis associated with clozapine or olanzapine therapy, there have been relatively few case reports of diabetes or hyperglycemia associated with risperidone treatment in the literature (Croarkin et al. 2000; Fukui and Murai 2002; Mallya et al. 2002; Wirshing et al. 2001). Wirshing et al. (2001) reported a retrospective analysis of two cases in which patients with schizophrenia developed diabetes while receiving risperidone treatment. In both cases, antipsychotic therapy was associated with weight gain. For one patient, the development of diabetes necessitated ongoing treatment with insulin. In other reports, Mallya et al. (2002) documented the resolution of hyperglycemia following discontinuation of risperidone treatment, and Croarkin et al. (2000) reported a case of diabetic ketoacidosis in a patient with HIV infection, with HIV possibly contributing to risk in this individual (Haupt and Newcomer 2001b).

Risperidone therapy was also associated with minimal changes in FBG levels from pretreatment in a review of 47 patients treated for 1 year (Meyer 2002). The mean increases in glucose were 0.68 mg/dL for all patients and 0.74 mg/dL for the subgroup of patients younger than 60 years ($n=39$). These changes were not statistically significant compared with baseline. The increase seen in a non-elderly subgroup was significantly less than the increase with olanzapine therapy

(10.8 mg/dL; $P=0.03$; $n=37$). A significant increase in body weight from baseline was observed with risperidone treatment for all patients (10.7 lb; $P<0.001$) and for the non-elderly subgroup (11.9 lb; $P<0.001$).

Quetiapine

Data from MedWatch (January 1997 to end July 2002) and published reports (Medline, January 1997 to end of July 2002) identified 46 cases of quetiapine-associated diabetes or hyperglycemia (Koller et al. 2004). Of these reports, 34 cases (74%) involved newly diagnosed hyperglycemia, and 8 cases (17%) involved exacerbation of preexisting diabetes; in the remaining 4 cases, this distinction was unclear. Of the 34 patients with newly diagnosed hyperglycemia, 23 met diagnostic criteria for diabetes based on blood glucose levels (fasting, ≥ 126 mg/dL; postload, ≥ 200 mg/dL) or HbA_{1c} levels, and 5 were receiving antidiabetic medication. In addition, there were 9 reports of acidosis with quetiapine treatment that were not associated with hyperglycemia.

The mean age at onset for patients with newly diagnosed diabetes (31.2 ± 14.8 years; 30 patients with available data) tended to be younger than for patients with exacerbation of existing diabetes (mean age$=43.5 \pm 16.4$ years; $n=8$). The time from initiation of quetiapine therapy to diagnosis of hyperglycemia ranged from 1 day to 21 months in the 36 patients with available data, with 27 patients (75%) experiencing onset of hyperglycemia within 6 months of starting quetiapine treatment. Among patients with newly diagnosed hyperglycemia, onset occurred within 6 months of starting therapy in 11 of the 27 patients with available data (41%). Time to onset tended to be shorter for patients experiencing exacerbation of existing disease, with 6 of 7 patients (86%) experiencing exacerbation within 3 months of starting therapy. Quetiapine therapy was reduced in one patient and discontinued in 15 patients. The limited outcomes data available reported improved glycemic control for 7 of these patients. One patient reported a recurrence of hyperglycemia and ketosis within 2 weeks of a rechallenge.

The severity of hyperglycemia associated with quetiapine therapy ranged from mild glucose intolerance to diabetic ketoacidosis or hyperosmolar coma. Nineteen patients experienced blood glucose levels of 500 mg/dL or above, and there were 21 reports of diabetic acidosis or ketosis. There were 11 deaths among quetiapine-treated patients; 7 occurred among patients with newly diagnosed hyperglycemia, and 1 occurred following a rechallenge in a patient with preexisting disease. Seven of the patients who died had had acidosis or ketosis. In an addendum to the paper, the authors reported on a further 23 cases of hyperglycemia (newly diagnosed, $n=15$; exacerbation, $n=6$; not clear, $n=2$) identified by extending their search to the end of November 2003. There were eight reported cases of acidosis or ketosis associated with hyperglycemia and two reports of pancreatitis. In all, there were 3 deaths among the 23 patients.

A few case reports of diabetes, diabetic ketoacidosis, or hyperglycemia associated with quetiapine treatment have appeared in the literature (Domon and Cargile 2002; Procyshyn et al. 2000; Sneed and Gonzalez 2003; Sobel et al. 1999). In two published reports (Procyshyn et al. 2000; Sobel et al. 1999), quetiapine therapy was associated with development of new-onset diabetes mellitus. In a third report (Sneed and Gonzalez 2003), addition of quetiapine to existing risperidone therapy led to highly elevated blood glucose levels (300–400 mg/dL). Blood glucose levels normalized with gradual discontinuation of quetiapine therapy and did not increase with subsequent initiation of ziprasidone therapy. In the other report (Domon and Cargile 2002), hyperglycemia and hypertriglyceridemia were observed in a patient receiving quetiapine therapy. In addition, Wilson et al. (2003) reported a patient developing diabetic ketoacidosis with quetiapine treatment, identified from a retrospective chart review of patients receiving second-generation antipsychotic treatment and evaluated or treated for diabetes. The patient experienced acute diabetic ketoacidosis 2 months after switching from risperidone to quetiapine.

Ziprasidone and Aripiprazole

Changes in FPG levels have been examined in a retrospective chart review of patients treated with ziprasidone (Cohen et al. 2003). In all, 40 patients with mental retardation and behavioral disturbances who had received at least 6 months of ziprasidone treatment were included in the study. Of these, 36 were switched to ziprasidone after excessive weight gain or inadequate response with other second-generation antipsychotics. The majority of patients ($n=28$; 70%) had received prior risperidone treatment; 5 had received quetiapine, 2 were treated with olanzapine, and 1 was treated with haloperidol/clozapine. Mean fasting glucose levels showed minimal changes during the first 6 months of ziprasidone therapy (baseline = 87.0 ± 21.5 mg/dL; 6 months = 83.4 ± 16.8 mg/dL). Changes in body weight were also reported over the analysis period. Mean body weight increased (mean = 1.8 kg) in the 6 months prior to the initiation of ziprasidone, then showed a significant mean decrease of 3.6 kg during the first 6 months of ziprasidone treatment ($P < 0.001$). In a switching study, nonfasting (random) plasma glucose levels showed no statistically significant change from baseline following 6 weeks of ziprasidone therapy (Kingsbury et al. 2001). Limited case reporting of abnormal glucose levels associated with ziprasidone therapy has appeared in the literature (Yang and McNeely 2002). Currently, only one case report of diabetic ketoacidosis associated with aripiprazole has been published (Church et al. 2005), and in no reports has diabetic ketoacidosis been associated with amisulpride or ziprasidone. The case involving aripiprazole concerned a 34-year-old African American woman with a 10-year history of T2DM without previously reported episodes of diabetic ketoacidosis. Four days before admission, aripiprazole 30 mg/day was added to her ongoing regimen of olanzapine 20 mg/day. One case involving rhabdomyolysis, hyperglycemia, and pancreatitis has been associated with ziprasidone treatment (Yang and McNeely 2002).

CHART REVIEWS AND UNCONTROLLED OBSERVATIONAL STUDIES INVOLVING MULTIPLE ANTIPSYCHOTICS

In a retrospective chart review of patients treated with first- or second-generation antipsychotic therapy (including clozapine, olanzapine, risperidone, and quetiapine), Wirshing et al. (2002) examined the changes in glucose levels that occurred in 215 patients after the initiation of antipsychotic treatment. Analysis of clozapine-treated patients showed a significant increase from baseline in mean FBG level (+14%; $P=0.05$) and maximum blood glucose level (+31%; $P=0.03$). In addition, 5 patients (13%) started treatment with a glucose-lowering agent following the initiation of clozapine therapy, and 44% of clozapine-treated patients with normal baseline glucose values experienced elevated FBG levels (≥ 126 mg/dL) during therapy. Data available for 32 patients receiving olanzapine therapy (mean treatment duration = 13.5 months) showed a significant increase in mean glucose levels (21%; $P=0.03$) and maximum glucose levels (37%; $P=0.04$) from baseline. Two patients who had been receiving glucose-lowering agents at baseline required a dosage increase to control glucose levels after initiating olanzapine. Of patients with normal FBG levels at baseline, 27% of patients receiving olanzapine developed a clinically significant increase in plasma glucose (≥ 126 mg/dL) during treatment. No significant changes in either mean or maximum fasting glucose levels, compared with pretreatment values, occurred with risperidone treatment. Among the 49 risperidone-treated patients (mean treatment duration = 19.2 months), mean glucose levels increased from 118.3 mg/dL at baseline to 122.3 mg/dL on therapy—an increase of 3%. Significant increases in mean, but not maximum, fasting glucose values were also observed with haloperidol. Excluding patients with abnormal FBG values at baseline, 36% of patients developed clinically significant elevated glucose levels (≥ 126 mg/dL) during risperidone therapy—an elevation similar to that seen with haloperidol. The 13 quetiapine-treated patients showed a small change in FBG levels from a mean baseline level of 106.6 mg/dL to 115.7 mg/dL, an increase of 9%. Mean maximum glucose levels remained virtually unchanged (pretreatment = 133.4 mg/dL; treatment = 133.3 mg/dL). The mean duration of quetiapine treatment was 7.3 months.

In a smaller, naturalistic study of 75 patients with schizophrenia or related psychotic disorders receiving first- or second-generation antipsychotic therapy (Kurt and Oral 2002), FBG levels also increased significantly from pretreatment levels after at least 2 months of clozapine treatment. In contrast, patients receiving typical therapy showed significant decreases in FBG levels from baseline. An open-label, nonrandomized study by Chae and Kang (2001) used weekly oral glucose tolerance tests (OGTTs) to assess blood glucose levels during 8 weeks of clozapine or haloperidol treatment in patients with psychotic disorders. Six of the 17 patients (35%) in the clozapine group developed impaired glucose tolerance (World Health Organization criteria) during treatment compared with none of 10 patients in the haloperidol group ($P=0.056$). Seven patients (41%) in the clozapine group and one (10%) in the haloperidol group developed glycemic peak delay. None of the patients in either group developed diabetes.

A case series study (Rubio and Gomez de la Camara 2002) examined the incidence of diabetes or hyperglycemia in patients with schizophrenia who had received second-generation antipsychotic treatment (olanzapine, $n=45$; clozapine, $n=38$; or risperidone, $n=51$) for 1–3 years. FBG measures showed that three cases of new-onset diabetes (FBG >126 mg/dL) occurred in the olanzapine group after the start of therapy compared with none in the clozapine or risperidone groups. In addition, four cases of hyperglycemia (FBG >110–126 mg/dL) occurred in the olanzapine group, four in the clozapine group, and none with risperidone therapy.

A chart review examined changes in the use of antidiabetic medication to assess the relationship between diabetic control and antipsychotic medication use in patients treated with first- or second-generation (olanzapine, clozapine, risperidone, or quetiapine) antipsychotics for at least 1 year (Casey and Matchett 2002). Among olanzapine-treated patients, 15 of 38 (39%) patients experienced an increase in antidiabetic medication of at least 50% at an average of 8 months of treatment, and 11 individuals (29%) required additional antidiabetic medication to control their diabetes. This finding compares with the 50% increase in antidiabetic medication found for 1 of 12 patients (8%) receiving typical antipsychotics (average of 276 months of treatment) and 2 of 11 patients (18%) receiving risperidone (22 months), and the additional antidiabetic medications for 3 (25%) and 5 (45%) patients receiving typical antipsychotic or risperidone therapy, respectively.

Two retrospective analyses of patient records reported significant increases in fasting glucose levels from pretreatment values with olanzapine. A retrospective study of patient records at Oregon State Hospital (Meyer 2002) compared metabolic outcomes after 1 year of treatment with either olanzapine ($n=47$) or risperidone ($n=47$) therapy. FBG levels in olanzapine-treated patients showed significant mean increases from baseline for all patients (7.3 mg/dL; $P=0.031$) and those younger than 60 years (10.8 mg/dL; $P=0.009$; $n=37$). These changes were greater than those observed with risperidone (+0.68 and +0.74 mg/dL, respectively), although the difference between the groups only reached statistical significance for non-elderly patients ($P=0.03$). Mean body weight increased significantly from baseline with olanzapine therapy for all patients (17.5 lb; $P\leq0.001$) and for non-elderly patients (20.4 lb; $P\leq0.001$). One case of new-onset diabetes occurred in the olanzapine group during the study period.

In contrast to studies reporting adverse metabolic events during olanzapine treatment, a study involving 75 patients with schizophrenia or related psychotic disorders treated with first- or second-generation antipsychotic therapy (Kurt and Oral 2002) showed no significant change in fasting or 2-hour postchallenge blood glucose levels from pretreatment values after at least 2 months of olanzapine treatment. No statistically significant change in peripheral insulin resistance was observed with olanzapine therapy. Data for eight individuals given quetiapine showed no significant changes in FBG levels from pretreatment values. However, significant increases were observed in blood glucose levels taken 2 hours after a standard OGTT. No statistically significant changes in peripheral insulin resistance were seen with quetiapine treatment. Similarly, a chart review of glucose and lipid parameters in 208 patients with psychotic illness (Gupta et al. 2003) showed no statistically significant difference in the prevalence of diabetes or mean FPG levels among patients treated with clozapine, risperidone, olanzapine, quetiapine, or typical antipsychotic monotherapy.

Changes in fasting insulin levels have also been examined in patients receiving olanzapine, clozapine, or typical antipsychotic therapy, mostly for schizophrenia, schizoaffective, or schizophreniform disorder (Melkersson and Hulting 2001). Patients treated with olanzapine had significantly higher median insulin levels than those receiving typical antipsychotics ($P<0.05$). Median insulin levels were above the upper limit of normal (>144 pmol/L) in the olanzapine group (234 pmol/L) but not in the clozapine (130 pmol/L) or typical antipsychotic (115 pmol/L) treatment groups. Ten patients (71%) in the olanzapine group had elevated insulin levels compared with seven (50%) in the clozapine group and six patients (32%) treated with typical agents. Two other studies have also examined fasting glucose and fasting insulin levels in patients with schizophrenia or related psychoses treated with olanzapine (Melkersson and Dahl 2003; Melkersson et al. 2000). Elevated fasting insulin levels were reported for 5 (31%) of the 16 olanzapine-treated outpatients included in the study (mean treatment duration = 1.2 years) (Melkersson and Dahl 2003). In addition, 7 patients (44%) had elevated fasting C-peptide levels, whereas 5 patients (31%) had elevated FBG levels. Increasing insulin and C-peptide levels both correlated with an increasing ratio between olanzapine and its metabolite *N*-desmethylolanzapine but showed an inverse correlation with *N*-desmethylolanzapine concentration. The earlier study reported elevated fasting insulin levels for 10 (71%) of the 14 patients treated with olanzapine (Melkersson et al. 2000). Three of the patients had elevated FBG levels (>6.0 mmol/L [108.1 mg/dL]), while values were normal for the remaining 11 patients. In addition, significant improvements in insulin resistance and β-cell function were reported for 40 patients with schizophrenia following a switch from olanzapine to risperidone therapy (Berry and Mahmoud 2002); data from 7 individuals showed a significant decrease in FBG levels after the switch (87.7 to 82.3 mg/dL; $P<0.04$) and a trend toward statistical significance for 2-hour postprandial blood glucose levels (105.5 to 80.0 mg/dL; $P < 0.09$) (Litman and Peterson 2002).

In another open-label, nonrandomized study, metabolic parameters were examined in patients with schizophrenia treated continuously with antipsychotic therapy for at least 3 months (Chue et al. 2003). Patients receiving clozapine therapy ($n = 34$) had significantly higher FPG levels ($P < 0.05$) and insulin resistance ($P < 0.05$) than those treated with typical antipsychotic therapy ($n = 17$). The proportions of patients with diabetes and hyperinsulinemia were highest among patients treated with clozapine. In contrast, clozapine treatment had no significant effect on insulin resistance in a prospective study of 20 patients initiating clozapine treatment (Howes et al. 2004). Mean insulin resistance and mean levels of other factors affecting glucose homeostasis did not differ significantly from baseline after an average of 2.5 months of clozapine therapy. However, baseline assessments suggested that these patients may have already had long-term insulin resistance at the start of clozapine therapy.

Level 2 Evidence: Observational Database Analyses

There are a growing number of reported observational analyses that used large administrative or health plan databases to test the strength of the association between treatment with specific antipsychotic medications and the presence of T2DM (Buse et al. 2003; Caro et al. 2002; Citrome and Jaffe 2003; Citrome et al. 2004; Farwell et al. 2002; Fuller et al. 2003; Gianfrancesco et al. 2002, 2003; Grogg et al. 2003; Koro et al. 2002; Lambert et al. 2005; Leslie and Rosenheck 2004; Lund et al. 2001; Ollendorf et al. 2004; Sernyak et al. 2002; Sumiyoshi et al. 2004; Wang et al. 2002). The approach common to all these studies has been to measure the association within a database between the use of specific antipsychotic medications and the presence of one or more surrogate indicators of T2DM (e.g., prescription of a antidiabetes agent, relevant ICD-9 codes). Approximately two-thirds of these studies reported to date had findings suggesting that drugs associated with greater weight gain (e.g., olanzapine) were also associated with an increased risk for T2DM compared with either no treatment, conventional treatment, or a drug producing less weight gain (e.g., risperidone). Although explicit tests of the relationship between diabetes risk and weight gain were not possible in these studies, none of the studies indicated that any drug with high weight-gain potential was associated with a lower risk for T2DM compared with an alternative treatment. Approximately one-third of the studies reported to date detected no difference between groups or a nonspecific increase in the association for all treated groups with risk for diabetes compared with untreated control subjects.

These studies have a number of methodological limitations related to the common use of medical claims databases. These limitations included lack of verification of psychiatric diagnosis and whether treatments were actually received, high rates of polypharmacy, and limited, if any, knowledge of earlier treatment conditions that can contribute to current levels of adiposity and insulin resistance. Most importantly, these studies lack direct measures of metabolism, relying on surrogate markers for the presence of diabetes, such as the prescription of a antidiabetes drug or an ICD code for diabetes. Such surrogate markers require the successful diagnosis of diabetes in the study sample, but underdiagnosis of diabetes is common. The American Diabetes Association estimates that approximately one-third of cases of diabetes are undiagnosed in the United States (Harris et al. 1998). Given that these database studies may involve samples that underestimate the prevalence of diabetes and that the hypothesized difference in prevalence rates across treatment conditions may be less than the prevalence of undiagnosed diabetes, this type of retrospective database analysis may face signal-to-noise challenges, which may explain some of the variability in studies of this kind.

In an effort to address some of this interstudy variability in results and to clarify the interpretation of findings in this area, investigators recently conducted a meta-analytic review of the relevant literature to quantify the relationship between various antipsychotic treatments and risk for diabetes in these large data sets (Newcomer 2005). The published data make it possible to 1) quantitatively examine the relationship between use of atypical antipsychotics and the development of new-onset diabetes across multiple studies; 2) apply a common referent group to these effect estimates (e.g., conventional antipsychotics); and 3) compare these summary measures by agent.

A search of Medline and Current Contents for all relevant publications from January 1990 to September 2004 was conducted, seeking studies in which atypical antipsychotics were used to treat schizophrenia or related disorders and that calculated summary odds ratios (ORs), relative risk, or hazard ratios. Fourteen primary studies were analyzed (Buse et al. 2003; Caro et al. 2002; Citrome et al. 2004; Farwell et al. 2002; Fuller et al. 2003; Gianfrancesco et al. 2002, 2003; Grogg et al. 2003; Koro et al. 2002; Lambert et al. 2005; Leslie and Rosenheck 2004; Ollendorf et al. 2004; Sernyak et al. 2002; Sumiyoshi et al. 2004). All of the included studies were retrospective analyses of existing databases, with 11 retrospective cohort studies that comprised the vast majority of patients (*n*=232,871) and 5 case-control studies (*n*=40,084). The study settings were primarily healthcare plans (e.g., Medicaid, Blue Cross and Blue Shield, Veterans Affairs). Six studies (*n*=122,270) selected only patients with a schizophrenia diagnosis, whereas 10 studies included patients receiving antipsychotic treatment for various psychoses (*n*=150,685). Data were available for clozapine, olanzapine, quetiapine, and risperidone but not for aripiprazole or ziprasidone because of the time frame of the included studies. Random effects models were used in the meta-analyses. Meta-analyses on the association of diabetes incidence among patients treated with atypical antipsychotics were performed using conventional antipsychotics or no antipsychotic treatment as the comparator groups. All odds ratios, relative risks, and hazard ratios included in the meta-analyses had been adjusted by the study authors for a variety of covariates, with the most common being treatment duration, age, and gender.

Clozapine was consistently associated with increased risk for diabetes (vs. conventional agents: OR=1.37, 95% CI=1.25–1.52; vs. no antipsychotics: OR=7.44, 95% CI=1.59–34.75). Olanzapine was also associated with increased risk for diabetes (vs. conventional agents: OR=1.26, 95% CI=1.10–1.46; vs. no antipsychotic: OR=2.31, 95% CI=0.98–5.46). Neither risperidone (vs. conventional agents: OR=1.07, 95% CI=1.00–1.13; vs. no antipsychotic: OR=1.20, 95% CI=0.51–2.85) nor quetiapine (vs. conventional agents: OR=1.22, 95% CI=0.92–1.61; vs. no antipsychotic: OR=1.00, 95% CI=0.83–1.20) was associated with an increase in risk for diabetes. These results of this quantitative analysis of the association between atypical antipsychotic use and incident diabetes in large, real-world databases suggest that the risk of diabetes varies among atypical antipsychotics, ranging from increases in risk relative to multiple comparators to no increase in risk for diabetes relative to any tested comparator.

Level 3 Evidence: Controlled Experimental Studies, Including Randomized Clinical Trials

The final level of evidence for an association between some antipsychotic medications and adverse metabolic outcomes is derived from controlled experimental studies and randomized clinical trials. There is a growing body of evidence supporting the key observation that treatments producing the greatest increases in body weight and adiposity are also associated with a consistent pattern of clinically significant adverse effects on insulin sensitivity and related changes in blood glucose and lipid levels. The effect of antipsychotic treatment on insulin resistance, rather than insulin secretion, may be most important for most patients.

In general, increases in insulin resistance are anticipated to occur secondary to increases in adiposity (Ebenbichler et al. 2003; Eder et al. 2001). The principle that increasing adiposity is associated with increasing insulin resistance is based on the association between these variables consistently observed in many studies in humans and other mammals that are reviewed elsewhere in this book, with a similar association not surprisingly observed in persons with schizophrenia who are taking antipsychotic medications (Fucetola et al. 2000).

Increased evidence of insulin resistance is manifested in a number of clinical trials reviewed in the following discussion, most often in the context of weight gain. It should be noted that statistical correlations between weight change and change in insulin resistance are often—but not always—significant because of contributions to insulin resistance from factors beyond just adiposity. In general, variation in adiposity (e.g., BMI or waist circumference) accounts for approximately 30%–50% of the variance in insulin resistance (Farin et al. 2005), with fitness (Rosenthal et al. 1983) and genetic or familial effects (Lillioja et al. 1987) each contributing to an additional 25%–30% of variance in insulin resistance. Simple correlations between change in weight and change in plasma glucose values should be expected to be weaker than correlations between weight change and change in insulin resistance, based on the potential for compensatory hyperinsulinemia to buffer plasma glucose when insulin resistance increases with increasing adiposity. The reduced probability of a simple correlation between these variables has not stopped some investigators from testing for correlations between weight changes and changes in plasma glucose and—upon finding no significant effect—interpreting the result as an indication that weight gain may be uncoupled from the risk of diabetes in persons taking antipsychotic medications. It remains prudent to understand the established risks posed by increasing adiposity. The well-established relationship between adiposity and insulin resistance and the host of changes in physiology associated with insulin resistance, including the potential for a progressive loss of glucose tolerance, remain important clinical considerations (Reaven 1999). From the standpoint of predictive value, an overweight or obese individual (BMI≥25) has a 50% probability of having insulin resistance (top tertile), increasing to 70% probability when this increased adiposity occurs along with a fasting plasma triglyceride of more than 130 mg/dL and to a 78% probability of insulin resistance when this individual also meets National Cholesterol Education Program–Adult Treatment Panel III (NCEP-ATP III) criteria for the metabolic syndrome (McLaughlin et al. 2003).

Although drug-induced increases in adiposity may be the most common mechanism contributing to drug-induced changes in glucose metabolism, a significant minority of patients may experience glucose dysregulation independent of weight or adiposity differences (Ebenbichler et al. 2003; Kemner et al. 2002; Koller and Doraiswamy 2002; Koller et al. 2001, 2003; Newcomer et al. 2002), suggesting the hypothesis that some antipsychotic medications may have a direct effect on insulin sensitivity or secretion. A recent study using euglycemic hyperinsulinemic clamps to study the effect of antipsychotics on insulin sensitivity in freely running Wistar rats found a highly significant dose-dependent reduction in insulin sensitivity within 2 hours of initial exposure to clozapine or olanzapine but not to ziprasidone or risperidone (Houseknecht et al. 2005).

A small number of clinical studies with schizophrenia patients have used oral and intravenous glucose tolerance tests to assess drug-related variation in glucose metabolism that occurs independent of variation in adiposity. Using a frequently sampled modified OGTT, Newcomer et al. (2002) compared glucose regulation in nondiabetic patients with schizophrenia treated with first- or second-generation (clozapine, olanzapine, or risperidone) therapy and untreated healthy subjects. Patient groups were well matched for age and BMI and balanced for gender and ethnicity. Despite the exclusion of patients with diabetes and matching for adiposity, the clozapine-treated subjects ($n=9$) showed significant elevations in plasma glucose levels at fasting and at 75 minutes post–glucose load compared with those treated with typical antipsychotics ($n=17$) and untreated healthy subjects ($n=31$) (all comparisons, $P<0.005$). Calculation of insulin resistance, based on FPG and insulin levels, showed a significant increase in insulin resistance associated with clozapine treatment compared with typical antipsychotics. Significant elevations in plasma glucose levels were observed in the olanzapine group at fasting and at all time points (15, 45, and 75 minutes) after the glucose load compared with untreated healthy subjects and with patients treated with typical antipsychotics (all comparisons, $P<0.005$). Insulin resistance, again calculated from FPG and insulin levels, was increased significantly in association with olanzapine compared with typical antipsychotic treatment ($P<0.05$).

Similar findings were reported by Henderson et al. (2005), who used frequent sampling of intravenous glucose tolerance tests to study nondiabetic patients chronically treated with clozapine, olanzapine, or risperidone. Treatment groups were carefully matched for adiposity, age, gender, and ethnicity. Patients treated with clozapine and olanzapine showed significant insulin resistance, as measured by minimal model–derived insulin sensitivity S_I, compared with subjects treated with risperidone (clozapine vs. risperidone, $t_{33}=-4.29$; $P=0.001$; olanzapine vs. risperidone, $t_{33}=-3.62$; $P=0.001$). There was no significant difference in S_I-measured insulin resistance between clozapine and olanzapine ($t_{33}=-0.67$; $P=0.51$). However, there were significant differences between clozapine and risperidone ($t_{33}=2.94$; $P=0.006$) and olanzapine and risperidone ($t_{33}=2.42$; $P=0.02$) in insulin resistance calculated by homeostasis model assessment of insulin resistance (HOMA-IR). Both of these studies were limited by adiposity matching that used BMI values, which may fail to capture potentially treatment-related differences in abdominal fat mass (i.e., despite equal BMI, some treatment groups might have larger abdominal fat mass), leading to differences in insulin sensitivity that might be driven by differences in fat mass rather than an adiposity-independent mechanism.

RANDOMIZED CLINICAL TRIALS

An increasing number of randomized clinical trials have included measures of weight or adiposity, fasting or postload plasma glucose, plasma lipids, and various indicators of insulin resistance. Treatment-induced changes in insulin resistance have typically been estimated using indirect indicators such as fasting plasma insulin, homeostasis model assessment (HOMA-IR = [fasting insulin (μU/mL) × fasting glucose (mmol/L)]/22.5; Haffner et al. 1997), fasting plasma triglyceride, or the ratio of triglycerides to high-density lipoprotein (HDL) cholesterol. There are a number of studies under way that estimate insulin resistance by means of more sensitive techniques, such as a frequently sampled OGTT, or via direct and sensitive measures, such as minimal model–derived insulin sensitivity values from frequently sampled intravenous glucose tolerance tests or gold-standard measurements based on hyperinsulinemic euglycemic clamp techniques. In general, the review of studies that follows is organized along the lines of increasing duration of drug exposure, increasing sample size, and/or increasing sensitivity of measures.

Howes et al. (2004) reported a prospective assessment of clozapine's effects on insulin resistance, measured by OGTT, in 20 schizophrenia patients switched to clozapine from a variety of other medications. There was no control group. After a mean 2.5 ± 0.95 months of treatment, mean fasting glucose level increased by 0.55 mmol/L ($t=-2.9$, $df=19$, $P=0.01$), and mean 2-hour glucose level increased by 1.4 mmol/L ($t=-3.5$, $df=19$, $P=0.002$). There was no significant change in insulin level ($t=0.128$, $df=14$, $P=0.9$) or insulin resistance level measured by the HOMA-IR ($t=-0.9$, $df=14$, $P=0.37$). Mean BMI increased by 0.82 kg/m^2, although the increase was not statistically significant ($t=-1.325$, $df=17$, $P=0.2$).

A nonblinded crossover study of 15 schizophrenia patients who were experiencing poor treatment response assessed the differential effects of olanzapine versus risperidone on weight and fasting lipid profile after 3 months of treatment (Su et al. 2005). Seven patients were switched from risperidone to olanzapine, and 8 patients were switched from olanzapine to risperidone. Mean overall dosages were 8.3 ± 2.4 mg of olanzapine and 2.7 ± 1.0 mg of risperidone. BMI decreased from 25.7 ± 3.1 kg/m^2 to 24.2 ± 3.1 kg/m^2 in the group switched to risperidone and increased from 24.8 ± 4.0 kg/m^2 to 25.9 ± 4.3 kg/m^2 in the group switched to olanzapine ($P=0.015$). Plasma triglycerides decreased from 211.8 ± 134.9 to 125.8 ± 90.8 mg/dL in patients switched to risperidone and increased from 112.4 ± 76.3 to 196.7 ± 154.8 mg/dL in patients switched to olanzapine ($P=0.001$). The study failed to detect significant differences in other lipid parameters.

A randomized, double-blind trial in 157 schizophrenia patients consisted of an 8-week fixed-dosage period and a 6-week variable-dosage period of treatment with clozapine, olanzapine, risperidone, or haloperidol (Lindenmayer et al. 2003). There were significant increases from baseline in mean glucose levels at the end of the 6-week variable-dosage period in patients who received olanzapine ($n=22$; $P<0.02$) and at the end of the 8-week fixed-dosage period in patients who received clozapine ($n=27$; $P<0.01$) or haloperidol ($n=25$; $P<0.03$). The authors indicated that a trend-level difference was seen between treatments at the end of the 8-week fixed-dosage period ($P=0.06$) but not at the end of the 6-week variable-dosage phase. Mean cholesterol levels were increased at the end of the 6-week variable-dosage period in patients who received olanzapine ($P<0.01$) and at the end of the 8-week fixed-dosage period in patients who received clozapine or olanzapine ($P<0.02$ and $P<0.04$, respectively). This study was complicated by baseline and endpoint body weights in some groups that are not typically seen in clinical practice or in other trials, underscoring the need to control for previous treatments and baseline status in future trials.

Glucose, insulin, and lipid parameters were assessed in a randomized, double-blind, 6-week study comparing olanzapine and ziprasidone therapy in 269 inpatients with acute exacerbation of schizophrenia or schizoaffective disorder (Glick and Romano 2001). No statistically significant changes in FPG levels from baseline were observed with olanzapine or ziprasidone treatment during the study. Significant increases from baseline in median fasting plasma insulin levels ($P<0.0001$) and HOMA-IR–calculated insulin resistance ($P<0.0001$) were observed with olanzapine therapy but not with ziprasidone. Median body weight increased by 7.2 lb (3.3 kg) from baseline with olanzapine treatment compared with 1.2 lb (0.5 kg) with ziprasidone—median body weight was significantly higher in the olanzapine group than the ziprasidone group at endpoint ($P<0.0001$). In this relatively young sample, with a significant compensatory hyperinsulinemia, plasma glucose in the olanzapine-treated subjects did not increase significantly. Statistically significant adverse changes in lipid parameters in the olanzapine group are discussed later. In a 6-month, blinded follow-up study comparing olanzapine ($n=71$) and ziprasidone ($n=62$) therapy in patients with schizophrenia or schizoaffective disorder (Simpson and Weiden 2002), statistically significant increases from baseline in median fasting glucose and insulin levels were seen with olanzapine therapy. No statistically significant changes were observed with ziprasidone after 6 months of treatment.

The comparative efficacy and safety of olanzapine and ziprasidone were again assessed in a prospective, randomized, double-blind study of 28 weeks' duration (Breier et al. 2005; Hardy et al. 2003). Patients with DSM-IV (American Psychiatric Association 1994) schizophrenia were randomly assigned to olanzapine 10–20 mg/day (mean = 15.27 ± 4.52 mg/day) or ziprasidone 80–160 mg/day (mean = 115.96 ± 39.91 mg/day) at a standardized initial dosage of each, with any further clinically determined dosage changes performed using standardized increments. The patients were randomly assigned to either olanzapine ($n=277$) or ziprasidone ($n=271$). The proportion of patients with treatment-emergent hyperglycemia (i.e., those with baseline FPG levels < 126 mg/dL who experienced levels ≥ 126 mg/dL during treatment) did not differ significantly between the two groups (olanzapine = 11.5%; ziprasidone = 7.4%; $P=0.159$). Thirty-five percent of olanzapine-treated patients, compared with 5% of ziprasidone-treated patients, experienced weight gain, presumed in this report to reflect a increase over baseline weight of 7% or more ($P<0.001$), with a mean weight gain of 3.06 ± 6.87 kg in the olanzapine group and −1.12 ± 4.70 kg in the ziprasidone group. A subjective increase in appetite was reported by 20% of the olanzapine group versus 2.6% of the ziprasidone group ($P=0.02$). The olanzapine group versus the ziprasidone group showed, respectively, +5.04 ± 30.24 versus −0.18 ± 21.42 mg/dL change in fasting glucose ($P=0.38$); $+3.1\pm36.74$ versus -12.76 ± 31.32 mg/dL change in total cholesterol ($P=0.002$); $+34.54\pm105.4$ versus -21.26 ± 96.54 mg/dL change in triglyceride level ($P<0.001$); $+0.77\pm29.8$ versus -10.44 ± 25.91 mg/dL change in low-density lipoprotein (LDL; $P=0.02$); and -2.32 ± 10.05 versus $+0.77\pm9.67$ mg/dL change in HDL (all values converted from mmol/L to mg/dL).

A pooled analysis of safety data from short-term (4–6 week) controlled trials of aripiprazole in patients with schizophrenia found that changes in fasting serum glucose concentrations were similar between patients who received aripiprazole ($n=860$) and those who received placebo ($n=392$) (Kroeze et al. 2003). A 26-week controlled study of aripiprazole for relapse prevention in 310 patients with schizophrenia found no clinically or statistically significant change from baseline in fasting glucose concentration ($+0.13$ mg/dL) (Reynolds et al. 2002).

Changes in FBG were examined in a 6-week, placebo-controlled study of aripiprazole treatment in patients with schizophrenia (Marder et al. 2003). Analysis of pooled data from three aripiprazole groups (10 mg/day, 15 mg/day, or 20 mg/day) showed minimal mean changes in blood glucose from baseline (-0.37 mg/dL; $n=120$), similar to those observed with placebo (-5.03 mg/dL; $n=34$). Random blood glucose measurements pooled from five short-term (4- or 6-week), controlled aripiprazole studies showed that only a small number of patients with normal blood glucose baseline levels (<160 mg/dL) had on-study values of 200 mg/dL or above with aripiprazole treatment (9/648; 1.4%) (Marder et al. 2003). Similar findings were observed with haloperidol treatment (5/182; 2.7%) and with placebo (4/309, 1.3%). Comparable effects on fasting serum glucose with aripiprazole and placebo have also been seen in patients with bipolar I disorder. The rates of patients with clinically significant levels of fasting serum glucose (≥110 mg/dL) were similar in both groups (Keck et al. 2003).

Data from long-term trials in schizophrenia demonstrate similar effects. In a 26-week relapse prevention study involving patients with chronic stable schizophrenia (Pigott et al. 2003), there was no clinically significant change from baseline in the fasting glucose levels of patients given aripiprazole or those given placebo (aripiprazole, $+0.13$ mg/dL change; placebo, $+2.1$ mg/dL). A 26-week, multicenter, double-blind, randomized trial (McQuade et al. 2004) compared weight change and metabolic indices during treatment with olanzapine ($n=161$) with those during treatment with aripiprazole ($n=156$); 37% of olanzapine-treated patients experienced significant weight gain (7% of baseline weight) compared with 14% of aripiprazole-treated patients ($P<0.001$). There was a mean weight gain of 4.23 kg in the olanzapine group and a mean weight loss of 1.37 kg in the aripiprazole group ($P<0.001$). The olanzapine group experienced statistically significant differences compared with the aripiprazole group in mean changes in triglycerides ($+79.4$ mg/dL vs. -6.5 mg/dL, respectively; $P<0.05$) and HDL levels (-3.39 mg/dL vs. $+3.61$ mg/dL, respectively; $P<0.05$). Changes in the groups in total cholesterol ($+16.3$ mg/dL for the olanzapine group vs. -1.13

mg/dL for the aripiprazole group) and LDL levels (+2.27 mg/dL vs. −3.86 mg/dL, respectively) did not reach statistical significance. In addition, 47% of olanzapine-treated patients with normal baseline lipids demonstrated total cholesterol values above 200 mg/dL at endpoint compared with 17% of aripiprazole-treated patients. Similar differences between groups among patients with normal baseline lipids were seen for LDL levels of more than 130 mg/dL at endpoint (38% with olanzapine and 19% with aripiprazole) and triglyceride levels of more than 150 mg/dL at endpoint (50% with olanzapine and 18% with aripiprazole). The change in mean FPG from baseline to endpoint was +7 mg/dL in the olanzapine group and +5 mg/dL in the aripiprazole group; the difference between the groups was not statistically significant. Despite the significant weight gain and dyslipidemia, there was no statistically significant difference in mean change in fasting glucose in this 26-week trial. This finding might be explained by a compensatory increase in insulin secretion in the olanzapine-treated subjects over the period of study, but no plasma insulin values were reported to validate this hypothesis. In general, pancreatic β-cells can hypersecrete insulin to compensate for reductions in insulin sensitivity. This compensatory effect might be sustained over the life span in those individuals with no family or personal history of risk for diabetes, whereas individuals at risk can typically sustain the compensatory hyperinsulinemia for only a limited period of time prior to experiencing a gradual, progressive failure of β-cell function that results in the progressive onset of plasma glucose elevations (American Diabetes Association et al. 2004).

Results from a prospective 16-week study showed elevated glucose levels both at fasting and following an OGTT in 7 of 13 patients receiving clozapine treatment (Rettenbacher et al. 2004). Significant increases in insulin resistance indices were also reported with clozapine therapy. In contrast, no elevations in fasting or post-OGTT glucose levels or in insulin resistance measures were observed among the 12 patients receiving amisulpride treatment.

OGTTs were used to assess changes in glucose levels from baseline to endpoint in a small ($n = 30$), randomized, 21-day study of olanzapine therapy given at a dosage of 20–40 mg/day (Hardy et al. 2004). Changes in mean 2-hour OGTT glucose values from baseline during olanzapine treatment did not appear to be dose dependent (20 mg/day, 4.68±38.37 mg/dL; 30–40 mg/day, 6.4±21.20 mg/dL; 40 mg/day, −4.58±33.76 mg/dL). Glucose tolerance worsened in one patient (from impaired glucose tolerance to diabetes) and improved in two patients (from impaired glucose tolerance to normal) during the study. Other postload time points for glucose (i.e., prior to the 2-hour values) and postload insulin values were not reported.

At least five studies have reported statistically significant increases in plasma insulin levels during olanzapine treatment compared with various control conditions ($P < 0.05$ for all) (Barak et al. 2002; Cuijpers and Smit 2002; Gallagher et al. 2000; Sikich et al. 2004; Visser et al. 2003), suggesting increased insulin resistance; two of these studies reported a significant increase in calculated insulin resistance from baseline during olanzapine therapy ($P<0.05$) (Gallagher et al. 2000; Visser et al. 2003). Other agents have not been reported to have this effect, with the exception of clozapine. Two studies reported elevated insulin levels in 31%–71% of patients receiving olanzapine treatment ($P<0.05$) (Barak 2002; Goldberg 2001). The findings of these studies are consistent with the evidence from general-population samples (Montague and O'Rahilly 2000; Resnick et al. 1998), suggesting that conditions that increase adiposity tend to be associated with increases in insulin resistance, potentially leading to compensatory insulin secretion in persons with pancreatic β-cell reserve and to hyperglycemia in individuals with relative β-cell failure.

A study of briefly treated healthy subjects showed an increased insulin response and decreased insulin sensitivity with both olanzapine and risperidone treatments compared with placebo (Sowell et al. 2002). The change in insulin response correlated with a change in BMI. After use of regression analyses to adjust for the effects of weight gain seen with active treatment, no statistically significant changes in insulin response or sensitivity were detected with olanzapine or risperidone therapy, suggesting that the adverse effects were largely related to changes in adiposity. A more recent study examining insulin sensitivity in healthy volunteers receiving olanzapine ($n=22$), risperidone ($n=14$), or placebo ($n=19$) for 3 weeks with restricted access to food showed no statistically significant changes in the insulin sensitivity index from baseline with olanzapine or risperidone therapy (Sowell et al. 2003). In this report, using two-step, hyperinsulinemic euglycemic clamp methodology, Sowell and colleagues showed no statistically significant difference in the mean change in insulin sensitivity index from baseline among the olanzapine, risperidone, and placebo groups at either low or high insulin steady states. Fasting insulin and fasting glucose levels both increased statistically significantly from baseline to endpoint in the olanzapine group but showed small decreases in the risperidone group. Another study in patients with schizophrenia or related psychotic disorders showed no statistically significant changes in peripheral insulin resistance after at least 2 months of olanzapine treatment (Kurt and Oral 2002). Finally, Berry and Mahmoud (2002) reported significant improvements in insulin resistance and β-cell function in schizophrenia patients following a change from olanzapine to risperidone treatment.

Limited findings to date suggest that quetiapine therapy is not associated with a consistent increase in the risk for T2DM or related dyslipidemia. However, a possible increase in metabolic risk would be predicted in association with any treatment that produces increases in body weight and adiposity, and quetiapine typically produces modest (e.g., approximately 2–3 kg long term) weight gain. A 6-week randomized study of atypical antipsychotics in 56 patients with schizophrenia (clozapine, olanzapine, quetiapine, and risperidone; $n=14$ each) found significant changes from baseline in triglyceride levels with quetiapine therapy (Atmaca et al. 2003). In quetiapine recipients, the mean increase in triglyceride levels from baseline was significant at week 6 (11.64 mg/dL; $P<0.05$), although this mean increase was approximately three times less than that observed in clozapine recipients (36.28 mg/dL; $P<0.01$) or olanzapine recipients (31.23 mg/dL; $P<0.01$). No significant increase from baseline in triglyceride levels was observed in risperidone-treated patients ($P=0.76$).

Using pooled data from two 26-week, randomized, double-blind, controlled trials (McQuade and Jody 2003; Pigott et al. 2003), a prospective study compared the effects of aripiprazole, olanzapine, and placebo on the incidence of worsening metabolic syndrome in 624 subjects (L'Italien 2003). The cumulative incidence of metabolic syndrome worsening varied across treatments, from a mean (standard error) incidence of 19.2% (4.0%) with olanzapine to 12.8% (4.5%) with placebo and 7.6% (2.3%) with aripiprazole. A log-rank test indicated a significant difference between the three rates ($P=0.003$), with a 69% relative risk reduction for aripiprazole versus olanzapine (Casey and L'Italien 2003; L'Italien 2003).

The Clinical Antipsychotic Trials of Intervention Effectiveness (CATIE) study is a major ongoing National Institute of Mental Health–sponsored prospective trial designed to assess the efficacy of the second-generation antipsychotic agents olanzapine, quetiapine, risperidone, and ziprasidone, with perphenazine included as a representative first-generation agent. The trial comprises 1,493 patients with schizophrenia at 57 sites in the United States. The primary outcome measure is time to all-cause discontinuation, chosen because, in the words of the study's authors, "stopping or changing medication is a frequent occurrence and major problem in the treatment of schizophrenia. In addition, this measure integrates patients' and clinicians' judgments of efficacy, safety, and tolerability into a global measure of effectiveness that reflects their evaluation of therapeutic benefits in relation to undesirable effects" (Lieberman et al. 2005, p. 1211). Secondary outcome measures include assessment of the reasons for discontinuation, for example, lack of efficacy versus intolerability due to side effects such as weight gain and metabolic disturbances.

Phase I results were published in September 2005. Patients in the olanzapine group gained more weight than patients in any other group (mean weight gain = 2 lb per month), and 30% of patients in the olanzapine group gained 7% or more of their baseline body weight (vs. 7%–16% in the other groups; $P<0.001$). Olanzapine-treated patients also showed the greatest increases in total cholesterol (mean increase = 9.7 ± 2.1 mg/dL), triglycerides (mean increase = 42.9 ± 8.4 mg/dL), and glycosylated hemoglobin (mean increase = 9.7 ± 2.1 mg/dL), with statistically significant differences between treatment groups in each of these indices (Lieberman et al. 2005).

In summary, evidence from various trial designs, data sources, and levels of evidence shows that there is a difference in risk for changes in glucose and lipid metabolism among the second-generation antipsychotics. A range of evidence suggests clozapine and olanzapine have a higher propensity to cause these changes compared with quetiapine, risperidone, ziprasidone, and aripiprazole.

Monitoring and Treatment Considerations

Individuals with mental illnesses such as schizophrenia have an increased prevalence of risk factors for diabetes mellitus and cardiovascular disease, such as obesity, dyslipidemia, hyperglycemia, and hypertension (McEvoy et al. 2005). Growing concerns about the impact of antipsychotic treatment on these risk factors and the implications for the overall health of a vulnerable patient population have led to increased interest in careful screening and monitoring of patients to improve their long-term health. This issue was discussed at the recent American Diabetes Association (ADA)/American Psychiatric Association (APA) Consensus Development Conference, and their published statement provides recommendations for the monitoring of patients receiving antipsychotic medications (American Diabetes Association et al. 2004). Recommended baseline screening measures include weight and height (for BMI calculation), waist circumference, blood pressure, fasting glucose and lipid profile, and personal and family history of obesity, diabetes, dyslipidemia, hypertension, or cardiovascular disease (see Table 7–2). Follow-up weight monitoring is recommended 4, 8, and 12 weeks after initiating or switching antipsychotic therapy, then quarterly at routine visits. FBG and lipid assessments are recommended at least 3 months after treatment initiation, then every year for glucose or every 5 years for lipids (although the 5-year interval is not consistent with NCEP-ATP III guidelines for individuals with anything above minimal risk, a status not characteristic of this population, suggesting the need for annual assessment along with glucose). However, increased baseline risk or treatment-emergent events may indicate the need for increased attention to some or all of these parameters, with more frequent monitoring or more sensitive assessments (e.g., OGTT in place of fasting glucose). The current review suggests that elevated baseline risk and treatment-emergent adverse metabolic events can be expected in many treated patients, implying that many patients will have clinical indications for closer and more detailed monitoring. For those patients who show weight gain ($\geq$5% increase) or worsening glycemia or dyslipidemia, a switch to another second-generation agent not associated with significant weight gain or diabetes risk should be considered along with other interventions.

Similar recommendations for weight, glucose, and lipid monitoring come from the 2002 Mount Sinai Conference, which brought together psychiatrists, endocrinologists, and other medical experts to develop guidelines for the routine

TABLE 7–2. Guidelines for monitoring patients receiving second-generation antipsychotics based on the Consensus Development Conference co-sponsored by the American Diabetes Association, the American Psychiatric Association, the American Association of Clinical Endocrinologists, and the North American Association for the Study of Obesity

	Baseline	4 weeks	8 weeks	12 weeks	Quarterly	Annually
Personal/family history	X					X
Body mass index/weight	X	X	X	X	X	
Waist circumference	X					X
Blood pressure	X			X		X
Fasting plasma glucose	X			X		X
Fasting lipid profile	X			X		

Source. Adapted from American Diabetes Association et al. 2004, p. 270.

monitoring of adult schizophrenia patients receiving antipsychotic therapy (Marder et al. 2004). These guidelines do, notably, recommend that patients with schizophrenia should be considered at high risk for coronary heart disease. Therefore, based on the NCEP guidelines, their lipid profile might need to be monitored more frequently (i.e., every 2 years for normal LDL cholesterol levels and every 6 months for LDL cholesterol >130 mg/dL) than is recommended by the ADA/APA consensus statement. The Mount Sinai guidelines suggest that fasting glucose or glycosylated hemoglobin (e.g., HbA_{1c}) could be used for glucose monitoring, whereas the ADA recommendations for screening in the general population advise against the use of glycosylated hemoglobin due to its relative insensitivity as a screening measure. An alternate proposal is to use glycosylated hemoglobin measurement along with a random glucose for persons in whom fasting assessments are not possible. In this case, abnormal glycosylated hemoglobin or a random glucose greater than 140 mg/dL could be used as an indicator of hyperglycemia that would warrant more definitive standardized evaluation using either fasting or postload glucose determinations. The introduction of regular routine monitoring should allow for the early detection of changes in these important risk factors and thus improve the overall long-term health of patients with schizophrenia and other mental illnesses.

Conclusion

Data from various sources on the use of atypical antipsychotics indicate that some drugs in this class are associated with a significant risk for weight gain and disordered glucose metabolism. Adverse effects on glucose metabolism have more frequently and consistently been associated with clozapine and olanzapine treatment, with discrepant reports for quetiapine and risperidone treatment (American Diabetes Association et al. 2004). Reports detailing limited short- and long-term weight gain with ziprasidone and aripiprazole are consistent with little or no evidence of adverse effects on metabolic outcomes (American Diabetes Association et al. 2004; Casey et al. 2004; Haupt and Newcomer 2001b; Yang and McNeely 2002). Notably, weight gain is not an absolute prerequisite for the development of insulin resistance, impaired glucose tolerance, or T2DM during antipsychotic treatment. Additional research is needed to examine the pharmacological factors that contribute to these adverse effects in vulnerable individuals.

KEY CLINICAL CONCEPTS

- A range of evidence, from case reports to controlled experimental studies, indicates that clozapine and olanzapine are associated with adverse changes in lipid and glucose metabolism.
- There are cases of glucose dysregulation associated with quetiapine and risperidone in the FDA MedWatch drug monitoring system, but there is a relative paucity of published case reports, observational database analyses, and randomized and nonrandomized observational studies linking these two agents directly to changes in glucose and lipid metabolism.
- There is little to no evidence that aripiprazole and ziprasidone are associated with changes in glucose and lipid metabolism.
- Antipsychotic-associated changes in glucose metabolism are associated with weight gain most of the time (approximately 75%), but some patients (approximately 25%) can develop hyperglycemia independent of weight gain.
- Patients receiving treatment with atypical antipsychotics should have their weight, lipids, glucose, and blood pressure monitored on a regular basis.

References

Amdisen A: Drug-produced obesity: experiences with chlorpromazine, perphenazine and clopenthixol. Dan Med Bull 11:182–189, 1964

American Diabetes Association, American Psychiatric Association, American Association of Clinical Endocrinologists, North American Association for the Study of Obesity: Consensus Development Conference on Antipsychotic Drugs and Obesity and Diabetes. Diabetes Care 27:596–601, 2004

Ananth J, Venkatesh R, Burgoyne K, et al: Atypical antipsychotic drug use and diabetes. Psychother Psychosom 71:244–254, 2002

Atmaca M, Kuloglu M, Ustundag B: Serum leptin and triglyceride levels in patients on treatment with atypical antipsychotics. J Clin Psychiatry 64:598–604, 2003

Azriel Mira S: Uncontrolled hyperglycemia with ketosis associated with olanzapine therapy [in Spanish]. Rev Clin Esp 202:672, 2002

Barak Y: No weight gain among elderly schizophrenia patients after 1 year of risperidone treatment. J Clin Psychiatry 63:117–119, 2002

Barak Y, Shamir E, Weizman R: Would a switch from typical antipsychotics to risperidone be beneficial for elderly schizophrenic patients? A naturalistic, long-term, retrospective, comparative study. J Clin Psychopharmacol 22:115–120, 2002

Bechara CI, Goldman-Levine JD: Dramatic worsening of type 2 diabetes mellitus due to olanzapine after 3 years of therapy. Pharmacotherapy 21:1444–1447, 2001

Beliard S, Valero R, Vialettes B: Atypical neuroleptics and diabetes. Diabetes Metab 29:296–299, 2003

Berry S, Mahmoud R: Improvement of insulin indices after switch from olanzapine to risperidone. Eur Neuropsychopharmacol 12(suppl):316, 2002

Bettinger TL, Mendelson SC, Dorson PG, et al: Olanzapine-induced glucose dysregulation. Ann Pharmacother 34:865–867, 2000

Bonanno DG, Davydov L, Botts SR: Olanzapine-induced diabetes mellitus. Ann Pharmacother 35:563–565, 2001

Breier AP, Berg H, Thakore JH, et al: Olanzapine versus ziprasidone: results of a 28-week double-blind study in patients with schizophrenia. Am J Psychiatry 162:1879–1887, 2005

Buse JB, Cavazzoni P, Hornbuckle K, et al: A retrospective cohort study of diabetes mellitus and antipsychotic treatment in the United States. J Clin Epidemiol 56:164–170, 2003

Caro JJ, Ward A, Levinton C, et al: The risk of diabetes during olanzapine use compared with risperidone use: a retrospective database analysis. J Clin Psychiatry 63:1135–1139, 2002

Casey DE, L'Italien GJ: Metabolic syndrome comparison between olanzapine, aripiprazole, and placebo. Poster presented at the annual meeting of the American Psychiatric Association. San Francisco, CA, May 2003

Casey D, Matchett JL: The effect of antipsychotic drugs in managing diabetes. Int J Neuropsychopharmacol 5(suppl):167, 2002

Casey DE, Haupt DW, Newcomer JW, et al: Antipsychotic-induced weight gain and metabolic abnormalities: implications for increased mortality in patients with schizophrenia. J Clin Psychiatry 65(suppl):4–18, 2004

Chae BJ, Kang BJ: The effect of clozapine on blood glucose metabolism. Hum Psychopharmacol 16:265–271, 2001

Chang HY, Ridky TW, Kimball AB, et al: Eruptive xanthomas associated with olanzapine use. Arch Dermatol 139:1045–1048, 2003

Chue P, Welch R, Lind J: Investigation of the metabolic effects of antipsychotics in patients with schizophrenia. J Eur Coll Neuropsychopharmacol 13 (suppl 4):S300, 2003

Church CO, Stevens DL, Fugate SE: Diabetic ketoacidosis associated with aripiprazole. Diabet Med 22:1440–1443, 2005

Citrome LA, Jaffe A: Antipsychotic medication treatment and new prescriptions for insulin and oral hypoglycemics (NR222), in New Research Program and Abstracts, American Psychiatric Association 156th Annual Meeting, San Francisco, CA, May 17–22, 2003. Washington, DC, American Psychiatric Association, 2003

Citrome L, Jaffe A, Levine J, et al: Relationship between antipsychotic medication treatment and new cases of diabetes among psychiatric inpatients. Psychiatr Serv 55:1006–1013, 2004

Clark M, Dubowski K, Colmore J: The effect of chlorpromazine on serum cholesterol in chronic schizophrenic patients. Clin Pharmacol Ther 11:883–889, 1970

Cohen S, Fitzgerald B, Okos A, et al: Weight, lipids, glucose, and behavioral measures with ziprasidone treatment in a population with mental retardation. J Clin Psychiatry 64: 60–62, 2003

Croarkin PE, Jacobs KM, Bain BK: Diabetic ketoacidosis associated with risperidone treatment (letter). Psychosomatics 41:369–370, 2000

Cuijpers P, Smit F: Excess mortality in depression: a meta-analysis of community studies. J Affect Disord 72:227–236, 2002

DeFronzo RA, Tobin JD, Andres R. Glucose clamp technique: a method for quantifying insulin secretion and resistance. Am J Physiol 237:E214–E223, 1979

Dewan V: Potential risk of diabetes mellitus with the use of atypical antipsychotic medication. Can J Psychiatry 48:351–352, 2003

Domon SE, Cargile CS: Quetiapine-associated hyperglycemia and hypertriglyceridemia. J Am Acad Child Adolesc Psychiatry 41:495–496, 2002

Domon SE, Webber JC: Hyperglycemia and hypertriglyceridemia secondary to olanzapine. J Child Adolesc Psychopharmacol 11:285–288, 2001

Ebenbichler CF, Laimer M, Eder U, et al: Olanzapine induces insulin resistance: results from a prospective study. J Clin Psychiatry 64:1436–1439, 2003

Eder U, Mangweth B, Ebenbichler C, et al: Association of olanzapine-induced weight gain with an increase in body fat. Am J Psychiatry 158:1719–1722, 2001

Farin HM, Abbasi F, Reaven GM: Body mass index and waist circumference correlate to the same degree with insulin-mediated glucose uptake. Metabolism 54:1323–1328, 2005

Farwell W, Stump T, Wang J, et al: Do olanzapine and risperidone cause weight gain and diabetes? Poster presented at the 23rd Collegium Internationale Neuro-Psychopharmacologium Congress, Montreal, Quebec, Canada, June 23–27, 2002

Fertig MK, Brooks VG, Shelton PS, et al: Hyperglycemia associated with olanzapine (letter). J Clin Psychiatry 59:687–689, 1998

Fucetola RJ, Newcomer JW: Influence of oral glucose administration on working memory in schizophrenia. Abstr Soc Neurosci 26:2013, 2000

Fukui H, Murai T: Severe weight gain induced by combination treatment with risperidone and paroxetine. Clin Neuropharmacol 25:269–271, 2002

Fuller MA, Shermock KM, Secic M, et al: Comparative study of the development of diabetes mellitus in patients taking risperidone and olanzapine. Pharmacotherapy 23:1037–1043, 2003

Gallagher D, Ruts E, Visser M, et al: Weight stability masks sarcopenia in elderly men and women. J Physiol Endocrinol Metab 279:E366–375, 2000

Gatta B, Rigalleau V, Gin H: Diabetic ketoacidosis with olanzapine treatment (letter). Diabetes Care 22:1002–1003, 1999

Gianfrancesco FD, Grogg AL, Mahmoud R, et al: Differential effects of risperidone, olanzapine, clozapine and conventional antipsychotics on type 2 diabetes: findings from a large health plan database. J Clin Psychiatry 63:920–930, 2002

Gianfrancesco F, White R, Wang RH, et al: Antipsychotic-induced type 2 diabetes: evidence from a large health plan database. J Clin Psychopharmacol 23:328–335, 2003

Glick ID, Romano SJ: Insulin resistance in olanzapine-and ziprasidone-treated patients: results of a double-blind, controlled 6-week trial. Presentation at the annual meeting of the American Psychiatric Association, New Orleans, LA, May 2001

Goldberg RJ: Weight variance associated with atypical neuroleptics in nursing home dementia patients. J Am Med Dir Assoc 2:26–28, 2001

Goldstein LE, Sporn EJ, Brown S, et al: New-onset diabetes mellitus and diabetic ketoacidosis associated with olanzapine treatment. Psychosomatics 40:438–443, 1999

Grogg AJ, Markowitz J: Risk of diabetes in medical patients prescribed atypical antipsychotics (NR209), in New Research Program and Abstracts, American Psychiatric Association 156th Annual Meeting, San Francisco, CA, May 17–22, 2003. Washington, DC, American Psychiatric Association, 2003

Gupta S, Steinmeyer C, Frank B, et al: Hyperglycemia and hypertriglyceridemia in real world patients on antipsychotic therapy. Am J Ther 10:348–355, 2003

Haffner SM, Miettinen H, Stern MP: The homeostasis model in the San Antonio Heart Study. Diabetes Care 20:1087–1092, 1997

Hardy MI, Flegal KM, Cowie CC, et al: Prevalence of diabetes, impaired fasting glucose, and impaired glucose tolerance in U.S. adults. The Third National Health and Nutrition Examination Survey, 1988–1994. Diabetes Care 21:518–524, 1998

Hardy TA, Poole-Hoffmann V: Fasting glucose and lipid changes in patients with schizophrenia treated with olanzapine or ziprasidone. Poster presented at the 42nd Annual Meeting of the American College of Neuropsychopharmacology, San Juan, Puerto Rico, December 2003

Hardy TA, Earley AW, Marquez E: : Oral glucose tolerance in patients treated with risperidone 20, 30, or 40 mg/day (abstract). Schizophr Res 67(184):abstract #373, 2004

Harris MI, Flegal KM, Cowie CC, et al: Prevalence of diabetes, impaired fasting glucose, and impaired glucose tolerance in U.S. adults. The Third National Health and Nutrition Examination Survey, 1988–1994. Diabetes Care 21(4):518–524, 1998

Haupt DW, Newcomer JW: Hyperglycemia and antipsychotic medications. J Clin Psychiatry 62(suppl):15–26, 2001a

Haupt DW, Newcomer JW: Risperidone-associated diabetic ketoacidosis. Psychosomatics 42:279–280, 2001b

Haupt DW, Newcomer JW: Abnormalities in glucose regulation associated with mental illness and treatment. J Psychosom Res 53:925–933, 2002

Henderson DC, Cagliero E, Gray C, et al: Clozapine, diabetes mellitus, weight gain, and lipid abnormalities: a five-year naturalistic study. Am J Psychiatry 157:975–981, 2000

Henderson DC, Cagliero E, Copeland PM, et al: Glucose metabolism in patients with schizophrenia treated with atypical antipsychotic agents: a frequently sampled intravenous glucose tolerance test and minimal model analysis. Arch Gen Psychiatry 62:19–28, 2005

Houseknecht K, et al: Diabetogenic effects of some atypical antipsychotics: rapid, whole body insulin resistance following a single dose. Diabetologia 48(suppl):A212, 2005

Howes OD, Bhatnagar A, Gaughran FP, et al: A prospective study of impairment in glucose control caused by clozapine without changes in insulin resistance. Am J Psychiatry 161: 361–363, 2004

Kasanin J: The blood sugar curve in mental disease. Arch Neurol Psychiatry 16:414–419, 1926

Keck PE Jr, Marcus R, Tourkodimitris S, et al: A placebo-controlled, double-blind study of the efficacy and safety of aripiprazole in patients with acute bipolar mania. Am J Psychiatry 160:1651–1658, 2003

Kemner C, Willemsen-Swinkels SH, de Jonge M, et al: Open-label study of olanzapine in children with pervasive developmental disorder. J Clin Psychopharmacol 22:455–460, 2002

Kingsbury SJ, Fayek M, Trufasiu D, et al: The apparent effects of ziprasidone on plasma lipids and glucose. J Clin Psychiatry 62:347–349, 2001

Koller EA, Doraiswamy PM: Olanzapine-associated diabetes mellitus. Pharmacotherapy 22:841–852, 2002

Koller E, Schneider B, Bennett K, et al: Clozapine-associated diabetes. Am J Med 111:716–723, 2001

Koller EA, Cross JT, Doraiswamy PM, et al: Risperidone-associated diabetes mellitus: a pharmacovigilance study. Pharmacotherapy 23:735–744, 2003

Koller EA, Weber J, Doraiswamy PM, et al: A survey of reports of quetiapine-associated hyperglycemia and diabetes mellitus. J Clin Psychiatry 65:857–863, 2004

Koro CE, Fedder DO, L'Italien GJ, et al: Assessment of independent effect of olanzapine and risperidone on risk of diabetes among patients with schizophrenia: population based nested case-control study. BMJ 325:243, 2002

Kozian R: Olanzapine-induced diabetes mellitus. Psychiatr Prax 29:318–320, 2002

Kroeze WK, Hufeisen SJ, Popadak BA, et al: H1-histamine receptor affinity predicts short-term weight gain for atypical antipsychotic drugs. Neuropsychopharmacology 28:519–526, 2003

Kropp S, Emrich HM, Bleich S, et al: Olanzapine-related hyperglycemia in a nondiabetic woman. Can J Psychiatry 46:457, 2001

Kurt E, Oral ET: Antipsychotics and glucose, insulin, lipids, prolactin, uric acid metabolism in schizophrenia. Eur Neuropsychopharmacol 12(suppl):276, 2002

Lambert BL, Chou CH, Chang KY, et al: Antipsychotic exposure and type 2 diabetes among patients with schizophrenia: a matched case-control study of California Medicaid claims. Pharmacoepidemiol Drug Saf 14:417–425, 2005

Leslie DL, Rosenheck RA: Incidence of newly diagnosed diabetes attributable to atypical antipsychotic medications. Am J Psychiatry 161:1709–1711, 2004

Lieberman JA, Stroup TS, McEvoy JP, et al: Effectiveness of antipsychotic drugs in patients with chronic schizophrenia. N Engl J Med 353:1209–1223, 2005

Lillioja S, Mott DM, Zawadzki JK, et al: In vivo insulin action is familial characteristic in nondiabetic Pima Indians. Diabetes 36:1329–1335, 1987

Lindenmayer JP, Patel R: Olanzapine-induced ketoacidosis with diabetes mellitus (letter). Am J Psychiatry 156:1471, 1999

Lindenmayer JP, Czobor P, Volavka J, et al: Changes in glucose and cholesterol levels in patients with schizophrenia treated with typical or atypical antipsychotics. Am J Psychiatry 160:290–296, 2003

L'Italien GJ: Pharmacoeconomic impact of antipsychotic-induced metabolic events. Am J Manag Care 3:38–42, 2003

Litman R, Peterson SW: Glucose metabolism, lipid levels, and body mass indices in olanzapine-treated schizophrenia patients before and after switching to risperidone: a prospective trial. Int J Neuropsychopharmacol 5(suppl):170, 2002

Lund BC, Perry PJ, Brooks JM, et al: Clozapine use in patients with schizophrenia and the risk of diabetes, hyperlipidemia, and hypertension: a claims-based approach. Arch Gen Psychiatry 58:1172–1176, 2001

Mallya A, Chawla P, Boyer SK, et al: Resolution of hyperglycemia on risperidone discontinuation: a case report. J Clin Psychiatry 63:453–454, 2002

Malyuk R, Gibson B, Procyshyn RM, et al: Olanzapine associated weight gain, hyperglycemia and neuroleptic malignant syndrome: case report. Int J Geriatr Psychiatry 17:326–328, 2002

Marder SR, McQuade RD, Stock E, et al: Aripiprazole in the treatment of schizophrenia: safety and tolerability in short-term, placebo-controlled trials. Schizophr Res 61:123–136, 2003

Marder SR, Essock SM, Miller AL, et al: Physical health monitoring of patients with schizophrenia. Am J Psychiatry 161:1334–1349, 2004

Matthews DR, Hosker JP, Rudenski AS, et al: Homeostasis model assessment: insulin resistance and beta-cell function from fasting plasma glucose and insulin concentrations in man. Diabetologia 28:412–419, 1985

McEvoy JP, Meyer JM, Goff DC, et al: Prevalence of the metabolic syndrome in patients with schizophrenia: baseline results from the Clinical Antipsychotic Trials of Intervention Effectiveness (CATIE) schizophrenia trial and comparison with national estimates from NHANES III. Schizophr Res 80:19–32, 2005

McLaughlin T, Abbasi F, Cheal K, et al: Use of metabolic markers to identify overweight individuals who are insulin resistant. Ann Intern Med 139:802–809, 2003

McQuade RD, Jody D: Long-term weight effects of aripiprazole versus olanzapine. Poster presented at the annual meeting of the American Psychiatric Association, San Francisco, CA, May 2003

McQuade RD, Stock E, Marcus R, et al: A comparison of weight change during treatment with olanzapine or aripiprazole: results from a randomized, double-blind study. J Clin Psychiatry 65(suppl):47–56, 2004

Meatherall R, Younes J: Fatality from olanzapine induced hyperglycemia. J Forensic Sci 47: 893–896, 2002

Melkersson KI, Dahl ML: Relationship between levels of insulin or triglycerides and serum concentrations of the atypical antipsychotics clozapine and olanzapine in patients on treatment with therapeutic doses. Psychopharmacology (Berl) 170:157–166, 2003

Melkersson KI, Hulting AL: Insulin and leptin levels in patients with schizophrenia or related psychoses: a comparison between different antipsychotic agents. Psychopharmacol (Berl) 154:205–212, 2001

Melkersson K, Hulting AL: Recovery from new-onset diabetes in a schizophrenic man after withdrawal of olanzapine. Psychosomatics 43:67–70, 2002

Melkersson KI, Hulting AL, Brismar KE: Different influences of classical antipsychotics and clozapine on glucose-insulin homeostasis in patients with schizophrenia or related psychoses. J Clin Psychiatry 60:783–791, 1999

Melkersson KI, Hulting AL, Brismar KE: Elevated levels of insulin, leptin, and blood lipids in olanzapine-treated patients with schizophrenia or related psychoses. J Clin Psychiatry 61:742–749, 2000

Meyer JM: A retrospective comparison of weight, lipid, and glucose changes between risperidone- and olanzapine-treated inpatients: metabolic outcomes after 1 year. J Clin Psychiatry 63:425–433, 2002

Montague CT, O'Rahilly S: The perils of portliness: causes and consequences of visceral adiposity. Diabetes 49:883–888, 2000

Muench J, Carey M: Diabetes mellitus associated with atypical antipsychotic medications: new case report and review of the literature. J Am Board Fam Pract 14:278–282, 2001

Newcomer JW: Second-generation (atypical) antipsychotics and metabolic effects: a comprehensive literature review. CNS Drugs 19(suppl):1–93, 2005

Newcomer JW, Rasgon N: Insulin resistance and metabolic risk during antipsychotic treatment. Presentation at the annual meeting of the American Psychiatric Association, Atlanta, GA, May 2005

Newcomer JW, Haupt DW, Fucetola R, et al: Abnormalities in glucose regulation during antipsychotic treatment of schizophrenia. Arch Gen Psychiatry 59:337–345, 2002

Ober SK, Hudak R, Rusterholtz A: Hyperglycemia and olanzapine (letter). Am J Psychiatry 156:970, 1999

Ollendorf DA, Joyce AT, Rucker M: Rate of new-onset diabetes among patients treated with atypical or conventional antipsychotic medications for schizophrenia. Med Gen Med 6:5, 2004

Opp D, Hildebrandt C: Olanzapine-associated type 2 diabetes mellitus. Schizophr Res 56:195–196, 2002

Pigott TA, Carson WH, Saha AR, et al: Aripiprazole for the prevention of relapse in stabilized patients with chronic schizophrenia: a placebo-controlled 26-week study. J Clin Psychiatry 64:1048–1056, 2003

Procyshyn RM, Pande S, Tse G: New-onset diabetes mellitus associated with quetiapine (letter). Can J Psychiatry 45:668–669, 2000

Ragucci KR, Wells BJ: Olanzapine-induced diabetic ketoacidosis. Ann Pharmacother 35:1556–1558, 2001

Ramankutty G: Olanzapine-induced destabilization of diabetes in the absence of weight gain. Acta Psychiatr Scand 105:235–237, 2002

Reaven G: Syndrome X: 10 years after. Drugs 58(suppl):19–20, 1999

Resnick HE, Valsania P, Halter JB, et al: Differential effects of BMI on diabetes risk among black and white Americans. Diabetes Care 21:1828–1835, 1998

Rettenbacher MA, Hummer M, Fleischhacker WW, et al: Transient hyperproinsulinemia during treatment with clozapine and amisulpride. J Clin Psychiatry 65:878–879, 2004

Reynolds GP: Metabolic syndrome and schizophrenia. Br J Psychiatry 188:86–87, 2006

Reynolds GP, Zhang ZJ, Zhang XB: Association of antipsychotic drug-induced weight gain with a 5-HT2C receptor gene polymorphism. Lancet 359:2086–2087, 2002

Riccitelli G, Baker N: Weight gain and hyperglycemia associated with olanzapine. Aust N Z J Psychiatry 36:270–271, 2002

Rigalleau V, Gatta B, Bonnaud S, et al: Diabetes as a result of atypical antipsychotic drugs: a report of three cases. Diabet Med 17:484–486, 2000

Roefaro J, Mukherjee SM: Olanzapine-induced hyperglycemic nonketonic coma. Ann Pharmacother 35:300–302, 2001

Rojas P, Arancibia P, Bravo V, et al: Diabetes mellitus induced by olanzapine: a case report. Rev Med Chil 129:1183–1185, 2001

Rosenthal M, Haskell WL, Solomon R, et al: Demonstration of a relationship between level of physical training and insulin-stimulated glucose utilization in normal humans. Diabetes 32:408–411, 1983

Rubio G, Gomez de la Camara A: The risk of developing diabetes in users of atypical antipsychotics: a feasibility pilot study. Int J Neuropsychopharmacol 5(suppl):168, 2002

Ryan MC, Collins P, Thakore JH: Impaired fasting glucose tolerance in first-episode, drug-naïve patients with schizophrenia. Am J Psychiatry 160:284–289, 2003

Seaburg HL, McLendon BM, Doraiswamy PM: Olanzapine-associated severe hyperglycemia, ketonuria, and acidosis: case report and review of literature. Pharmacotherapy 21:1448–1454, 2001

Selva KA, Scott SM: Diabetic ketoacidosis associated with olanzapine in an adolescent patient. J Pediatr 138:936–938, 2001

Sernyak MJ, Leslie DL, Alarcon RD, et al: Association of diabetes mellitus with use of atypical neuroleptics in the treatment of schizophrenia. Am J Psychiatry 159:561–566, 2002

Sernyak MJ, Gulanski B, Leslie DL, et al: Undiagnosed hyperglycemia in clozapine-treated patients with schizophrenia. J Clin Psychiatry 64:605–608, 2003

Sikich L, Hamer RM, Bashford RA, et al: A pilot study of risperidone, olanzapine, and haloperidol in psychotic youth: a double-blind, randomized, 8-week trial. Neuropsychopharmacology 29:133–145, 2004

Simpson G, Weiden P: Ziprasidone vs olanzapine in schizophrenia: 6-month continuation study. Eur Neuropsychopharmacol 12(suppl):310, 2002

Sneed KB, Gonzalez EC: Type 2 diabetes mellitus induced by an atypical antipsychotic medication. J Am Board Fam Pract 16:251–254, 2003

Sobel M, Jaggers ED, Franz MA: New-onset diabetes mellitus associated with the initiation of quetiapine treatment (letter). J Clin Psychiatry 60:556–557, 1999

Sowell M, Mukhopadhyay N, Cavazzoni P, et al: Hyperglycemic clamp assessment of insulin secretory responses in normal subjects treated with olanzapine, risperidone, or placebo. J Clin Endocrinol Metab 87:2918–2923, 2002

Sowell M, Mukhopadhyay N, Cavazzoni P, et al: Evaluation of insulin sensitivity in healthy volunteers treated with olanzapine, risperidone, or placebo: a prospective, randomized study using the two-step hyperinsulinemic, euglycemic clamp. J Clin Endocrinol Metab 88:5875–5880, 2003

Straker D, Mendelowitz A, Karlin L: Near fatal ketoacidosis with olanzapine treatment. Psychosomatics 43:339–340, 2002

Su KP, Wu PL, Pariante CM: A crossover study on lipid and weight changes associated with olanzapine and risperidone. Psychopharmacology (Berl) 183:383–386, 2005

Sumiyoshi T, Roy A, Anil AE, et al: A comparison of incidence of diabetes mellitus between atypical antipsychotic drugs: a survey for clozapine, risperidone, olanzapine, and quetiapine. J Clin Psychopharmacol 24:345–348, 2004

Tavakoli SA, Arguisola MS: Diabetic ketoacidosis in a patient treated with olanzapine, valproic acid, and venlafaxine. South Med J 96:729–730, 2003

Thakore JH: Metabolic syndrome and schizophrenia. Br J Psychiatry 186:455–456, 2005

Thonnard-Neumann E: Phenothiazines and diabetes in hospitalized women. Am J Psychiatry 124:978–982, 1968

Torrey EF, Swalwell CI: Fatal olanzapine-induced ketoacidosis. Am J Psychiatry 160:2241, 2003

Visser M, Pahor M, Tylavsky F, et al: One-and two year change in body composition as measured by DXA in a population-based cohort of older men and women. J Appl Physiol 94:2368–2374, 2003

Von Hayek D, Huttl V, Reiss J, et al: Hyperglycemia and ketoacidosis associated with olanzapine. Nervenarzt 70:836–837, 1999

Wang PS, Glynn RJ, Ganz DA, et al: Clozapine use and risk of diabetes mellitus. J Clin Psychopharmacol 22:236–243, 2002

Wilson DR, D'Souza L, Sarkar N, et al: New-onset diabetes and ketoacidosis with atypical antipsychotics. Schizophr Res 59:1–6, 2003

Wirshing DA, Spellberg BJ, Erhart SM, et al: Novel antipsychotics and new onset diabetes. Biol Psychiatry 44:778–783, 1998

Wirshing DA, Pierre JM, Eyeler J, et al: Risperidone-associated new-onset diabetes. Biol Psychiatry 50:148–149, 2001

Wirshing DA, Boyd JA, Meng LR, et al: The effects of novel antipsychotics on glucose and lipid levels. J Clin Psychiatry 63:856–865, 2002

Yang SH, McNeely MJ: Rhabdomyolysis, pancreatitis, and hyperglycemia with ziprasidone. Am J Psychiatry 159:1435, 2002

Yazici KM, Erbas T, Yazici AH: The effect of clozapine on glucose metabolism. Exp Clin Endocrinol Diabetes 106:475–477, 1998

Zajecka JM, Weisler R, Sachs G, et al: A comparison of the efficacy, safety, and tolerability of divalproex sodium and olanzapine in the treatment of bipolar disorder. J Clin Psychiatry 63:1148–1155, 2002

Zhang ZJ, Yao ZJ, Liu W, et al: Effects of antipsychotics on fat deposition and changes in leptin and insulin levels: magnetic resonance imaging study of previously untreated people with schizophrenia. Br J Psychiatry 184:58–62, 2004

Chapter 8

SERUM LIPIDS

Effects of Antipsychotics

Jonathan M. Meyer, M.D.

Patients with severe mental illnesses, such as bipolar disorder and schizophrenia, are a medically vulnerable population at high risk for cardiovascular mortality, with standardized mortality ratios from cardiovascular disease two times greater than the general population (Osby et al. 2000, 2001). Much of psychiatric care is focused on suicide prevention, yet cardiovascular disease remains the single largest cause of death among males and females with schizophrenia.

Given this sobering data, it is imperative that those who care for the severely mentally ill have a working knowledge of the risks associated with cardiovascular disease, and the patterns of risk factors seen in this patient population. Recognition and treatment of diabetes mellitus has been covered elsewhere in this volume (see Chapter 1, "Diabetes: An Overview," and Chapter 4, "Severe Mental Illness and Diabetes Mellitus," this volume), but the importance of diabetes relates not only to the adverse effects of hyperglycemia but also to its impact on cardiovascular risk. Diabetes mellitus is now a condition considered equivalent in future risk for major cardiovascular events (e.g., myocardial infarction [MI], sudden death) to having established coronary heart disease (CHD) (Expert Panel on Detection, Evaluation, and Treatment of High Blood Cholesterol in Adults 2001). This view of diabetes-related CHD risk is based on data that show patients with established diabetes have the same future MI incidence as patients without diabetes who have had an MI (Haffner et al. 1998).

239

For nondiabetic persons, the focus remains on modifying the traditional risk factors of hypertension, hyperlipidemia, and smoking. Baseline data from the Clinical Antipsychotic Trials of Intervention Effectiveness (CATIE) study provide the most timely and complete picture of the risk patterns in chronic schizophrenia patients residing in the United States (Goff et al. 2005). Among the 1,460 schizophrenia patients assessed upon study entry, 10-year CHD risk, calculated by using Framingham scores, was significantly elevated in males (9.4% vs. 7.0%) and females (6.3% vs. 4.2%), with schizophrenia patients compared with age-, gender-, and race/ethnicity-matched control subjects from a general population database ($P=0.0001$). In particular, schizophrenia patients had significantly higher rates of smoking (68% vs. 35%), diabetes (13% vs. 3%), and hypertension (27% vs. 17%) and lower high-density lipoprotein (HDL) cholesterol levels (43.7 vs. 49.3 mg/dL) compared with control subjects ($P<0.001$). Moreover, CATIE subjects also had greater prevalence of central adiposity and elevated serum triglycerides, both of which are components of the metabolic syndrome and are associated with insulin resistance and future diabetes risk (McEvoy et al. 2005). The importance of monitoring serum triglyceride values during antipsychotic treatment will become readily apparent, because this is the lipid parameter most greatly affected by offending medications.

Induction of hyperlipidemia during antipsychotic therapy thus represents a serious condition not only because of its inherent impact on cardiovascular risk but also because it is occurring in a group that possesses considerable risk (Saari et al. 2004). What has become evident in recent years is that the atypical antipsychotics have a decreased liability for neurological side effects, but certain agents in this class have a marked propensity for adverse metabolic outcomes, especially hyperlipidemia (Meyer and Koro 2004). Given the widespread use of atypical antipsychotics for disorders beyond schizophrenia and bipolar disorder, this review is intended to guide the clinician in choice of medications and appropriate monitoring strategies for hyperlipidemia, presenting the best available data. This discussion is bolstered by the recent publication of the double-blind, controlled data from Phases I and II of the CATIE Schizophrenia Trial (Lieberman et al. 2005; Stroup et al. 2006). The large population under study in the CATIE study is one of the best sources of prospective information for certain compounds, especially quetiapine, for which prospective data were sorely lacking.

There is increased interest in improving medical outcomes for severely mentally ill patients (Marder et al. 2004; Meyer et al. 2006), so minimization of iatrogenically induced lipid problems and appropriate monitoring of those at risk are increasingly becoming the standards of care for this patient population. Recognition of which antipsychotics impose the greatest risk for hyperlipidemia and an understanding of the common dyslipidemia patterns seen during use of these antipsychotics are necessities for providing high-quality care to antipsychotic-treated patients.

Hyperlipidemia and Typical Antipsychotics

Typical antipsychotics are used in the treatment of only 5%–10% of schizophrenia patients in the United States but are commonly available throughout the world and represent an important class of psychotropic medications. Moreover, a review of the lipid effects of typical antipsychotics illustrates an important concept seen in the atypical antipsychotic data: medications with similar modes of therapeutic action can have disparate metabolic profiles. Within a decade after the widespread use of chlorpromazine and other low-potency phenothiazines, several studies emerged examining the metabolic profiles of this class of antipsychotics (Clark and Johnson 1960; Clark et al. 1967; Mefferd et al. 1958). In general, these compounds were found to elevate serum triglycerides and total cholesterol, but with greater effects on triglyceride concentrations. Subsequent studies of the phenothiazine chlorpromazine and related compounds in 1970 and 1972 by Clark et al. (1970, 1972) confirmed these findings that high serum triglycerides seemed to be the primary significant lipid abnormality, but elevated total cholesterol could also be found. What also emerged from this early literature was the fact that not all dopamine D_2 receptor antagonists had similar lipid effects as the phenothiazine class.

The lipid neutrality of high-potency typical antipsychotics was seen in the early uncontrolled studies of butyrophenone derivatives published in the mid-1960s (Braun and Paulonis 1967; Clark et al. 1968; Simpson and Cooper 1966; Simpson et al. 1967) and a placebo-controlled trial in 1971 (Serafetinides et al. 1971). Comparative trials of low-potency phenothiazines and butyrophenones (primarily haloperidol) published in the 1970s confirmed the lipid neutrality of high-potency agents, whereas low-potency phenothiazine treatment was associated with hyperlipidemia, primarily in the form of hypertriglyceridemia (Serafetinides et al. 1972; Vaisanen et al. 1979).

Surprisingly, there has been only a limited amount of work published since that time covering lipid changes during typical antipsychotic therapy. The appendix to this chapter summarizes studies, case reports, and case series related to lipids and antipsychotics that have been published from 1984 onward and demonstrates the paucity of controlled data on typical antipsychotics after 1980. Two papers were published by a Japanese group in 1984 and 1985 that analyzed serum total cholesterol and triglycerides in male chronic schizophrenia inpatients receiving phenothiazines or butyrophenones who were compared with age- and sex-matched control subjects (Sasaki et al. 1984, 1985). The cohort exposed to phenothiazines had mean serum triglyceride of 163 mg/dL compared with 104 mg/dL for the butyrophenone group and 127 mg/dL for control subjects, with no significant differences in total cholesterol between the three groups. The phenothiazine cohort also had higher serum low-density lipoprotein (LDL) cholesterol, and decreased HDL cholesterol concentrations compared with the other study arms. Cross-sectional studies from Pakistan (Shafique et al. 1988) and a psychiatric hospital in Spain (Martinez et al. 1994) substantiated earlier findings, although specific analysis on the basis of type of neuroleptic prescribed was not performed in the Spanish study. Last, the CATIE Schizophrenia Trial employed a medium-potency phenothiazine, perphenazine, as one of its treatment arms in Phase I, thus providing controlled comparative data versus atypical antipsychotics in a randomized, double-blind study (Lieberman et al. 2005). As shown in Table 8–1, use of perphenazine was associated with modest increases in serum triglycerides and total cholesterol, with a greater effect on triglycerides. The extent of lipid changes related to perphenazine use in neuroleptic-naïve patients might actually be greater than seen in CATIE Phase I, because 22% of the CATIE sample at baseline was taking olanzapine. Given olanzapine's known effects on serum lipids, olanzapine-exposed patients switched to perphenazine in Phase I would likely have minimal further increases in serum triglycerides. Further analyses of the CATIE Phase I data set will provide more definitive answers about the effect of switching to perphenazine from more lipid-neutral agents. With the increasing use of atypical antipsychotics throughout the world, this may be the last randomized, controlled data on the lipid effects of a typical antipsychotic published.

Hyperlipidemia and Atypical Antipsychotics

Atypical antipsychotics have been primarily designed to mimic the identifiable features of clozapine's pharmacology: weaker dopamine D_2 antagonism than typical antipsychotics combined with potent serotonin 5-HT_{2A} antagonism (Meyer and Simpson 1997). A recurring theme related to the metabolic effects of this antipsychotic class echoes the earlier findings for typical agents, namely, that drugs with similar mechanisms of action may have disparate metabolic adverse effects. This analogy is more than superficial, because the structurally related dibenzodiazepine-derived atypicals (clozapine, olanzapine, and quetiapine) all appear to have significantly greater effects on serum triglycerides than on total cholesterol, much as do the low-potency phenothiazines, whereas other atypicals (risperidone, ziprasidone, and aripiprazole) have minimal lipid effects, as do the high-potency typical antipsychotics.

CLOZAPINE

Through 2002 there were virtually no randomized, prospective, controlled data on the lipid effects of the atypical antipsychotics, so the early literature is replete with case reports and retrospective studies, primarily focused on clozapine, the only atypical antipsychotic available until 1994. The first reports of hyperlipidemia with atypical antipsychotics were small studies of fluperlapine, a dibenzodiazepine-derived compound never marketed. Two trial reports published in the mid-1980s documented elevated triglycerides, in one case as high as 900 mg/dL (Fleis-

TABLE 8–1. Mean exposure-adjusted lipid changes for Clinical Antipsychotic Trials of Intervention Effectiveness (CATIE) Schizophrenia Trial Phases I, IIa, and IIb

	Clozapine	Olanzapine	Quetiapine	Risperidone	Perphenazine	Ziprasidone
Cholesterol (mg/dL)						
Phase I, mean ± SE (n=1,460)	—	9.4 ± 2.4	6.6 ± 2.4	−1.3 ± 2.4	1.5 ± 2.7	−8.2 ± 3.2
Phase IIa, mean ± SE (n=444)	—	17.5 ± 5.2	6.5 ± 5.3	−3.1 ± 5.2	—	−10.7 ± 5.1
Phase IIb, mean ± SE (n=99)[a]	5.9 ± 4.7	1.0 ± 7.1	−11.0 ± 8.1	7.4 ± 8.7	—	—
Triglycerides (mg/dL)						
Phase I, mean ± SE (n=1,460)	—	40.5 ± 8.9	21.2 ± 9.6	−2.4 ± 9.1	9.2 ± 10.1	−16.5 ± 12.2
Phase IIa, mean ± SE (n=444)	—	94.1 ± 21.8	39.3 ± 22.1	−5.2 ± 21.6	—	−3.5 ± 20.9
Phase IIb, mean ± SE (n=99)[a]	43.8 ± 21.2	−5.3 ± 32.0	7.1 ± 36.2	30.0 ± 39.0	—	—

[a]Blood chemistry change from Phase II baseline to average of two largest values.

chhacker et al. 1986; Muller-Oerlinghausen 1984). Despite clozapine's use from the 1960s onward, the first case report of hyperlipidemia (presenting as hyper-triglyceridemia) occurred in 1994 (Vampini et al. 1994) and was followed in 1995 by a report of four clozapine-treated patients with hypertriglyceridemia whose triglycerides normalized upon switching to risperidone (Ghaeli and Dufresne 1995). The following year the authors of that case series published a chart review comparing serum lipids in patients exposed to clozapine or typical antipsychotics (primarily butyrophenones) for at least 1 year with no prior history of hyper-lipidemia or use of lipid-lowering agents (Ghaeli and Dufresne 1996). This retro-spective study found serum triglycerides 114 mg/dL higher in the clozapine cohort ($P<0.001$), but nearly identical total cholesterol levels: clozapine = 217.0 ± 52.9 mg/dL versus typicals = 215.0 ± 43.2 mg/dL. A 1998 study comparing 30 patients taking clozapine with 30 taking typical antipsychotics for at least 1 year also found higher triglyceride levels in the clozapine group (202.9 ± 131.1 mg/dL) compared with the typicals group (134.4 ± 51.9 mg/dL), but again without significant differ-ences in total cholesterol (clozapine = 197.1 ± 46.4 mg/dL vs. typicals = 194.9 ± 51.5 mg/dL) (Spivak et al. 1998). A small, prospective study (Dursun et al. 1999) and two subsequent chart reviews of long-term clozapine-treated patients, one with 70 patients (Spivak et al. 1999) and the other with 222 patients (Gaulin et al. 1999), demonstrated that the mean increase in serum triglycerides ranged from 11% to 45%.

More recent cross-sectional and short- and long-term prospective clozapine studies have noted the same pattern of marked elevations of serum triglycerides with modest increases in total cholesterol (Atmaca et al. 2003a; Baymiller et al. 2003; Henderson et al. 2000; Leonard et al. 2002; Wirshing et al. 2002) com-pared with baseline and with those receiving typical antipsychotics (Lund et al. 2001). A 1-year prospective study of 50 clozapine-treated patients (Baymiller et al. 2003) found mean increases of 41.7% in serum triglycerides, exactly in the range predicted by prior retrospective data, and only a 7.5% increase in total cho-lesterol. The authors also noted no significant changes in HDL and LDL and that triglyceride elevations peaked between days 41 and 120 and then declined but still remained elevated at the 1-year interval. As part of a 5-year naturalistic study of 82 clozapine-treated patients with schizophrenia, Henderson et al. (2000) found ongoing increases in serum triglycerides (linear coefficient 2.75 mg/dL per month; $P=0.04$). A subsequent 10-year follow-up study of clozapine-treated patients found that triglyceride levels had plateaued significantly, with the linear coeffi-cient over that time frame now 0.5 mg/dL/month ($P=0.04$) (Henderson et al. 2005). In neither study were total cholesterol changes significant.

There are other cross-sectional, retrospective and other nonprospective cloza-pine studies noted in the appendix to this chapter, but the recently published "nonresponse" portion of the CATIE Phase II (hereafter referred to as Phase IIb), generated prospective randomized data on a sample of 49 schizophrenia patients compared with 50 subjects assigned to other agents (McEvoy et al. 2006). As seen in Table 8–1, the exposure-adjusted mean increases in serum lipids for clozapine-treated subjects were greatest for triglycerides and substantially less for total cholesterol. The samples for each of the other Phase IIb drug arms are extremely small (<15), so the findings for the other atypicals in Phase IIb are of limited reliability.

OLANZAPINE

The first published studies of olanzapine-associated hypertriglyceridemia appeared in 1999 and revealed patterns of dyslipidemia similar to those reported for clozapine. A study of nine patients receiving olanzapine who were followed for an average of 16 months (mean age=41 years; mean olanzapine dosage=19 mg/day), showed a mean increase in serum triglycerides of 41%, with no significant changes in total cholesterol levels and a mean weight gain of 22 lb (Sheitman et al. 1999). A subsequent report on 25 inpatients followed prospectively for 12 weeks found a mean fasting triglyceride increase of 37%. Both weight and triglyceride increases were significant ($P<0.05$), and there was a significant association between weight gain and triglyceride changes ($P<0.02$); however, after controlling for baseline weight, analysis of covariance showed no independent increase in triglycerides (Osser et al. 1999).

More recent work involving olanzapine illustrates not only its much greater effect on serum triglycerides than on total cholesterol but also the risk of severe hypertriglyceridemia. Melkersson et al. (2000) followed a group of 14 schizophrenia patients receiving olanzapine monotherapy for an average of 5 months and noted that 62% had elevated fasting triglyceride level (mean=273.45 mg/dL) and 85% exhibited hypercholesterolemia (mean=257.14 mg/dL). Although these lipid changes were comparable with those reported for clozapine, the issue of severe hypertriglyceridemia was noted in Meyer's (2001b) case series of 12 olanzapine and 2 quetiapine patients with fasting triglyceride levels exceeding 500 mg/dL, including 1 patient taking olanzapine whose fasting serum triglyceride level was measured at 7,688 mg/dL and a subsequent case of olanzapine-associated severe hypertriglyceridemia (triglyceride level=5,093 mg/dL) reported by Stoner et al. (2002) in a patient who also developed new-onset type 2 diabetes mellitus (T2DM). As is discussed later in the chapter, one concern with serum triglyceride levels of 1,000 mg/dL or greater is the development of acute pancreatitis, with the majority of cases associated with atypical antipsychotic treatment related to olanzapine or clozapine exposure (Koller et al. 2003).

The cases of severe hypertriglyceridemia noted above are extreme findings, but the majority of studies published since 2002 have confirmed the greater effects of olanzapine on serum lipids, primarily on triglycerides, compared with more lipid-neutral medications, such as high-potency typicals or risperidone, ziprasidone, and aripiprazole. The earlier comparative literature was composed of retrospective, cross-sectional, or small prospective studies but confirmed the greater effects of olanzapine on serum lipids compared with other atypical antipsychotic medications (with the exception of clozapine) (Atmaca et al. 2003a, 2003b; Bouchard et al. 2001; Garyfallos et al. 2003; Kinon et al. 2001, 2004; Meyer 2002; Wirshing et al. 2002). There were also two retrospective, large-database studies performed using data from the England and Wales–based General Practice Research Database (Koro et al. 2002) or the state of California's Medi-Cal claims system (Lambert et al. 2005). Koro et al.'s (2002) case-control study of 18,309 schizophrenia patients, with 1,268 incident cases of hyperlipidemia, compared typical antipsychotics, risperidone, and olanzapine with no antipsychotic usage and found that risperidone was not associated with increased odds of hyperlipidemia compared with typicals or no antipsychotic exposure, whereas olanzapine use was associated with nearly a fivefold increase compared with no antipsychotic exposure and more than a threefold increase compared with those receiving typicals. Lambert et al.'s (2005) case-control study of Medi-Cal claims after schizophrenia diagnosis in those receiving antipsychotic monotherapy within 12 weeks prior to hyperlipidemia claim found greater risk for olanzapine compared with typicals or risperidone. Increasing the exposure window to 24 or 52 weeks did not affect the results.

One of the more recently published cross-sectional studies is noteworthy because other lipid parameters were studied besides triglyceride level and total cholesterol. The cross-sectional study by Almeras et al. (2004) of male schizophrenia patients in Quebec, Canada, examined only patients treated with olanzapine (n=42) or risperidone (n=45) for more than 6 months and compared the results of a comprehensive lipid panel with those from a reference group of non-diabetic males (mean ages=28.4 years for risperidone, 31.7 years for olanzapine, 32.8 years for control subjects). The olanzapine-treated cohort had significantly higher serum cholesterol, LDL, triglycerides, cholesterol-to-HDL ratio, and apolipoprotein B and significantly lower HDL, smaller LDL peak particle size, and lower apolipoprotein A₁. Interestingly, compared with the control group, the olanzapine subjects had no significant differences in total cholesterol, triglycerides, or LDL, but they did have lower HDL and a higher cholesterol-to-HDL ratio. Also, the risperidone cohort had lower total cholesterol and LDL but lower HDL than the reference group.

Given the modest sizes of the early prospective literature and the uncontrolled nature of many retrospective studies, questions were raised about the extent to which olanzapine induces greater dyslipidemia than risperidone. Phases I and IIa of the CATIE Schizophrenia Trial provided an answer, as shown in Table 8–1. This large, randomized study demonstrated convincingly that olanzapine is one of the greatest offending agents with respect to its effects on serum lipids, again mostly on serum triglycerides, whereas both risperidone and ziprasidone appear neutral. Phase IIa is likely more reflective of the true extent of olanzapine's effects, because the CATIE trial design mandated that those who entered that arm of the trial not be exposed to an agent to which they had been randomized in Phase I. Thus all of the subjects in the olanzapine arm of Phase IIa were new to that medication. This fact explains why the triglyceride increase in Phase IIa olanzapine subjects was 94.1 mg/dL compared with only a 40.5-mg/dL increase seen in the Phase I olanzapine cohort, 22% of which were taking olanzapine at study baseline. The differential impact of olanzapine compared with other agents can also be seen in switch studies (Meyer et al. 2005; Su et al. 2005).

Institutionalized populations may see lesser metabolic effects, as seen in a switch study of developmentally disabled adults (McKee et al. 2005) and two studies of olanzapine in elderly inpatient populations, one with schizophrenia or schizoaffective disorder (Barak and Aizenberg 2003) and the other for dementia of the Alzheimer type with behavioral disturbances or psychosis (De Deyn et al. 2004). For the latter two studies in particular, what is not known is whether subject age or being confined with a fixed dietary regimen mitigates the development of dyslipidemia.

QUETIAPINE

Quetiapine and zotepine are structurally related to the other dibenzodiazepine-derived antipsychotics clozapine and olanzapine, but there is limited published information on their metabolic effects. The extent of available information was so sparse that the American Diabetes Association (ADA)/American Psychiatric Association (APA) consensus paper on the metabolic effects of atypicals was unclear as to whether quetiapine could be differentiated from risperidone in its effects on serum lipids (American Diabetes Association et al. 2004). Unlike clozapine and olanzapine, quetiapine generally has a much lower risk of significant weight gain (Lieberman et al. 2005; Wetterling 2001). Nonetheless, the available data suggest that quetiapine shares the propensity of other benzodiazepine-derived atypical antipsychotics to elevate serum triglyceride levels, as illustrated by case reports from Meyer (2001b) and others as well as two 6-week prospective comparative studies by Atmaca et al. (2003a, 2003b) and an 8-week study by Shaw et al. (2001) (see also Domon and Cargile 2002). As with other dibenzodiazepine-derived atypicals, there were lesser effects on total cholesterol (Shaw et al. 2001). The extent of the lipid effects were best seen in the CATIE trials (Lieberman et al. 2005; Stroup et al. 2006), especially Phase IIa, in which quetiapine's nearly 40-mg/dL elevation in serum triglycerides was second only to olanzapine and more than the elevations caused by risperidone or ziprasidone, despite weight gain being only marginally greater than for risperidone.

Zotepine is associated with weight gain similar to that experienced with olanzapine and clozapine (Wetterling 2001), but the sum total of the published literature on lipid changes during zotepine therapy is one case report, in which serum triglycerides peaked at 1,247 mg/dL and normalized upon switch to a high-potency typical agent (Wetterling 2002).

NONDIBENZODIAZEPINE AGENTS: RISPERIDONE, ZIPRASIDONE, AND ARIPIPRAZOLE

The limited effects of the nonbenzodiazepine agents (risperidone, ziprasidone, and aripiprazole) on serum lipids have been demonstrated in large, prospective trials, because the pharmaceutical industry began to routinely include multiple lipid measures as part of study protocols. The more benign effects of risperidone were largely known from the comparative trials versus olanzapine and confirmed by the results from CATIE Phases I and IIa (Lieberman et al. 2005; Stroup et al. 2006). Although there may have been doubts about the differential effects of quetiapine and risperidone on serum lipids, as expressed in the ADA/APA consensus paper (American Diabetes Association et al. 2004), when quetiapine is prescribed in full therapeutic dosages for schizophrenia, it appears to elevate serum triglycerides in a manner not typically seen with risperidone.

Ziprasidone appears to have even fewer effects on serum lipids than risperidone, as evidenced by the statistically significant improvement in serum triglycerides and total cholesterol over 6 weeks when patients were switched to ziprasidone from risperidone (Kingsbury et al. 2001). The lipid neutrality of ziprasidone has been subsequently confirmed in a retrospective chart review (Brown and Estoup 2005) and multiple prospective trials of short (6 weeks) (Simpson et al. 2004; Weiden et al. 2003) and long (≥ 26 weeks) duration (Breier et al. 2005; Cohen et al. 2004; Simpson et al. 2005), including CATIE Phases I and IIa (Lieberman et al. 2005; Stroup et al. 2006), in which the net impact of ziprasidone treatment was to lower serum lipid levels.

The early clinical trials data on aripiprazole suggested that it also had nominal effects on serum lipids (Goodnick and Jerry 2002), a finding confirmed in a large, prospective trial. In a 26-week trial versus olanzapine (McQuade et al. 2004), the mean change in fasting triglycerides was +79.4 mg/dL for olanzapine but only +6.5 mg/dL for aripiprazole ($P<0.05$); HDL decreased by 3.39 mg/dL for olanzapine and increased 3.61 mg/dL for aripiprazole ($P<0.05$). Changes in serum LDL between the drug cohorts were not significant, but the incidence of new dyslipidemias was significantly greater for olanzapine, based on the proportion of new subjects with endpoint serum LDL above 130 mg/dL (38% olanzapine vs. 19% aripiprazole; $P<0.05$).

Patient Variables and Possible Mechanisms for Antipsychotic-Related Hyperlipidemia

In reviewing the data on certain metabolic outcomes, such as the development of T2DM or diabetic ketoacidosis, ethnicity and obesity stand out as important predictors of risk that are additive with the risk imposed by the antipsychotic medication itself (Jin et al. 2002, 2004). As of 2006, no important trends regarding patient risk for hyperlipidemia can be assigned on the basis of ethnicity, gender, patient weight, or even medication dosing within the range commonly used to treat schizophrenia. There are case reports of significant hypertriglyceridemia with low-dosage olanzapine (e.g., 5 mg/day) (Meyer 2001b), but there are no data for those medications employed at extremely low dosages (relative to their antipsychotic dosing), such as quetiapine, which is frequently used in the United States as a sedative at dosages of 25–100 mg/day. The only demographic variable that may be predictive of decreased risk for dyslipidemia is age, with the caveat that the olanzapine studies in older subjects previously cited were both performed among subjects in controlled settings, presumably with controlled diets as well (Barak and Aizenberg 2003; De Deyn et al. 2004). Conversely, reports exist of dyslipidemia in adolescents exposed to antipsychotic medications, primarily olanzapine, so younger age is not protective (Domon and Cargile 2002; Domon and Webber 2001; Martin and L'Ecuyer 2002; Nguyen and Murphy 2001; Shaw et al. 2001).

It is not entirely surprising that an antipsychotic agent can induce dyslipidemia, given that hyperlipidemia can occur with a variety of medications, including certain diuretics, progestins, β-adrenergic antagonists, immunosuppressive agents, protease inhibitors, and some anticonvulsants (Echevarria et al. 1999; Mantel-Teeuwisse et al. 2001). In their comprehensive review of the subject, Mantel-Teeuwisse et al. (2001) noted that global changes in serum lipids are described with some medications, whereas certain agents appear to have specific effects on particular lipid fractions. For example, isotretinoin, acitretin, certain protease inhibitors, low-potency phenothiazines, and dibenzodiazepine-derived antipsychotics primarily elevate serum triglyceride levels. Moreover, in a manner that parallels the differential metabolic effects of the atypical antipsychotics, the protease inhibitors also vary dramatically in their metabolic effects (Manfredi and Chiodo 2001).

There are several possible means by which any agent may induce hyperlipidemia, although none of these have been proved definitively for the atypical antipsychotics. Nonetheless, several biologically plausible hypotheses have been advanced that focus on weight gain, dietary changes, and the development of insulin resistance to explain the high incidence of hyperlipidemia with certain antipsychotic medications (Meyer 2001a).

The variation in weight gain liability is quite marked among the atypical agents (Allison et al. 1999; Lieberman et al. 2005), with clozapine and olanzapine associated with the greatest gains (Beasley et al. 1997; Bustillo et al. 1996; Cohen et al. 1990; Hummer et al. 1995; Lamberti et al. 1992; Umbricht et al. 1994). Obesity and weight gain have a demonstrable negative impact on serum lipid profiles, so it is not surprising that those atypical antipsychotics most likely to cause significant weight gain are also correlated with the greatest impact on serum lipids (American Diabetes Association et al. 2004). Nonetheless, recent switch data suggest that there may be direct, weight-independent effects of the more metabolically offending medications on serum lipids. A long-term ziprasidone switch study presented by Weiden et al. (2004) charted the time course of weight and lipid changes over 58 weeks after subjects had their medication switched from typical antipsychotics, risperidone, and olanzapine. Those switching from high-potency typicals experienced no significant lipid changes, but those previously taking olanzapine and risperidone experienced an immediate reduction in lipids (triglycerides more than total cholesterol) over the first 6 weeks after the switch, whereas weight loss progressed slowly but steadily over the course of the year. The rapid improvement in serum lipids during a time frame when weight loss had been minimal points to a direct, weight-independent effect of certain antipsychotic medications on serum lipids.

There have been accumulating data in the past to suggest that the metabolic pathway most likely to mediate the increase in serum triglycerides relates to the development of insulin resistance. In those who have become less sensitive to the action of insulin, the inability of insulin to adequately suppress lipolysis in adipose cells results in an outflow of free fatty acids and dyslipidemia characterized primarily by elevated serum triglyceride levels (Reaven 2005). The literature certainly supports the concept that some patients who develop new-onset T2DM experience hypertriglyceridemia (Meyer 2001b), often with reversal of these problems upon discontinuation of the offending agent (Domon and Cargile 2002; Domon and Webber 2001; Meyer et al. 2005). However, the majority of patients with elevated triglycerides related to antipsychotic treatment do not have overt T2DM, but many do show signs of insulin resistance, as seen in studies of glucose/insulin parameters in patients receiving clozapine or olanzapine (Melkersson and Dahl 2003).

Undoubtedly, weight gain contributes to insulin resistance, but there are compelling biological data that support the Weiden switch study findings (Weiden et al. 2004) and point to direct effects of the more metabolically offending medications on insulin sensitivity. Single doses of medications such as olanzapine and clozapine have now been shown to induce a dose-dependent loss of insulin sensitivity among laboratory animals in a manner not seen with risperidone or ziprasidone (Houseknecht et al. 2005). Evidence for this effect can be directly measured within 2 hours of drug exposure (using the hyperinsulinemic euglycemic clamp technique) as both decreased ability to metabolize glucose and failure to adequately suppress endogenous glucose production from the liver. The means by which clozapine and olanzapine induce these effects is not known, but the propensity to cause insulin resistance with single doses strongly suggests that these two agents have weight-independent effects on glucose/insulin homeostasis, effects that will be exacerbated by future medication-related weight gain.

Monitoring Recommendations for Hyperlipidemia During Antipsychotic Therapy

Multiple cardiovascular risk factors exist in patients with schizophrenia (Goff et al. 2005), so caution must be exercised in the choice of antipsychotic therapy in order to minimize the added morbidity and mortality of hyperlipidemia. Unfortunately, hyperlipidemia is undertreated in schizophrenia patients (Nasrallah et al. 2006), thereby exposing patients to ongoing substantial additional cardiovascular risk. For example, a normotensive smoker exposed to a dibenzodiazepine-derived atypical antipsychotic might have the 10-year risk for a major cardiovascular event (e.g., sudden death, acute myocardial infarction) increased two to four times from baseline (Meyer and Nasrallah 2003). Hyperlipidemia is associated with long-term cardiovascular consequences, yet monitoring for hyperlipidemia is not solely a long-term issue, because severe hypertriglyceridemia also represents a risk for acute pancreatitis (Koller et al. 2003; Meyer 2001b).

The following guidelines are based upon prior published recommendations (American Diabetes Association et al. 2004; Marder et al. 2004; Melkersson et al. 2004; Meyer et al. 2006) and my clinical experience. Some of the considerations inherent in these recommendations include the fact that schizophrenia patients have multiple risk factors for cardiovascular disease, that certain antipsychotics are associated with greater adverse effects on serum lipids, that many healthcare providers outside of the psychiatric arena are unaware of the potential metabolic complications of atypical antipsychotic therapy, and that schizophrenia patients often receive limited or no medical care outside of that provided by the mental health practitioner, so the burden of medical monitoring necessarily falls upon those who prescribe antipsychotic medications (Meyer and Nasrallah 2003). Although the following recommendations are specific to monitoring of serum lipids, these are understood to be part of the monitoring recommended elsewhere as part of routine medical care for those receiving atypical antipsychotics (Marder et al. 2004; Melkersson et al. 2004).

BASELINE ASSESSMENT

1. In all patients with schizophrenia, record smoking status and patient and first-degree family history of cardiovascular disease, hyperlipidemia, and glucose intolerance in the medical record.
2. Obtain weight, waist circumference, blood pressure, and (ideally) fasting lipid panel. Total cholesterol and HDL are valid on nonfasting specimens,

but triglycerides and LDL are not. This is recommended for all patients with schizophrenia, regardless of medication regimen, given the limited healthcare access for these patients.

FOLLOW-UP

1. For patients receiving agents associated with lower risk for hyperlipidemia (high-potency typicals, ziprasidone, risperidone, aripiprazole), an annual fasting lipid panel is sufficient unless dyslipidemia is suspected on the basis of baseline evaluation.

2. For patients receiving agents associated with higher risk for hyperlipidemia (low-potency typicals, quetiapine, olanzapine, clozapine), a quarterly fasting lipid panel is necessary for the first year to pick up cases of severe hypertriglyceridemia. This may be decreased to semiannually if fasting lipids remain normal but should continue on a quarterly basis in those identified with abnormal values.

3. All patients with persistent dyslipidemia should be referred for lipid-lowering therapy or considered for a switch to a less offending agent if possible.

KEY CLINICAL CONCEPTS

- Patients with severe mental illness have twice the risk for cardiovascular mortality versus their non–mentally ill counterparts. Thus the induction of hyperlipidemia secondary to antipsychotic treatment represents a serious condition not only for its impact on cardiovascular risk but for the fact that it is occurring in a group possessing considerable risk.

- High-potency typical antipsychotic agents (butyrophenones) are lipid neutral, whereas low-potency agents (phenothiazines) are associated with hyperlipidemia, primarily in the form of hypertriglyceridemia.

- The structurally related dibenzodiazepine-derived atypical antipsychotics (clozapine, olanzapine, and quetiapine) are associated with greater elevations in serum triglycerides than in total cholesterol, whereas the nondibenzodiazepine agents (risperidone, ziprasidone, and aripiprazole) have minimal effects on lipids.

- Mechanisms by which antipsychotics cause hyperlipidemia include weight gain, dietary changes, and the direct development of insulin resistance.

- A thorough baseline assessment in all patients should include a cardiovascular assessment. Subsequent yearly monitoring for hyperlipidemia is recommended in all patients prescribed antipsychotics; those prescribed higher-risk agents should be monitored as often as quarterly.

References

Allison DB, Mentore JL, Heo M, et al: Antipsychotic-induced weight gain: a comprehensive research synthesis. Am J Psychiatry 156:1686–1696, 1999

Almeras N, Despres JP, Villeneuve J, et al: Development of an atherogenic metabolic risk factor profile associated with the use of atypical antipsychotics (see comment). J Clin Psychiatry 65:557–564, 2004

American Diabetes Association, American Psychiatric Association, American Association of Clinical Endocrinologists, North American Association for the Study of Obesity: Consensus Development Conference on Antipsychotic Drugs and Obesity and Diabetes. Diabetes Care 27:596–601, 2004

Atmaca M, Kuloglu M, Tezcan E, et al: Serum leptin and triglyceride levels in patients on treatment with atypical antipsychotics. J Clin Psychiatry 64:598–604, 2003a

Atmaca M, Kuloglu M, Tezcan E, et al: Weight gain, serum leptin and triglyceride levels in patients with schizophrenia on antipsychotic treatment with quetiapine, olanzapine and haloperidol. Schizophr Res 60:99–100, 2003b

Ball MP, Hooper ET, Skipwith DF, et al: Clozapine-induced hyperlipidemia resolved after switch to aripiprazole therapy. Ann Pharmacother 39:1570–1572, 2005

Baptista T, Lacruz A, Angeles F, et al: Endocrine and metabolic abnormalities involved in obesity associated with typical antipsychotic drug administration. Pharmacopsychiatry 34:223–231, 2001

Barak Y, Aizenberg D: Effects of olanzapine on lipid abnormalities in elderly psychotic patients. Drugs Aging 20:893–896, 2003

Baymiller SP, Ball P, McMahon RP, et al: Serum glucose and lipid changes during the course of clozapine treatment: the effect of concurrent beta-adrenergic antagonist treatment. Schizophr Res 59:49–57, 2003

Beasley CM Jr, Tollefson GD, Tran PV: Safety of olanzapine. J Clin Psychiatry 58(suppl): 13–17, 1997

Bouchard RH, Demers M-F, Simoneau I, et al: Atypical antipsychotics and cardiovascular risk in schizophrenic patients. J Clin Psychopharmacol 21:110–111, 2001

Braun GA, Paulonis ME: Sterol metabolism: biochemical differences among the butyrophenones. Int J Neuropsychiatry 3(suppl):26–27, 1967

Breier A, Berg PH, Thakore JH, et al: Olanzapine versus ziprasidone: results of a 28-week double-blind study in patients with schizophrenia. Am J Psychiatry 162:1879–1887, 2005

Brown RR, Estoup MW: Comparison of the metabolic effects observed in patients treated with ziprasidone versus olanzapine. Int Clin Psychopharmacol 20:105–112, 2005

Bustillo JR, Buchanan RW, Irish D, et al: Differential effect of clozapine on weight: a controlled study. Am J Psychiatry 153:817–819, 1996

Clark M, Johnson PC: Amenorrhea and elevated serum cholesterol produced by a trifluoromethylated phenothiazine. J Clin Endocrinol Metab 20:641–646, 1960

Clark M, Ray TS, Paredes A, et al: Chlorpromazine in women with chronic schizophrenia: the effect on cholesterol levels and cholesterol-behavior relationships. Psychosom Med 29:634–642, 1967

Clark M, Braun GA, Hewson JR, et al: Trifluperidol and cholesterol in man. Clin Pharmacol Ther 9:333–340, 1968

Clark M, Dubowski K, Colmore J: The effect of chlorpromazine on serum cholesterol in chronic schizophrenic patients. Clin Pharmacol Ther 11:883–889, 1970

Clark ML, Huber WK, Sullivan J, et al: Evaluation of loxapine succinate in chronic schizophrenia. Dis Nerv Syst 33:783–791, 1972

Cohen S, Chiles J, MacNaughton A: Weight gain associated with clozapine (see comments). Am J Psychiatry 147:503–504, 1990

Cohen SA, Fitzgerald BJ, Khan SR, et al: The effect of a switch to ziprasidone in an adult population with autistic disorder: chart review of naturalistic, open-label treatment. J Clin Psychiatry 65:110–113, 2004

De Deyn PP, Carrasco MM, Deberdt W, et al: Olanzapine versus placebo in the treatment of psychosis with or without associated behavioral disturbances in patients with Alzheimer's disease. Int J Geriatr Psychiatry 19:115–126, 2004

Domon SE, Cargile CS: Quetiapine-associated hyperglycemia and hypertriglyceridemia. J Am Acad Child Adolescent Psychiatry 41:495–496, 2002

Domon SE, Webber JC: Hyperglycemia and hypertriglyceridemia secondary to olanzapine. J Child Adolesc Psychopharmacol 11:285–288, 2001

Dursun SM, Szemis A, Andrews H, et al: The effects of clozapine on levels of total cholesterol and related lipids in serum of patients with schizophrenia: a prospective study. J Psychiatry Neurosci 24:453–455, 1999

Echevarria KL, Hardin TC, Smith JA: Hyperlipidemia associated with protease inhibitor therapy. Ann Pharmacother 33:859–863, 1999

Expert Panel on Detection, Evaluation, and Treatment of High Blood Cholesterol in Adults: Executive Summary of the third report of the National Cholesterol Education Program (NCEP) Expert Panel on Detection, Evaluation, and Treatment of High Blood Cholesterol in Adults (Adult Treatment Panel III). JAMA 285:2486–2497, 2001

Fleischhacker WW, Stuppack C, Moser C, et al: Fluperlapine vs haloperidol: a comparison of their neuroendocrinological profiles and the influence on serum lipids. Pharmacopsychiatry 19:111–114, 1986

Garyfallos G, Dimelis D, Kouniakis P, et al: Olanzapine versus risperidone: weight gain and elevation of serum triglyceride levels. Eur Psychiatry 18:320–321, 2003

Gaulin BD, Markowitz JS, Caley CF, et al: Clozapine-associated elevation in serum triglycerides. Am J Psychiatry 156:1270–1272, 1999

Ghaeli P, Dufresne RL: Elevated serum triglycerides on clozapine resolve with risperidone. Pharmacotherapy 15:382–385, 1995

Ghaeli P, Dufresne RL: Serum triglyceride levels in patients treated with clozapine. Am J Health Syst Pharm 53:2079–2081, 1996

Goff DC, Sullivan L, McEvoy JP, et al: A comparison of ten-year cardiac risk estimates in schizophrenia patients from the CATIE study and matched controls. Schizophr Res 80:45–53, 2005

Goodnick PJ, Jerry JM: Aripiprazole: profile on efficacy and safety. Expert Opin Pharmacother 3:1773–1781, 2002

Graham KA, Perkins DO, Edwards LJ, et al: Effect of olanzapine on body composition and energy expenditure in adults with first-episode psychosis. Am J Psychiatry 162:118–123, 2005

Haffner SM, Lehto S, Ronnemaa T, et al: Mortality from coronary heart disease in subjects with type 2 diabetes and in nondiabetic subjects with and without prior myocardial infarction (see comment). N Engl J Med 339:229–234, 1998

Henderson DC, Cagliero E, Gray C, et al: Clozapine, diabetes mellitus, weight gain, and lipid abnormalities: a five-year naturalistic study. Am J Psychiatry 157:975–981, 2000

Henderson DC, Nguyen DD, Copeland PM, et al: Clozapine, diabetes mellitus, hyperlipidemia and cardiovascular risks and mortality: results of a 10-year naturalistic study. J Clin Psychiatry 66:1116–1121, 2005

Houseknecht KL, Robertson AS, Zavadoski W, et al: Diabetogenic effects of some atypical antipsychotics: rapid, whole body insulin resistance following a single dose. Diabetologia 48(suppl):A212, 2005

Hummer M, Kemmler G, Kurz M, et al: Weight gain induced by clozapine. Eur Neuropsychopharmacol 5:437–440, 1995

Jin H, Meyer JM, Jeste DV: Phenomenology of and risk factors for new-onset diabetes mellitus and diabetic ketoacidosis associated with atypical antipsychotics: an analysis of 45 published cases. Ann Clin Psychiatry 14:59–64, 2002

Jin H, Meyer JM, Jeste DV: Atypical antipsychotics and glucose dysregulation: a systematic review. Schizophr Res 71:195–212, 2004

Kingsbury SJ, Fayek M, Trufasiu D, et al: The apparent effects of ziprasidone on plasma lipids and glucose. J Clin Psychiatry 62:347–349, 2001

Kinon BJ, Basson BR, Gilmore JA, et al: Long-term olanzapine treatment: weight change and weight-related health factors in schizophrenia. J Clin Psychiatry 62:92–100, 2001

Kinon BJ, Liu-Seifert H, Ahl J, et al: Longitudinal effect of olanzapine on fasting serum lipids: a randomized, prospective, 4-month study. Ann N Y Acad Sci 1032:295–296, 2004

Koller E, Cross JT, Doraiswamy PM, et al: Pancreatitis associated with atypical antipsychotics: from the Food and Drug Administration's MedWatch surveillance system and published reports. Pharmacotherapy 23:1123–1130, 2003

Koro CE, Fedder DO, L'Italien GJ, et al: An assessment of the independent effects of olanzapine and risperidone exposure on the risk of hyperlipidemia in schizophrenic patients. Arch Gen Psychiatry 59:1021–1026, 2002

Lambert BL, Chang KY, Tafesse E, et al: Association between antipsychotic treatment and hyperlipidemia among California Medicaid patients with schizophrenia. J Clin Psychopharmacol 25:12–18, 2005

Lamberti JS, Bellnier T, Schwarzkopf SB: Weight gain among schizophrenic patients treated with clozapine. Am J Psychiatry 149:689–690, 1992

Leonard P, Halley A, Browne S: Prevalence of obesity, lipid and glucose abnormalities in outpatients prescribed clozapine. Ir Med J 95:119–120, 2002

Lieberman JA, Stroup TS, McEvoy JP, et al: Effectiveness of antipsychotic drugs in patients with chronic schizophrenia. N Engl J Med 353:1209–1223, 2005

Lund BC, Perry PJ, Brooks JM, et al: Clozapine use in patients with schizophrenia and the risk of diabetes, hyperlipidemia, and hypertension: a claims-based approach. Arch Gen Psychiatry 58:1172–1176, 2001

Manfredi R, Chiodo F: Disorders of lipid metabolism in patients with HIV disease treated with antiretroviral agents: frequency, relationship with administered drugs, and role of hypolipidaemic therapy with bezafibrate. J Infect 42:181–188, 2001

Mantel-Teeuwisse AK, Kloosterman JM, Maitland-van der Zee AH, et al: Drug-induced lipid changes: a review of the unintended effects of some commonly used drugs on serum lipid levels. Drug Saf 24:443–456, 2001

Marder SR, Essock SM, Miller AL, et al: Physical health monitoring of patients with schizophrenia. Am J Psychiatry 161:1334–1349, 2004

Martin A, L'Ecuyer S: Triglyceride, cholesterol and weight changes among risperidone-treated youths: a retrospective study. Eur Child Adolesc Psychiatry 11:129–133, 2002

Martinez JA, Velasco JJ, Urbistondo MD: Effects of pharmacological therapy on anthropometric and biochemical status of male and female institutionalized psychiatric patients. J Am Coll Nutr 13:192–197, 1994

McEvoy JP, Meyer JM, Goff DC, et al: Prevalence of the metabolic syndrome in patients with schizophrenia: baseline results from the Clinical Antipsychotic Trials of Intervention Effectiveness (CATIE) Schizophrenia Trial and comparison with national estimates from NHANES III. Schizophr Res 80:19–32, 2005

McEvoy JP, Lieberman JA, Stroup TS, et al: Effectiveness of clozapine versus olanzapine, quetiapine, and risperidone in patients with chronic schizophrenia who did not respond to prior atypical antipsychotic treatment. Am J Psychiatry 163:600–610, 2006

McKee JR, Bodfish JW, Mahorney SL, et al: Metabolic effects associated with atypical antipsychotic treatment in the developmentally disabled. J Clin Psychiatry 66:1161–1168, 2005

McQuade RD, Stock E, Marcus R, et al: A comparison of weight change during treatment with olanzapine or aripiprazole: results from a randomized, double-blind study. J Clin Psychiatry 65(suppl):47–56, 2004

Mefferd RB, Labrosse EH, Gawienowski AM, et al: Influence of chlorpromazine on certain biochemical variables of chronic male schizophrenics. J Nerv Ment Dis 127:167–179, 1958

Melkersson KI, Dahl ML: Relationship between levels of insulin or triglycerides and serum concentrations of the atypical antipsychotics clozapine and olanzapine in patients on treatment with therapeutic doses. Psychopharmacology 170:157–166, 2003

Melkersson KI, Hulting AL, Brismar KE: Elevated levels of insulin, leptin, and blood lipids in olanzapine-treated patients with schizophrenia or related psychoses. J Clin Psychiatry 61:742–749, 2000

Melkersson KI, Dahl ML, Hulting AL: Guidelines for prevention and treatment of adverse effects of antipsychotic drugs on glucose-insulin homeostasis and lipid metabolism. Psychopharmacology (Berl) 175:1–6, 2004

Meyer JM: Effects of atypical antipsychotics on weight and serum lipid levels. J Clin Psychiatry 62(suppl):27–34; discussion 40–1, 2001a

Meyer JM: Novel antipsychotics and severe hyperlipidemia (comment). J Clin Psychopharmacol 21:369–374, 2001b

Meyer JM: A retrospective comparison of weight, lipid, and glucose changes between risperidone- and olanzapine-treated inpatients: metabolic outcomes after 1 year. J Clin Psychiatry 63:425–433, 2002

Meyer JM, Koro CE: The effects of antipsychotic therapy on serum lipids: a comprehensive review. Schizophr Res 70:1–17, 2004

Meyer JM, Nasrallah HA (eds): Medical Illness and Schizophrenia. Washington, DC, American Psychiatric Press, 2003

Meyer JM, Simpson GM: Psychopharmacology from chlorpromazine to olanzapine: a brief history of antipsychotics. Psychiatr Serv 48:1137–1140, 1997

Meyer JM, Pandina G, Bossie CA, et al: Effects of switching from olanzapine to risperidone on the prevalence of the metabolic syndrome in overweight or obese patients with schizophrenia or schizoaffective disorder: analysis of a multicenter, rater-blinded, open-label study. Clin Ther 27:1930–1941, 2005

Meyer JM, Loh C, Leckband SG, et al: Prevalence of the metabolic syndrome in veterans with schizophrenia. J Psychiatr Pract 12:5–10, 2006

Muller-Oerlinghausen B: A short survey on untoward effects of fluperlapine. Arzneimittel-Forschung 34:131–134, 1984

Nasrallah HA, Meyer JM, Goff DC, et al: Low rates of treatment for hypertension, dyslipidemia and diabetes in schizophrenia: data from the CATIE Schizophrenia Trial sample at baseline. Schizophr Res 86:15–22, 2006

Nguyen M, Murphy T: Olanzapine and hypertriglyceridemia. J Am Acad Child Adolesc Psychiatry 40:133, 2001

Osby U, Correia N, Brandt L, et al: Mortality and causes of death in schizophrenia in Stockholm county, Sweden. Schizophr Res 45:21–28, 2000

Osby U, Brandt L, Correia N, et al: Excess mortality in bipolar and unipolar disorder in Sweden. Arch Gen Psychiatry 58:844–850, 2001

Osser DN, Najarian DM, Dufresne RL: Olanzapine increases weight and serum triglyceride levels. J Clin Psychiatry 60:767–770, 1999

Reaven GM: Compensatory hyperinsulinemia and the development of an atherogenic lipoprotein profile: the price paid to maintain glucose homeostasis in insulin-resistant individuals. Endocrinol Metab Clin North Am 34:49–62, 2005

Saari K, Koponen H, Laitinen J, et al: Hyperlipidemia in persons using antipsychotic medication: a general population-based birth cohort study. J Clin Psychiatry 65:547–550, 2004

Sasaki J, Kumagae G, Sata T, et al: Decreased concentration of high density lipoprotein cholesterol in schizophrenic patients treated with phenothiazines. Atherosclerosis 51:163–169, 1984

Sasaki J, Funakoshi M, Arakawa K: Lipids and apolipoproteins in patients treated with major tranquilizers. Clin Pharmacol Ther 37:684–687, 1985

Serafetinides EA, Colmore JP, Rahhal DK, et al: Trifluperidol in chronic male psychiatric patients. Behav Neuropsychiatry 3:10–12, 1971

Serafetinides EA, Collins S, Clark ML: Haloperidol, clopenthixol, and chlorpromazine in chronic schizophrenia. Chemically unrelated antipsychotics as therapeutic alternatives. J Nerv Ment Dis 154:31–42, 1972

Shafique M, Khan IA, Akhtar MH, et al: Serum lipids and lipoproteins in schizophrenic patients receiving major tranquilizers. J Pak Med Assoc 38:259–261, 1988

Shaw JA, Lewis JE, Pascal S, et al: A study of quetiapine: efficacy and tolerability in psychotic adolescents. J Child Adolesc Psychopharmacol 11:415–424, 2001

Sheitman BB, Bird PM, Binz W, et al: Olanzapine-induced elevation of plasma triglyceride levels (letter). Am J Psychiatry 156:1471–1472, 1999

Simpson GM, Cooper TB: The effect of three butyrophenones on serum cholesterol levels. Curr Ther Res Clin Exp 8:249–255, 1966

Simpson GM, Cooper TB, Braun GA: Further studies on the effect of butyrophenones on cholesterol synthesis in humans. Curr Ther Res Clin Exp 9:413–418, 1967

Simpson GM, Glick ID, Weiden PJ, et al: Randomized, controlled, double-blind multicenter comparison of the efficacy and tolerability of ziprasidone and olanzapine in acutely ill inpatients with schizophrenia or schizoaffective disorder. Am J Psychiatry 161:1837–1847, 2004

Simpson GM, Weiden P, Pigott T, et al: Six-month, blinded, multicenter continuation study of ziprasidone versus olanzapine in schizophrenia. Am J Psychiatry 162:1535–1538, 2005

Spivak B, Roitman S, Vered Y, et al: Diminished suicidal and aggressive behavior, high plasma norepinephrine levels, and serum triglyceride levels in chronic neuroleptic-resistant schizophrenic patients maintained on clozapine. Clin Neuropharmacol 21: 245–250, 1998

Spivak B, Lamschtein C, Talmon Y, et al: The impact of clozapine treatment on serum lipids in chronic schizophrenic patients. Clin Neuropharmacol 22:98–101, 1999

Stoner SC, Dubisar BM, Khan R, et al: Severe hypertriglyceridemia associated with olanzapine. J Clin Psychiatry 63:948–949, 2002

Stroup TS, Lieberman JA, McEvoy JP, et al: Effectiveness of olanzapine, quetiapine, risperidone, and ziprasidone in patients with chronic schizophrenia following discontinuation of a previous atypical antipsychotic. Am J Psychiatry 163:611–622, 2006

Su KP, Wu PL, Pariante CM: A crossover study on lipid and weight changes associated with olanzapine and risperidone. Psychopharmacology 183:383–386, 2005

Umbricht DS, Pollack S, Kane JM: Clozapine and weight gain. J Clin Psychiatry 55(suppl): 157–160, 1994

Vaisanen K, Rimon R, Raisanen P, et al: A controlled double-blind study of haloperidol versus thioridazine in the treatment of restless mentally subnormal patients: serum levels and clinical effects. Acta Psychiatr Belg 79:673–685, 1979

Vampini C, Steinmayr M, Bilone F, et al: The increase of plasma levels of triglyceride during clozapine treatment: a case report. Neuropsychopharmacology 10(suppl):249s, 1994

Virkkunen M, Wahlbeck K, Rissanen A, et al: Decrease of energy expenditure causes weight increase in olanzapine treatment: a case study. Pharmacopsychiatry 35:124–126, 2002

Waage C, Carlsson H, Nielsen EW: Olanzapine-induced pancreatitis: a case report. JOP 5:388–391, 2004

Weiden PJ, Daniel DG, Simpson G, et al: Improvement in indices of health status in outpatients with schizophrenia switched to ziprasidone. J Clin Psychopharmacol 23:595–600, 2003

Weiden PJ, Loebel A, Yang R, et al: Course of weight and metabolic benefits 1 year after switching to ziprasidone. Abstract presented at the annual meeting of the American Psychiatric Association, New York, May 2004

Wetterling T: Bodyweight gain with atypical antipsychotics: a comparative review. Drug Saf 24:59–73, 2001

Wetterling T: Hyperlipidemia: side-effect of the treatment with an atypical antipsychotic (zotepine)? Psychiatr Prax 29:438–440, 2002

Wirshing DA, Boyd JA, Meng LR, et al: The effects of novel antipsychotics on glucose and lipid levels. J Clin Psychiatry 63:856–865, 2002

Wu G, Dias P, Chun W, et al: Hyperglycemia, hyperlipidemia, and periodic paralysis: a case report of new side effects of clozapine. Prog Neuropsychopharmacol Biol Psychiatry 24:1395–1400, 2000

Appendix: Lipid Changes During Antipsychotic Therapy: 1984–2006

Lipid changes during antipsychotic therapy: 1984–2006

Reference	Study design	Findings
Sasaki et al. 1984	Chart review in chronic phenothiazine users (mean exposure = 8 years) 10-week prospective data in eight new phenothiazine-treated patients	Patients chronically treated with phenothiazines (chlorpromazine, levomepromazine, perphenazine) had significantly lower HDL ($P<0.001$) and higher triglyceride levels ($P<0.05$) than normal control subjects. HDL decreased 24% within 1 week of new phenothiazine exposure, with no significant changes in total cholesterol and triglyceride levels after 10 weeks.
Muller-Oerlinghausen 1984	Multicenter fluperlapine trial in 43 schizophrenia and depression patients	In 16 of 28 patients triglycerides increased significantly, with notable increases in serum total cholesterol.
Sasaki et al. 1985	Chart review in males with chronic schizophrenia Excluded patients with diabetes mellitus or those taking lipid-lowering medication 17 phenothiazine 14 haloperidol 14 healthy control subjects	After a mean 8 years of antipsychotic exposure, there was no effect of butyrophenones on lipids but significantly elevated mean fasting triglyceride levels for the phenothiazine group (163 mg/dL) compared with the butyrophenone group (104 mg/dL) and control subjects (127 mg/dL). No significant differences in total cholesterol or LDL or HDL values among the three groups.
Fleischhacker et al. 1986	Double-blind, prospective 6-week study 6 haloperidol 6 fluperlapine	No significant differences in mean HDL or total cholesterol between groups or compared with baseline by day 28. One fluperlapine subject developed a serum triglyceride level of 900 mg/dL on day 7 that required treatment on day 28.

Lipid changes during antipsychotic therapy: 1984–2006 *(continued)*

Reference	Study design	Findings
Shafique et al. 1988	Chart review in males with chronic schizophrenia treated for 6–12 months 35 phenothiazine 30 butyrophenone 22 combined drug classes	Total cholesterol, VLDL, and LDL levels were significantly elevated in patients given phenothiazines, and LDL was elevated in patients given butyrophenone. VLDL and LDL levels were significantly higher and HDL levels lower in patients given combined therapy.
Vampini et al. 1994	Case report of 1 patient given clozapine 400 mg/day	Increased triglyceride levels were seen after 15 months.
Martinez et al. 1994	Chart review in 311 chronically hospitalized schizophrenia patients 225 neuroleptic exposed (mostly haloperidol, thioridazine, or fluphenazine) for prior 2 years 86 no psychotropic medications	Neuroleptic administration was associated with changes in HDL and triglycerides in males but not in females.
Ghaeli and Dufresne 1995	Case series of 4 clozapine-treated patients (dosages 600–900 mg/day) switched to risperidone	Patients given clozapine had increased serum triglyceride levels that decreased upon switching to risperidone and increased upon clozapine rechallenge.
Ghaeli and Dufresne 1996	Chart review in 67 schizophrenia patients 39 clozapine 21 high-potency typical antipsychotics 2 medium-potency typical antipsychotics 5 low-potency typical antipsychotics	Mean triglyceride level was significantly higher in the clozapine vs. the typicals groups (264.6 mg/dL vs. 149.8 mg/dL; $P<0.001$). This difference was not explained by concomitant illness or medication, age, or gender. No significant difference was found in total cholesterol.

Lipid changes during antipsychotic therapy: 1984–2006 *(continued)*

Reference	Study design	Findings
Spivak et al. 1998	Chart review in schizophrenia patients 30 clozapine (mean=295.0±165 mg/day) 30 typical antipsychotics (mean=348.9±298.8 mg/day in CPZ equivalents)	Mean triglyceride levels were significantly higher in the clozapine vs. the typicals group after 1 year of treatment (202.9 mg/dL vs. 134.4 mg/dL; $P<0.01$). No significant difference was found in serum total cholesterol.
Spivak et al. 1999	Chart review in schizophrenia patients 70 clozapine (mean=332.9±168.1 mg/day) 30 typical antipsychotics (mean=347.3±247.3 mg/day in CPZ equivalents)	Mean triglyceride levels increased in the clozapine group and decreased in the typicals group after 6 months of treatment ($P<0.005$).
Sheitman et al. 1999	Prospective study in schizophrenia patients 9 olanzapine (mean=19 mg/day)	After 16 months, a mean increase in serum triglycerides of 70 mg/dL was reported. No significant change was found in total cholesterol, HDL, or LDL. Five patients had a >50% increase in triglycerides.
Osser et al. 1999	Prospective study in schizophrenia patients 25 olanzapine (mean=13.8±4.4 mg/day)	37% (60 mg/dL) increase in fasting triglycerides from baseline ($P<0.05$) with no increase in fasting total cholesterol.
Gaulin et al. 1999	Chart review in schizophrenia patients 222 treated with clozapine or haloperidol	45% increase in serum triglycerides in clozapine-treated patients ($P<0.01$); insignificant decrease in serum triglycerides in haloperidol-treated patients after a mean treatment period of 590 days for clozapine and 455 for haloperidol.
Dursun et al. 1999	Prospective 12-week study 8 clozapine (mean=352±73 mg/day)	Small increase in triglyceride levels (11%) but no significant changes in other lipid levels after 12 weeks
Wu et al. 2000	Case report of 25-year-old Chinese male taking clozapine	Dose-dependent increases in fasting serum triglycerides and glucose.

Lipid changes during antipsychotic therapy: 1984–2006 *(continued)*

Reference	Study design	Findings
Melkersson et al. 2000	Prospective cohort study 14 olanzapine (median dosage = 12.5 mg/day)	62% prevalence of hypertriglyceridemia (mean = 273.45 mg/dL) and 85% prevalence of hypercholesterolemia (mean = 257.14 mg/dL) after a median exposure of 5 months (range, 2.4–16.8 months).
Henderson et al. 2000	5-year naturalistic study 82 clozapine	Significant changes in serum triglycerides in patients treated with clozapine over 60 months (P = 0.04); linear coefficient = 2.75 mg/dL per month, SE = 1.28.
Shaw et al. 2001	8-week open trial 15 quetiapine (300–800 mg/day)	Total cholesterol remained unchanged in this group of adolescents with psychosis.
Nguyen and Murphy 2001	Case report of 10-year-old boy given olanzapine 5 mg/day for attention-deficit/ hyperactivity disorder	Over 3 months, patient experienced 20-lb weight gain with resulting total cholesterol of 193 mg/dL and triglyceride level of 183 mg/dL. Olanzapine was discontinued, and 5 weeks later total cholesterol was 151 mg/dL and triglycerides were 61 mg/dL, with more than 20 lb weight loss.
Meyer 2001b	Case series 12 olanzapine (5–20 mg/day) 2 quetiapine (200–250 mg/day)	Hypertriglyceridemia up to 7,668 mg/dL on olanzapine and 1,932 mg/dL on quetiapine reported. Time to peak triglyceride level ranged from 1 to 23.5 months.
Lund et al. 2001	Retrospective cohort study 2,461 typical antipsychotics 552 clozapine	In patients ages 20–34 years, clozapine significantly increased relative risk of hyperlipidemia (RR = 2.4; 95% CI = 1.1–5.2), but not in older patients.

Lipid changes during antipsychotic therapy: 1984–2006 *(continued)*

Reference	Study design	Findings
Kingsbury et al. 2001	Prospective 6-week switch study 37 ziprasidone (mean=124.3 mg/day) Prior medications 15 from olanzapine 12 from risperidone 10 from typical antipsychotics	Serum total cholesterol decreased significantly (−17.57 mg/dL; $P<0.001$), as did serum triglycerides (−62.38 mg/dL; $P=0.018$). Change in triglycerides correlated with weight change ($r=0.409$; $P=0.018$; $r^2=0.167$). Change in total cholesterol did not correlate with weight change.
Kinon et al. 2001	Retrospective cohort 573 olanzapine (5–20 mg/day) 103 haloperidol (5–20 mg/day)	Median nonfasting endpoint serum total cholesterol significantly higher for olanzapine than for haloperidol (205.7 mg/dL vs. 189.9 mg/dL; $P=0.002$).
Domon and Webber 2001	Case report of 15-year-old African American male given olanzapine 20 mg/day	After 3 months, the patient's weight was 91 kg, fasting glucose 90 mg/dL, fasting triglycerides 155 mg/dL, and fasting total cholesterol 131 mg/dL; 5 months later, his weight peaked at 108 kg but declined with onset of type 2 diabetes. The maximum triglyceride level was 298 mg/dL on olanzapine. Both the diabetes and hyperlipidemia resolved over 8 weeks after olanzapine was discontinued.

Lipid changes during antipsychotic therapy: 1984–2006 *(continued)*

Reference	Study design	Findings
Bouchard et al. 2001	Retrospective study 22 olanzapine (mean = 12.8 ± 4.4 mg/day) 22 risperidone (mean = 2.8 ± 1.8 mg/day)	After mean exposure of 17.9 months (olanzapine) and 17.4 months (risperidone), olanzapine patients had significantly higher triglycerides (185 mg/dL vs. 115 mg/dL; $P<0.01$), significantly higher VLDL (0.9 mol/L vs. 0.5 mol/L; $P<0.03$), and a trend for a higher cholesterol:HDL ratio (5.3 vs. 4.3; $P=0.06$) and lower HDL ($P=0.08$). No significant differences were found in total cholesterol, fasting glucose, or insulin.
Baptista et al. 2001	Cross-sectional cohort study in women matched for age, BMI, and day of menses 26 typical antipsychotics (>6 consecutive months of treatment) 26 control subjects	Antipsychotic-treated subjects had a trend for lower HDL and increased insulin resistance.
Virkkunen et al. 2002	Case report of 48-year-old male receiving olanzapine 10–15 mg/day for 1 month	6-kg weight gain and 3.6% decrease in basal and 11.4% decrease in 3-hour energy expenditure; HDL decreased, and triglycerides and LDL increased; no change in insulin sensitivity using hyperinsulinemic euglycemic clamp.

Lipid changes during antipsychotic therapy: 1984–2006 *(continued)*

Reference	Study design	Findings
Wirshing et al. 2002	Chart review 39 clozapine 42 olanzapine 49 risperidone 13 quetiapine 41 haloperidol 41 fluphenazine	Clozapine was associated with greatest increase in total cholesterol, whereas risperidone and fluphenazine were associated with decreases. Clozapine and olanzapine had greatest increase in triglyceride levels.
Wetterling 2002	Case report of 1 patient taking zotepine	Maximum triglyceride level of 1,247 mg/dL, which normalized on switch to high-potency typical antipsychotic.
Stoner et al. 2002	Case report of 42-year-old African American male with treated hyperlipidemia taking olanzapine 15 mg/day	Baseline lipid panel: total cholesterol 227 mg/dL, triglycerides 134 mg/dL, HDL 38 mg/dL. After 8 weeks of olanzapine: serum triglyceride level 5,093 mg/dL and total cholesterol 375 mg/dL, with evidence of new-onset type 2 diabetes (fasting glucose=395 mg/dL, HbA$_{1c}$=11.9%).
Meyer 2002	Retrospective chart review of 1-year exposure 47 risperidone 47 olanzapine	After 52 weeks, total cholesterol increased 24 mg/dL for olanzapine vs. 7 mg/dL for risperidone ($P=0.029$) and fasting triglyceride increased 88 mg/dL for olanzapine vs. 30 mg/dL for risperidone ($P=0.042$). In the nongeriatric cohort, total cholesterol increased 31 mg/dL for olanzapine vs. 7 mg/dL for risperidone ($P=0.004$) and fasting triglycerides increased 105 mg/dL for olanzapine vs. 32 mg/dL for risperidone ($P=0.037$).

Lipid changes during antipsychotic therapy: 1984–2006 *(continued)*

Reference	Study design	Findings
Martin and L'Ecuyer 2002	Retrospective chart review of child and adolescent inpatients (mean age = 12.8 years) 22 risperidone (mean = 2.7 ± 2.2 mg/day)	After mean exposure of 4.9 ± 1.0 months, no significant changes in serum triglycerides or total cholesterol levels were seen in the group as a whole.
Leonard et al. 2002	Chart review study in 13 males and 8 females 21 clozapine (mean = 485 mg/day)	11 patients (52%) had hypertriglyceridemia, 3 (14%) had hypercholesterolemia. Mean total cholesterol = 193 ± 46 mg/dL (range = 131–309), mean triglycerides = 196 ± 142 mg/dL (range = 39–665 mg/dL).
Koro et al. 2002	Case-control database study of 18,309 schizophrenia patients with 1,268 incident cases of hyperlipidemia. Typical or atypical antipsychotic use analyzed.	Olanzapine use was associated with nearly a fivefold increase in the odds of developing hyperlipidemia compared with no antipsychotic exposure and more than a threefold increase compared with those receiving typicals.
Goodnick and Jerry 2002	Meta-analysis of trial data comprising 1,919 patients treated with aripiprazole, olanzapine, risperidone, haloperidol, or placebo	Meta-analysis of short-term trial data showed that increases in total cholesterol after aripiprazole administration were lower than for haloperidol, risperidone, or placebo. A 26-week trial comparing aripiprazole with olanzapine found significant differences after 4 weeks; olanzapine increased total cholesterol, whereas aripiprazole decreased it. Data from a 1-year study found that aripiprazole produced less of an increase in total cholesterol than haloperidol.

Lipid changes during antipsychotic therapy: 1984–2006 *(continued)*

Reference	Study design	Findings
Domon and Cargile 2002	Case report of 17-year-old African American female taking quetiapine 600 mg/day and metformin 1,000 mg orally twice a day for type 2 diabetes	Total cholesterol 235 mg/dL, triglycerides 456 mg/dL on admission; quetiapine discontinued with complete resolution of diabetes and hyperlipidemia; 6 weeks post-quetiapine (and 4 weeks without metformin), total cholesterol 226 mg/dL and triglycerides 163 mg/dL.
Barak and Aizenberg 2003	Prospective 6-month study of elderly inpatients (mean age=71.7 years) with schizophrenia or schizoaffective disorder (16 female, 5 male) 21 olanzapine (mean=12.9 mg/day)	After a mean duration of 289 days of olanzapine treatment, no significant change from baseline serum lipid levels were found for triglycerides or total cholesterol.
Garyfallos et al. 2003	8-week prospective randomized study of acute schizophrenia spectrum inpatients 25 olanzapine (mean=18.0 mg/day) 25 risperidone (mean=7.7 mg/day)	Compared with baseline, there were significant increases in fasting triglycerides (+43.5 mg/dL; $P<0.001$) for olanzapine but not risperidone (+7.5 mg/dL; $P>0.05$). There were nonsignificant increases in total cholesterol: +10.2 mg/dL for olanzapine and +0.7 mg/dL for risperidone. The between-group difference in change was significant for both triglycerides and cholesterol parameters ($P<0.001$ for each).

Lipid changes during antipsychotic therapy: 1984–2006 *(continued)*

Reference	Study design	Findings
Melkersson and Dahl 2003	Cross-sectional study of lipids and insulin parameters in long-term treatment (mean=8.2 years for clozapine and 1.2 years for olanzapine) 18 clozapine (median dosage=400 mg/day) 16 olanzapine (median dosage=10 mg/day)	Triglycerides were elevated in 44% of clozapine and 56% of olanzapine patients. Cholesterol was elevated in 39% of the clozapine and 63% of the olanzapine cohort. High LDL was found in 17% of clozapine- and 38% of olanzapine-treated patients. Normal HDL levels were reported in all but one patient of each drug group. No significant between-group differences were found in hyperlipidemia rates or median lipid levels.
Weiden et al. 2003	6-week ziprasidone switch study. All labs were nonfasting. Mean ziprasidone dosage=91 mg/day Prior medications 104 from olanzapine 58 from risperidone 108 from typical antipsychotics	Median changes from baseline for triglycerides: −50 mg/dL in those switched from olanzapine ($P<0.0001$) and −29 mg/dL in those switched from risperidone ($P<0.01$). Median changes in cholesterol: −17 mg/dL ($P<0.0001$) for olanzapine and −12 mg/dL ($P<0.005$) for risperidone. Cholesterol levels declined in 76% of patients switched from olanzapine and 72% switched from risperidone. Reductions in lipid levels in patients switched from typical antipsychotics were nonsignificant.

Lipid changes during antipsychotic therapy: 1984–2006 *(continued)*

Reference	Study design	Findings
Atmaca et al. 2003a	6-week prospective schizophrenia study 14 quetiapine (mean=535.7 mg/day) 14 olanzapine (mean=15.7 mg/day) 14 risperidone (mean=6.7 mg/day) 14 clozapine (mean=207.1 mg/day) 11 control subjects (no psychotropic medication)	Compared with control subjects, significant increases in fasting triglycerides were seen for olanzapine (+31.23 mg/dL; $P<0.001$), clozapine (+36.28 mg/dL; $P<0.001$), and quetiapine (+11.64 mg/dL; $P<0.05$) but not risperidone (+3.87 mg/dL; $P=0.76$).
Atmaca et al. 2003b	6-week prospective schizophrenia study 15 haloperidol 15 olanzapine 15 quetiapine	Serum triglyceride increases were much greater for olanzapine compared with quetiapine or haloperidol and for quetiapine compared with haloperidol.
Baymiller et al. 2003	Prospective 1 year open-label study 50 clozapine (mean=454±109 mg/day)	From baseline, 54.7 mg/dL (41.7%) increase in serum triglycerides ($P=0.001$) and 14.4 mg/dL (7.5%) increase in total cholesterol ($P<0.001$). No significant changes in HDL or LDL. Serum triglyceride level peaked between days 41 and 120 and then declined but remained elevated. Use of propranolol exacerbated increases in total cholesterol and triglycerides.

Lipid changes during antipsychotic therapy: 1984–2006 *(continued)*

Reference	Study design	Findings
Almeras et al. 2004	Cross-sectional study of male schizophrenia patients in Canada. All subjects on drug more than 6 months. Results compared with reference group of nondiabetic males (mean age=28.4 years for risperidone, 31.7 years for olanzapine, 32.8 years for control subjects) 42 olanzapine (mean dosage=12.4 mg/day) 45 risperidone (mean dose=2.9 mg/day)	Risperidone subjects had significantly lower serum cholesterol, LDL, triglycerides, cholesterol:HDL ratio, and apolipoprotein B. Risperidone cohort had significantly higher HDL, larger LDL peak particle size, and greater apolipoprotein A₁. Compared with reference group, no differences were found for olanzapine subjects in cholesterol, triglycerides, or LDL, but olanzapine subjects had lower HDL and higher cholesterol:HDL ratio. Risperidone cohort had lower cholesterol and LDL but also lower HDL than the reference group.
Cohen et al. 2004	Chart review of 10 autistic adults (mean age, 43 years) switched to ziprasidone and followed for more than 6 months 10 ziprasidone (mean dosage=128 mg/day)	Data on lipids available for only 5 subjects: 4 of 5 had a decrease in total cholesterol, but mean decrease (−2.6 mg/dL) was not significant; 3 of 5 had a decrease in serum triglycerides, but mean decrease (−21.8 mg/dL) was not significant.
De Deyn et al. 2004	Randomized, fixed-dosage, 10-week trial of olanzapine (1.0, 2.5, 5.0, 7.5 mg/day) vs. placebo for psychosis/behavioral disturbance in Alzheimer's disease (mean age=76.6 years) 520 olanzapine 129 placebo	Serum values not reported, but report states that cholesterol and triglyceride levels were not significantly different among or between treatment groups.

Lipid changes during antipsychotic therapy: 1984–2006 *(continued)*

Reference	Study design	Findings
Kinon et al. 2004	Randomized, prospective 4-month study comparing those who switched to olanzapine with those who continued prior medication 27 olanzapine 27 risperidone or typical antipsychotics	After 4 months, no significant within-group change was found at endpoint in mean total cholesterol (−4.7 mg/dL, $P=0.69$) or triglycerides (−6.6 mg/dL, $P=0.81$) in patients switched to olanzapine or those who continued taking risperidone or typical antipsychotics (cholesterol: −0.6 mg/dL, $P=0.69$; triglycerides: +13.6 mg/dL, $P=0.28$). Elevations in lipids were noted prior to month 4 in olanzapine cohort, but these declined over time.
McQuade et al. 2004	26-week, double-blind, randomized trial in acutely relapsed schizophrenia patients 156 aripiprazole (mean dosage=25.1 mg/day) 161 olanzapine (mean dosage=16.5 mg/day)	At week 26, mean change in fasting triglycerides +79.4 mg/dL for olanzapine, +6.5 mg/dL for aripiprazole ($P<0.05$); HDL −3.39 mg/dL for olanzapine, +3.61 mg/dL for aripiprazole ($P<0.05$). Changes in total cholesterol and LDL favored aripiprazole but were not significant: total cholesterol +16.3 mg/dL for olanzapine, −1.13 mg/dL for aripiprazole; LDL +2.27 mg/dL for olanzapine, −3.86 mg/dL for aripiprazole. Incidence of new dyslipidemias was significantly greater for olanzapine on the basis of elevated total cholesterol (> 200 mg/dL: 47% olanzapine vs. 17% aripiprazole), LDL (> 130 mg/dL: 38% vs. 19%), triglycerides (> 150 mg/dL: 50% vs. 18%) ($P<0.05$ for each).

Lipid changes during antipsychotic therapy: 1984–2006 *(continued)*

Reference	Study design	Findings
Simpson et al. 2004	6-week, double-blind, randomized trial in acute schizophrenia/schizoaffective disorder 136 ziprasidone (mean dosage=129.9 mg/day) 133 olanzapine (mean dosage=11.3 mg/day)	Endpoint change in fasting total cholesterol was significant for olanzapine (median=+19.5 mg/dL; $P<0.0001$) vs. ziprasidone (median=−1.0 mg/dL; $P=0.48$ from baseline); $P<0.0001$ between groups. Triglycerides increased a median 26 mg/dL for olanzapine ($P=0.0003$) and decreased a median of 2 mg/dL for ziprasidone ($P=0.77$); between-group difference was significant ($P<0.003$). LDL increased by a median of 13 mg/dL for olanzapine ($P<0.0001$) and decreased 1 mg/dL for ziprasidone ($P=0.78$); between-group difference was significant ($P<0.0004$). Apolipoprotein B increased 9.0 mg/dL for olanzapine ($P<0.0001$) and decreased 3.0 mg/dL for ziprasidone ($P=0.17$); between-group difference was significant ($P<0.0001$). There was no impact or between-group differences in HDL, apolipoprotein A₁, or lipoprotein A levels.
Waage et al. 2004	Case report of olanzapine-induced pancreatitis in a 42-year-old man with chronic paranoid psychosis	Baseline total cholesterol 189 mg/dL. After 7 months, total cholesterol 282 mg/dL. At time of admission with pancreatitis, 19 months after starting olanzapine, total cholesterol was 552 mg/dL and triglycerides 2,044 mg/dL.

Lipid changes during antipsychotic therapy: 1984–2006 *(continued)*

Reference	Study design	Findings
Ball et al. 2005	Case report of clozapine-induced hypercholesterolemia and hypertriglyceridemia that resolved after switch to aripiprazole in a 42-year-old male with schizoaffective disorder	Peak lipid levels: total cholesterol 477 mg/dL and triglycerides 4,758 mg/dL. Patient hospitalized subsequently due to noncompliance, with lipid levels at time of admission: cholesterol 213 mg/dL, triglycerides 298 mg/dL, and LDL 146 mg/dL while on simvastatin. Trial of aripiprazole, up to 45 mg/day for 5 weeks, with lipids (off of simvastatin): cholesterol 163 mg/dL, triglycerides 145 mg/dL, LDL 100 mg/dL.
Breier et al. 2005	28-week randomized, double-blind study in patients with schizophrenia 277 olanzapine (mean dosage=15.27 mg/day) 271 ziprasidone (mean dosage=115.96 mg/day)	All between-group lipid changes significantly favored ziprasidone. Endpoint change in fasting total cholesterol for olanzapine (+3.09 mg/dL; $P=0.07$) vs. ziprasidone (−12.74 mg/dL; $P=0.08$): $P<0.0001$ between groups. Triglycerides increased +34.52 mg/dL for olanzapine ($P=0.09$) and decreased 21.24 mg/dL for ziprasidone ($P=0.11$); between-group difference was significant ($P<0.001$). LDL increased by a median of 0.77 mg/dL for olanzapine ($P=0.06$) and decreased 10.42 mg/dL for ziprasidone ($P=0.07$); between-group difference was significant ($P<0.001$). HDL decreased 2.32 mg/dL for olanzapine ($P=0.02$) and increased 0.77 mg/dL for ziprasidone ($P=0.02$); between-group difference was significant ($P=0.001$).

Lipid changes during antipsychotic therapy: 1984–2006 *(continued)*

Reference	Study design	Findings
Brown and Estoup 2005	Chart review study from Portland, OR, Veterans Affairs Medical Center 88 ziprasidone 103 olanzapine	Olanzapine associated with significant increases in total cholesterol (+16 mg/dL; $P=0.01$) and triglycerides (+61 mg/dL; $P=0.05$) but not LDL or HDL. Ziprasidone associated with significant decrease in total cholesterol (−15 mg/dL; $P<0.01$) and LDL (−18 mg/dL; $P=0.001$) and increase in HDL (+3 mg/dL, $P<0.05$). Among those who switched between agents, significant differences were found for total cholesterol ($P<0.05$) and LDL ($P<0.01$).
Graham et al. 2005	Prospective study of resting energy expenditure and metabolic outcomes in 9 adults started on olanzapine and followed 12 weeks 9 olanzapine (dosage range = 2.5–20 mg/day)	Median changes were −7 mg/dL for HDL ($P=0.19$), +1 mg/dL for LDL ($P=0.47$), + 59 mg/dL for triglycerides ($P=0.04$). The triglyceride change was a 62.8% increase from baseline.
Henderson et al. 2005	Review of data on 96 subjects treated with clozapine and followed for 10 years	A significant linear increase in triglyceride levels was found for the duration of the follow-up (0.5 mg/dL/month; $P=0.04$) but was not found for total cholesterol ($P=0.13$). Elevations in triglycerides and total cholesterol were associated with new-onset diabetes but not cardiovascular mortality.

Lipid changes during antipsychotic therapy: 1984–2006 *(continued)*

Reference	Study design	Findings
Lambert et al. 2005	Case-control study of Medi-Cal claims after schizophrenia diagnosis and exposure to only one antipsychotic within 12 weeks prior to hyperlipidemia claim. Cases were matched for gender and age with patients with schizophrenia who did not develop hyperlipidemia.	For the 12-week exposure window, olanzapine (OR=1.20; 95% CI=1.08–1.33) was significantly associated with hyperlipidemia risk compared with typical agents but not exposure to clozapine, risperidone, or quetiapine. The odds ratio for olanzapine was greater than for risperidone (*P*=0.002). Increasing the exposure window to 24 or 52 weeks did not affect the results, although clozapine's association did become significant at 24 weeks (OR=1.22; 95% CI=1.03–1.45).
Lieberman et al. 2005	Phase I of CATIE Schizophrenia Trial	See Table 8–1 for Phase I results.
McKee et al. 2005	Chart review of 41 developmentally delayed adults switched from typical antipsychotics to olanzapine or risperidone (and some then to olanzapine) and followed up to 2 years. At endpoint: 33 olanzapine 8 risperidone	At endpoint, there were no significant changes in serum total cholesterol, LDL, or triglycerides.
Meyer et al. 2005	20-week switch study in overweight or obese olanzapine-treated patients with schizophrenia following metabolic syndrome parameters 71 risperidone	At endpoint, there was a nonsignificant decrease in serum triglycerides (−13.1 mg/dL) and HDL (−1.6 mg/dL). Overall, the prevalence of the metabolic syndrome decreased from 53.5% to 36.6% over 20 weeks (*P*<0.005).

Lipid changes during antipsychotic therapy: 1984–2006 *(continued)*

Reference	Study design	Findings
Simpson et al. 2005	6-month continuation of prior 6-week randomized, double-blind study of olanzapine vs. ziprasidone 55 ziprasidone (mean dosage = 135.2 mg/day) 71 olanzapine (mean dosage = 12.6 mg/day)	There were significant within-group median increases from baseline in total cholesterol (+13.0 mg/dL; $P=0.03$) and LDL (+17.0 mg/dL; $P=0.04$) with olanzapine and nonsignificant changes with ziprasidone in total cholesterol (−1.0 mg/dL; $P=0.98$) and LDL (9.0 mg/dL; $P=0.29$).
Su et al. 2005	Cross-over switch study in 15 schizophrenia patients followed for 3 months after switch 7 risperidone switched to olanzapine 8 olanzapine switched to risperidone	After switch to olanzapine there were nonsignificant changes in LDL (−1.0 mg/dL), HDL (+0.4 mg/dL), and total cholesterol (+20.5 mg/dL), but a significant increase in triglycerides (+84.3 mg/dL; $P<0.05$). In those switched to risperidone there were nonsignificant changes in LDL (+5.9 mg/dL), HDL (+6.8 mg/dL), and total cholesterol (−8.6 mg/dL), but a significant decrease in triglycerides (−86.0 mg/dL; $P<0.05$).
Stroup et al. 2006	Phase II intolerability arm of CATIE Schizophrenia Trial	See Table 8–1 for Phase IIa results.
McEvoy et al. 2006	Phase II nonresponse arm of CATIE Schizophrenia Trial	See Table 8–1 for Phase IIb results.

Note.   CATIE = Clinical Antipsychotic Trials of Intervention Effectiveness; CPZ = chlorpromazine; HbA$_{1c}$ = hemoglobin A$_{1c}$; HDL = high-density lipoprotein; LDL = low-density lipoprotein; VLDL = very-low-density lipoprotein.

Chapter 9

METABOLIC RISK ASSESSMENT, MONITORING, AND INTERVENTIONS

Translating What We Have Learned Into Practice

Richard A. Bermudes, M.D.
Paul E. Keck Jr., M.D.
Susan L. McElroy, M.D.

Clinicians are well informed of the metabolic risks of the atypical antipsychotics (American Diabetes Association et al. 2004; Expert Group 2004; Lambert et al. 2004; Marder et al. 2004). A recent survey indicated psychiatrists commonly identify the metabolic risks of weight gain and premature diabetes associated with atypical antipsychotics and regularly monitor patients' weight. However, psychiatrists differ as to whether they are responsible for monitoring the general medical conditions of the mentally ill and rarely report monitoring waist circumference, lipid profiles, or blood pressures of their patients (Newcomer et al. 2004). Although psychiatrists perceive their patients to be at significant risk for metabolic problems versus the general population, it is unclear how they come to this conclusion with individual patients. That is, which particular metabolic problems or parameters are used by psychiatrists in determining a patient's metabolic risk? Do psychiatrists consider a patient's lipid profile, blood pressure, or family history as part of this calculation? What metabolic parameters, data, or history do they have or gather prior to starting pharmacotherapy?

In this chapter we propose an assessment tool to evaluate patients' metabolic risk. In addition to the fact that many psychiatric medications are associated with metabolic problems, there are a number of reasons why we propose a thorough metabolic risk assessment of each patient:

- Cardiovascular disease (CVD) is the primary cause of death for both men and women in the United States and in most countries worldwide and correlates with other metabolic problems such as dyslipidemia, high blood pressure, and diabetes (Bonow et al. 2002).
- CVD is a leading cause of death in persons with mental disorders. Individuals with mental illness possess a substantial burden of metabolic morbidity and die at an earlier age from these conditions versus the general population (Kilbourne et al. 2004).
- There may be a correlation between the mechanisms leading to CVD and other metabolic problems and the mechanisms leading to mental illness, such as dysregulation of cortisol, coagulation, and inflammatory factors.
- Lifestyle changes in diet, exercise, and tobacco use improve mental health and well-being. One of the best ways to monitor the success of a patient's lifestyle changes is to monitor cardiovascular and diabetic risk markers.
- Despite the evidence that psychiatric patients are at high risk for metabolic problems and poor health outcomes secondary to complications from diabetes and CVD, this is not true for all patients. Certainly we do not want to deprive patients of efficacious agents out of a blanket fear of metabolic complications, especially when a number of patients do not carry this risk.

Predicting which patients will have medication-induced metabolic side effects is difficult. The majority of information in this area is on the atypical antipsychotics, although the studies are retrospective and involve secondary outcomes. Studies of olanzapine identify younger age, lower body mass index (BMI), positive clinical response, early rapid weight gain, and appetite increases to predict a final weight gain of 7% or more of premedication weight (Basson et al. 2001; Jones et al. 2001; Kinon et al. 2001). Similar factors predict weight gain associated with risperidone, clozapine, haloperidol, and other antipsychotics (Basson et al. 2001; Briffa and Meehan 1998; Hummer et al. 1995; Lamberti et al. 1992; Lane et al. 2003; Leadbetter et al. 1992; Meltzer et al. 2003; Umbricht et al. 1994; Wetterling and Mussigbrodt 1999). However, none of these studies controlled for diet, tobacco use, family history, or other baseline measures of metabolic status such as fasting glucose, waist circumference, or lipid profile. It is not known what predicts clinically significant weight gain ($\geq$7% baseline weight) or metabolic disturbances in ziprasidone- or aripiprazole-treated patients, although from studies and clinical use this appears to be an infrequent problem (Centorrino et al. 2005; Harvey and Bowie 2005). In addition, little is known about predictors of metabolic disturbances or weight gain with medications outside of the atypical antipsychotic class, such as valproic acid, lithium, and mirtazapine (Fawcett and Barkin 1998; Fisfalen and Hsiung 2003; Isojaryi et al. 1996; Livingstone and Rampes 2005).

Given the difficulty of predicting metabolic side effects and the propensity of patients with mental disorders to have metabolic problems, we propose a thorough cardiovascular and diabetic risk assessment prior to pharmacotherapy in order to better inform clinicians, patients, and their families of the particular cardiovascular or diabetic risk they may face.

Initial Assessment

The objective of the proposed assessment tool is to identify patients who are at highest risk for diabetes or CVD. The assessment begins by cataloging risk factors for diabetes and CVD as well as the metabolic disorders the patient has been diagnosed with to date (Step 1; see Table 9–1). Patients should be asked about current smoking status, physical activity levels, and family history of diabetes and coronary heart disease (CHD); although other risk factors are important in predisposing patients to diabetes or CVD, these particular risk factors have been identified by the National Cholesterol Education Program and the American Diabetes Association for predicting and quantifying patients' risk for these two disorders (Expert Panel on Detection, Evaluation, and Treatment of High Blood Cholesterol in Adults 2001; Herman et al. 1995). All patients should have BMI, blood pressure, and, if BMI≤ 35, waist circumference measured (Step 2). These anthropometric measures are simple, inexpensive, require no fasting blood work, and with proper training can be completed in outpatient settings with little to no impact on the time for psychiatric assessment. Waist circumference in particular is the single best anthropometric measure to use in identifying patients at high risk for CVD, and in combination with fasting glucose or blood pressure it is a cost-effective screening tool in psychiatric settings (Dobbelsteyn et al. 2001; Pouliot et al. 1994; Straker et al. 2005).

In Step 3 of the assessment we differentiate patients who should receive fasting blood work from those who do not require this monitoring. The following patients require a fasting glucose and lipid profile:

- Patients prescribed any of the atypical antipsychotics
- Patients with two or more risk factors or previously diagnosed metabolic conditions
- Patients with newly diagnosed hypertension or obesity or individuals with abnormal waist circumferences
- In the absence of any of these criteria, men older than 35 years of age and women older than 45 years of age who have not been monitored in the previous 5 years also are candidates for testing (U.S. Preventive Services Task Force 2001).

TABLE 9–1.   Assessing and assigning risk

Step 1:

Assess risk factors and history of metabolic problems	**History** Risk factors
	 • Age
	   Men ≥ 45 years
	   Women ≥ 55 years
	 • Cigarette smoking
	 • Family history of CHD
	   CHD in male first-degree relative <55 years of age
	   CHD in a female first-degree relative <65 years of age
	 • Family history of diabetes
	   Diabetes in first-degree relative
	 • Physical inactivity
	   Less than 30 minutes, 3 times a week of moderate activity such as walking
		Diagnosed metabolic disorders
		 • Hypertension
		 • CHD
		 • Hyperlipidemia
		 • Diabetes
		 • Gestational diabetes
		 • Obesity

Step 2

Physical examination to assess metabolic risk	• Measure weight and height (calculate BMI) • Measure blood pressure • Assess waist circumference if BMI≤35

Step 3

Assess need for further laboratory testing	Check fasting lipid panel and fasting glucose if any of the following exist: • Two or more risk factors are present • Previous or current diagnosis of a metabolic disorder • Age > 35 years in males or > 45 years in females and no testing in the previous 5 years • Blood pressure > 140/90 • BMI > 30 • Waist circumference > 40 inches in a male or > 35 inches in a female • Prescribing an atypical antipsychotic

TABLE 9–1. Assessing and assigning risk *(continued)*

Step 4	Age, years	Points
Assign patient risk level for CHD using Framingham point system	20–34	−9
	35–39	−4
	40–44	0
	45–49	3
	50–54	6
	55–59	8
	60–64	10
	65–69	11
	70–74	12
	75–79	13

TC, mg/dL	20–39 years	40–49 years	50–59 years	60–69 years	70–79 years
<160	0	0	0	0	0
160–199	4	3	2	1	0
200–239	7	5	3	1	0
240–279	9	6	4	2	1
≥280	11	8	5	3	1

Smoking status	20–39 years	40–49 years	50–59 years	60–69 years	70–79 years
Nonsmoker	0	0	0	0	0
Smoker	8	5	3	1	1

HDL, mg/dL	Points
≥ 60	−1
50–59	0
40–49	1
< 40	2

Systolic blood pressure, mm Hg	Untreated	Treated
< 120	0	0
120–129	0	1
130–139	1	2
140–159	1	2
≥ 160	2	3

TABLE 9–1. Assessing and assigning risk *(continued)*

Add points
  Age   _____
  TC   _____
  Smoking   _____
  HDL   _____
  Blood pressure   _____
  Total   _____

Total points and 10-year risk for CHD	Total points	10-year risk for CHD	Framingham risk level
	<12	<10%	Low
	12–15	10%–20%	Moderate
	>15	>20%	High

Step 5	Risk factors	Points
Assign patient risk level for diabetes	BMI ≥ 27	5
	< 65 years of age and physically inactive	5
	Age 46–64 years	5
	Age ≥ 65 years	9
	History of gestational diabetes or baby weighing >9 lb	1
	Parent with diabetes	1
	Sibling with diabetes	1
	If total points ≥9, patient at high risk for diabetes	

Note. BMI=body mass index; CHD=coronary heart disease; HDL=high-density lipoprotein; TC=total cholesterol.

In Steps 4 and 5, the clinician quantifies the patient's risk for CHD and diabetes. In Step 4, the Framingham risk calculation is performed for patients with two or more risk factors (abnormal values for two or more of the following measures): 1) total cholesterol, 2) systolic blood pressure, 3) high-density lipoprotein (HDL) level, 4) smoking status, and 5) age. When a patient has fewer than two risk factors, the calculation is unnecessary because the 10-year risk for CHD generally is low (<10% risk for CHD in 10 years) and pharmacotherapy or lifestyle interventions are generally not needed to meet low-density lipoprotein (LDL) treatment goals for patients in this category. The Framingham system divides individuals into three risk groups: 1) patients with a 10-year risk for CHD higher than 20% (high risk), 2) patients with a 10%–20% 10-year risk for CHD (moderate risk), and 3) patients with a 10-year risk for CHD that is less than 10% (low risk). For example consider, a 55-year-old female patient with a total cholesterol level of 220 mg/dL, HDL of 50 mg/dL, and an untreated systolic blood pressure of 120 mm Hg who also smokes. She would receive 8 points for her age, 3 points for her total cholesterol level, 3 points for her smoking status, 0 points for her HDL level, and 0 points for her systolic blood pressure. Her total score would be 14 points, placing her in the moderate-risk category (10%–20%) for CHD.

In Step 5, the patient's risk for diabetes is categorized by means of the Diabetes Risk Test. This score incorporates age, family history, activity level, BMI, and history of delivery of a macrosomic infant to categorize an individual's risk for diabetes. The Diabetes Risk Test is a simple, fast, inexpensive, noninvasive, self-administered, and reliable tool to identify individuals at high risk for type 2 diabetes (T2DM) and a useful alternative to indiscriminate fasting blood glucose measurement. In a representative U.S. sample ($N>3,000$), the test had a sensitivity of 79% and specificity of 65% for detecting diabetes (Herman et al. 1995). Individuals with scores of 10 or higher should be categorized at high risk for future development of diabetes and metabolic complications (American Diabetes Association 2005). Consider the case of a 49-year-old physically active woman with a BMI of 24, no family history of diabetes, and no history of gestational diabetes or a macrosomic infant. She would receive 5 points for age and 0 points for family history, normal birth history, and her physical activity level, placing her in the low-risk category.

Selection of Treatment

Once a patient's cardiovascular and diabetes risks are assessed, clinicians can customize pharmacotherapy, making treatment choices that minimize further metabolic complications (Figure 9–1). With a reliable metabolic risk profile for each patient, clinicians, patients, and families can weigh the benefits and risks of specific medications in order to minimize unwanted complications of weight gain, dyslipidemia, and hypertension. In patients at highest risk for CVD or diabetes or patients with established obesity, hypertension, dyslipidemia, CVD, or diabetes, medications associated with greater severity of metabolic side effects should be considered as a last resort. Furthermore, medications with fewer propensities for metabolic side effects should be considered in treatment-naïve patients and in patients without established history of response to a particular medication, given the high risk for metabolic disorders that psychiatric patients face, independent of treatment. Given the increasing number of agents available to treat psychiatric disorders with little to no metabolic side effects, our objective is to reduce the risk for CVD and diabetes for high-risk patients and help low-risk patients maintain their healthy status.

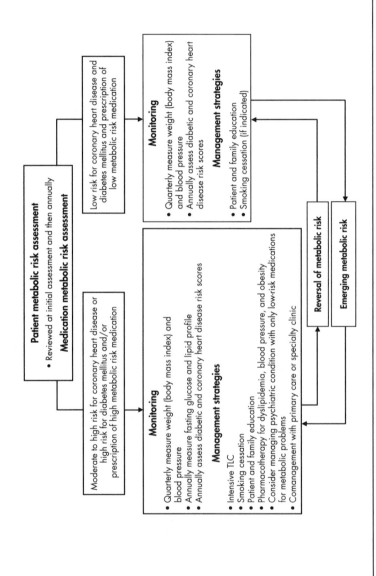

FIGURE 9–1.   Tailoring metabolic monitoring and management to metabolic risk.

Follow-up Monitoring

PUBLISHED CONSENSUS MONITORING GUIDELINES

Table 9–2 summarizes the monitoring guidelines for atypical antipsychotics from the different consensus documents published to date (American Diabetes Association et al. 2004; Expert Group 2004; Lambert et al. 2004; Marder et al. 2004). These guidelines recommend regular monitoring of weight, waist circumference, blood pressure, fasting blood glucose, and lipid profile. In general, the frequency of monitoring decreases as the duration of treatment increases. There are several unaddressed issues related to the guidelines. First, the guidelines do not address the increased risk psychiatric patients face independent of pharmacotherapy. Second, they do not address how to monitor or manage patients who already have a metabolic disorder. Should all patients, regardless of baseline metabolic status, be monitored at the same frequency? Third, the guidelines do not address monitoring for patients who are prescribed other medications (outside of the atypical class) that may have a high likelihood of causing weight gain or other metabolic problems. A number of psychiatric medications outside the atypical antipsychotic class are associated with weight gain and other metabolic disorders. In this regard, the current guidelines are too narrow and specific to atypical antipsychotic treatment despite the weight and metabolic liability of a number of psychotropic medications.

SPECIFIC METABOLIC MONITORING RECOMMENDATIONS FOR ALL PATIENTS WITH MENTAL DISORDERS

Given the risk psychiatric patients have for metabolic problems, we present guidelines for monitoring metabolic problems as well as criteria for management interventions (Table 9–3; Figure 9–2). The first assessment includes CHD risk scoring and diabetes risk scoring as well as measurement of weight (BMI), waist circumference, and blood pressure. Fasting glucose and lipid profile are measured according to the criteria outlined in Table 9–1. When a new medication with a high liability for weight or metabolic disturbance is initiated or added to a patient's regimen, follow-up monitoring of most parameters should occur sometime within the first 12 weeks. Low-risk patients with no emerging signs or symptoms of metabolic disturbances can then have their weight and blood pressure monitored quarterly, with an updated risk assessment renewed annually. Patients with moderate or high risk for CHD or high risk for diabetes should have their fasting glucose and lipid profile regularly monitored (annually). When patients are taking stable medication and when there are no changes in baseline metabolic parameters or risk categorization, these patients' weight and blood pressure should be monitored quarterly, and CHD risk, diabetes risk, fasting glucose, and lipid profile should be annually reassessed. Thus risk stratification for diabetes or CHD is es-

TABLE 9–2. Published monitoring protocols for patients prescribed atypical antipsychotics

Metabolic parameter	Baseline	Each visit for 6 months	4 weeks	8 weeks	12 weeks	4 months	Quarterly	Every 6 months	Annually	Every 2 years	Every 5 years
Weight	X[1,2]	X[2]	X[1]	X[1]	X[1,3]		X[1,2]				
Waist circumference	X[1,3]				X[3]				X[1]		
Blood pressure	X[1,3]				X[1]			X[3]	X[1]		
Fasting plasma glucose	X[1,2,3,4]		X[3]		X[1]	X[2,4]		X[3]	X[1,2,4]		
Glycosylated hemoglobin (HbA$_{1c}$) test	X[2,4]					X[2,4]			X[2]		
Fasting lipid profile	X[1,3]				X[1]			X[2,3]		X[2]	X[1]

[1]American Diabetes Association et al. 2004.
[2]Marder et al. 2004.
[3]Lambert et al. 2004.
[4]Expert Group 2004.

TABLE 9–3. Metabolic monitoring guidelines for patients with mental disorders

Metabolic parameter	Baseline	12 weeks[a]	Quarterly	Annually	Criteria for management interventions
CHD/DRS	X	X		X	DRS ≥ 9 or CHD risk score ≥ 12
Weight (BMI)	X	X	X	X	≥ 5% increase in baseline weight
Waist circumference	X	X		X	Male: > 102 cm (40 in) / Female: > 88 cm (35 in)
Fasting glucose	b	X		X[c]	Fasting glucose ≥ 100 mg/dL
Fasting lipid profile	b	X		X[c]	LDL ≥ 130, HDL < 40, triglycerides ≥ 200[d]
Blood pressure	X	X	X	X	Diastolic ≥ 90 or Systolic ≥ 160

Note.   BMI = body mass index; CHD = coronary heart disease; DRS = Diabetes Risk Score.

[a]Check parameters within 12 weeks of beginning new pharmacotherapy with high liability for metabolic problems, such as atypical antipsychotics or other medications with high risk for weight gain.

[b]See Table 9–1.

[c]Patients with moderate or high risk for CHD or high risk for diabetes or patients receiving pharmacotherapy with high liability for metabolic problems.

[d]See Figure 9–2 for detailed cut-off criteria.

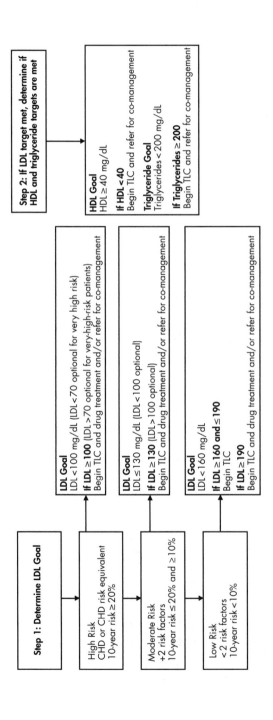

FIGURE 9–2.   Coronary heart disease (CHD) risk: low-density lipoprotein (LDL), high-density lipoprotein (HDL), and triglyceride goals.

CHD includes history of myocardial infarction, unstable angina, stable angina, coronary artery procedures (angioplasty or bypass surgery), or evidence of clinically significant myocardial ischemia. CHD risk equivalents include clinical manifestations of noncoronary forms of atherosclerotic disease (peripheral arterial disease, abdominal aortic aneurysm, and carotid artery disease [transient ischemic attacks or stroke of carotid origin or >50% obstruction of a carotid artery]), diabetes, and two or more risk factors with 10-year risk for hard CHD > 20%. TLC = therapeutic lifestyle changes.

Source.   Data from Grundy et al. 2004; Expert Panel on Detection, Evaluation, and Treatment of High Blood Cholesterol in Adults 2001.

sential not only for patients beginning new medications but also at the initial assessment and then annually in order to determine which patients get more intensive monitoring for metabolic problems.

Management of Metabolic Conditions

In monitoring for metabolic problems in psychiatric patients, it is important to define cutoff criteria for intensive management or referral. These criteria are listed in Table 9–3 and include values for weight gain, waist circumference, fasting glucose, lipids, and blood pressure. Although these parameters have not been studied as cutoff points to intensify management of metabolic problems in psychiatric patients, each is a potentially reversible risk factor that predicts poor metabolic outcomes (i.e., diabetes or CVD) and in some cases, when combined with other criteria, predicts mortality (Ford 2005).

The objective of treating and managing metabolic problems is to prevent T2DM and CHD. Three levels of intervention are 1) lifestyle interventions aimed at weight control, enhancing regular exercise, and promoting a healthy diet; 2) changing pharmacotherapy to minimize metabolic risks; and 3) managing individual conditions such as dyslipidemia, hypertension, obesity, and hyperglycemia.

Weight control, regular exercise, a healthy diet, and smoking cessation are the areas in which treatment should begin. Switching medication from the "offending agent" may be the first response, but this may not be the best option, particularly if the patient has responded to the agent despite metabolic side effects. For example, results from a national study of the effectiveness of atypical antipsychotics in schizophrenia suggest olanzapine may be more effective than other atypical antipsychotics despite its high liability for weight gain and associated metabolic abnormalities (Lieberman et al. 2005). Lifestyle interventions should be considered the first option of choice in patients taking an effective agent with metabolic side effects. Smoking cessation, weight loss, exercise, and switching to a diet low in fat and carbohydrates reverse metabolic abnormalities and delay the onset of T2DM and CVD. Even modest weight loss, such as 10% of initial body weight in individuals who are overweight (BMI≥25) or obese (BMI≥30) can significantly reduce weight-associated hypertension, hyperlipidemia, and hyperglycemia as well as decrease mortality (National Institutes of Health 1998).

There is no single diet that specifically reverses metabolic abnormalities. One approach is to tailor dietary advice to each patient's specific metabolic abnormality. The infeasibility of doing this in a psychiatric practice without access to specialized nutritional counseling makes the approach impractical. There is considerable debate about which diet (e.g., low-fat, low-carbohydrate) produces the best results for patients' overall metabolic profiles. However, if a patient is exercising and consuming fewer calories than he or she is expending, diet composition is secondary, because weight loss itself reverses metabolic abnormalities. Dansinger et al. (2005) compared adherence and the effectiveness of four popular diets (Atkins, Zone, Weight Watchers, and Ornish) for weight loss and cardiac risk factor reduction and found each had comparable adherence rates and reductions in weight and cardiac risk factors. Overall dietary adherence rates were low among the four diets. Contrary to popular belief, adherence best predicted weight and cardiac risk factor reduction for each diet group rather than the specific diet itself. This study also challenges the notion that one type of diet is best for everybody, as well as the suggestion that low-carbohydrate diets are better than standard diets. Thus in clinical practice emphasis should be placed on reducing caloric intake rather than on a specific diet. A broad spectrum of diet options to better match the individual patient's food preferences, lifestyle, and cardiovascular risk profile should be offered in clinical practice to maximize patient adherence and improve metabolic outcomes.

Regular exercise, even at modest levels, improves metabolic risk factors, including HDL and triglyceride levels, blood pressure, and hyperglycemia (Fagard 2001; Leon and Sanchez 2001; Thompson et al. 2001). Even exercise in the absence of dietary change can reverse metabolic abnormalities. In one prospective study, the prevalence of the metabolic syndrome was decreased by 30% in a cohort after 20 weeks of supervised aerobic training three times a week (Katzmarzyk et al. 2003). Participants received counseling at the initial visit and at midway through the study that they should not alter their usual health and lifestyle habits other than their exercise training. Among participants who no longer met criteria for the metabolic syndrome, 43% decreased triglycerides, 16% improved HDL cholesterol, 38% decreased blood pressure, 9% improved fasting glucose, and 28% decreased waist circumference. Modest changes in aerobic exercise and weight loss improve cardiac and diabetic risk factors and reverse metabolic abnormalities.

Despite the fact that cigarette smoking continues to be the single most important preventable cause of death and disability in the United States and that individuals with mental illness have high rates of tobacco dependence, psychiatrists rarely offer smoking cessation counseling to psychiatric patients (Himelhoch and Daumit 2003; Lasser et al. 2000; "A Clinical Practice Guideline for Treating Tobacco Use and Dependence" 2000). Although it is true that smoking cessation often leads to weight gain and may thereby lead to subsequent deleterious metabolic problems, smoking itself has far-reaching negative effects on metabolic parameters and continues to be the most important lifestyle variable and contributor to excess mortality from cardiovascular causes (Flegal et al. 1995; Liese et al. 2000; Williamson et al. 1991). Smokers have a lower mean BMI compared with nonsmokers; however, they have higher central adiposity, which is associated with more metabolic problems (Bamia et al. 2004; Barrett-Connor and Khaw 1989; Conoy et al. 2005; Lissner et al. 1992; Shimokata et al. 1989). A meta-analysis of cross-sectional studies on the association of lipid profiles and cigarette smoking status revealed that smokers had higher serum concentrations of total cholesterol (3.0%), triglycerides (9.1%), very-low-density lipoprotein cholesterol (10.4%) and LDL cholesterol (1.7%), and lower serum concentrations of HDL cholesterol (−5.7%) than nonsmokers (Craig et al. 1989). Prospective studies show smokers have an increased risk for impaired fasting glucose and T2DM (Manson et al. 2000; Nakanishi et al. 2000; Sairenchi et al. 2004). Despite the risk of weight gain with smoking cessation, smoking is the wrong way to stay slim (Califano 1995). Smoking cessation alone reduces metabolic problems such as low HDL, and it can decrease the risk for CHD by as much as 50% (Eliasson et al. 1997, 2001; Maeda et al. 2003; Villablanca et al. 2000).

Interest in smoking cessation among the mentally ill is often higher than assumed by clinicians. In some surveys 20%–30% of patients express a significant desire to quit (Addington et al. 1997, 1999). Standard approved smoking cessation medications and therapies are efficacious and tolerated in the chronically mentally ill, including those with primary psychotic disorders (Table 9–4) (Chengappa et al. 2001; Chou et al. 2004; Evins et al. 2001, 2004; George et al. 2000, 2002; Ziedonis and George 1997). Smoking cessation in this population with the nicotine transdermal patch produces quit rates of approximately 30%–40% and with bupropion of 10%–50% (George et al. 2003). Furthermore, specialized programs designed specifically for the mentally ill, such as integrated treatment of smoking cessation and mental illness and certain pharmacotherapies such as atypical antipsychotics, may improve abstinence rates in this population (Addington et al. 1998; George et al. 1995; McEvoy et al. 1995; McFall et al. 2005).

Motivating patients with chronic mental illness to reduce their weight, improve exercise habits, and stop smoking may seem like an impossible task. With deficits in attention, memory, and motivation, as well as high rates of substance abuse disorders, many clinicians assume mentally ill patients will not derive any benefit from recommended exercise or weight reduction programs. However, in a prospective 12-month trial, Menza et al. (2004) found patients with schizophrenia or schizoaffective disorder had significant improvements in weight, blood pressure, exercise level, nutrition level, and hemoglobin A_{1c} when enrolled in a 52-week multimodal program that incorporated nutrition, exercise, and behavioral interventions compared with patients given usual care. This intervention occurred in the context of a community mental health day program with real-world patients taking second-generation antipsychotics. Most successful programs incorporate a multidisciplinary educational approach that focuses on changes in diet, exercise, and other lifestyle factors over the long term (Littrell et al. 2003). By utilizing a multidisciplinary approach and teaming up with nurses, dieticians, recreational therapists, and self-help and specialized groups, community psychiatrists can be more effective in helping their patients make changes in diet and exercise.

TABLE 9–4.   Practical office-based treatments for smoking cessation

Medication	Dosage	Duration	Availability	Comments
Psychotropics				
Bupropion (SR)	150 mg each morning for 3 days then 150 mg twice daily	Begin treatment 1–2 weeks prior to quit date and continue up to 6 months	Prescription only	Considered to be first-line agent Can treat depression and smoking cessation Can be used in combination with NRT Appropriate for smokers with weight concerns
Clonidine	0.15–0.75 mg/day	Begin just prior to quit date (up to 3 days) or on quit date and continue for 3–10 weeks	Prescription only	Considered to be second-line agent Comes in patch or pill form
Nortriptyline	75–100 mg/day	Begin treatment 3–4 weeks prior to quit date and continue for 12 weeks	Prescription only	Considered to be second-line agent Can treat depression and smoking cessation

TABLE 9–4. Practical office-based treatments for smoking cessation *(continued)*

Medication	Dosage	Duration	Availability	Comments
NRT				
Nicotine gum	1–24 cigarettes/day: 2 mg gum (up to 24 pieces/day) >25 cigarettes/day: 4 mg gum (up to 24 pieces/day)	Up to 12 weeks	Over the counter only	Adverse effects can include dyspepsia and mouth soreness
Nicotine inhaler	6–16 cartridges a day	Up to 6 months	Prescription only	Adverse effects can include irritation of mouth and throat
Nicotine nasal spray	8–40 doses a day	3–6 months	Prescription only	Adverse effects can include nasal irritation
Nicotine patch	7–21 mg/24 hours	Up to 8 weeks	Prescription and over the counter	Adverse effects can include insomnia and local skin infection

Note. Please see package inserts for complete prescribing information. NRT=nicotine replacement therapy.

Source. Reprinted from "A Clinical Practice Guideline for Treating Tobacco Use and Dependence: A U.S. Public Health Service Report. The Tobacco Use and Dependence Clinical Practice Guideline Panel, Staff, and Consortium Representatives." *JAMA* 283:3244–3254, 2000. Copyright 2000, American Medical Association. All rights reserved.

If weight control and exercise do not reduce metabolic abnormalities after 6 months, consider switching to a medication with a lower propensity for causing metabolic effects. Debate exists regarding which agents generate the most improvement in the metabolic risk profile. Within the atypical antipsychotic medication class, preliminary evidence from switch studies indicates aripiprazole or ziprasidone may improve weight gain and cholesterol profiles (Casey et al. 2003; Cohen et al. 2004). Recent data published from phase 2T of the Clinical Antipsychotic Trials of Intervention Effectiveness (CATIE) Schizophrenia Trial confirm patients with atypical antipsychotic–associated weight gain can lose weight and improve cholesterol and triglyceride levels independent of other lifestyle interventions. In that study, 20%–40% of patients who had clinically significant weight gain (≥7% baseline weight) during phase 1 of the trial lost weight and improved their lipid profiles after being randomly assigned to either ziprasidone or risperidone (Stroup et al. 2006). These findings are consistent with the American Diabetes Association/American Psychiatric Association consensus guidelines that indicate that metabolic and weight risk varies among atypical antipsychotics (American Diabetes Association et al. 2004).

Medical management of hypertension, dyslipidemia, and obesity should begin in collaboration with a primary care physician if lifestyle and medication changes do not reverse metabolic problems (Table 9–5). Medications targeted at each metabolic abnormality reduce the risk for diabetes and CVD. For example, the risk for CHD can be reduced by more than 50% through proper control of blood pressure and HDL and LDL levels in patients with metabolic problems (Wong et al. 2003). Insulin-sensitizing agents and metformin, alone or in combination with lifestyle changes, have been shown to be effective in delaying the onset of T2DM. Studies indicate that this approach effectively delays the progression to T2DM and CVD in individuals with more than one metabolic abnormality.

Metabolic problems often co-occur and interact to confer a higher risk for CVD and diabetes in individuals with mental disorders. Because these disorders occur at high rates in the mentally ill and many psychotropic medications increase the prevalence of these disorders, a thorough metabolic risk assessment and regular monitoring of metabolic risk is the new standard of care for all psychiatric patients. Identification of metabolic problems should prompt intensive intervention and lifestyle changes for which weight loss, exercise, and smoking cessation are the foundation. Emerging secondary intervention for the metabolic problems consists of targeted pharmacotherapy for weight loss, hypertension, dyslipidemia, and hyperglycemia. Mild improvements in metabolic parameters such as waist circumference, blood pressure, fasting glucose, or lipid profile can reduce CVD, T2DM, and mortality.

TABLE 9–5. Treatment interventions and goals for metabolic abnormalities

Metabolic abnormality	Diet and physical activity interventions	Pharmacological intervention	Treatment goal
Abdominal obesity	Reduce weight Increase physical activity	Sibutramine[a,b] • Appetite suppressant indicated for patients with a BMI $\geq$30 kg/m^2 Orlistat[a,b] • Lipase inhibitor indicated for patients with a BMI $\geq$30 kg/m^2	Decrease waist size to <102 cm (40 in) in men, <88 cm (35 in) in women
Hypertriglyceridemia	Reduce weight Increase physical activity Increase intake of foods with low glycemic index Reduce intake of total carbohydrates Increase consumption of omega-3 fatty acids Limit alcohol consumption	Fibrates[a,b] • Reduce fasting and postprandial triglyceride levels (20%–50%) • Shift small, dense LDL to large, buoyant particles • Increase HDL particles Nicotinic acid • Reduces triglycerides (20%–50%) Statins • Reduce fasting and postprandial triglyceride levels (7%–30%) • Reduce LDL particles • Increase HDL particles • Reduce major coronary vascular events	Decrease triglycerides to <150 mg/dL

TABLE 9–5. Treatment interventions and goals for metabolic abnormalities *(continued)*

Metabolic abnormality	Diet and physical activity interventions	Pharmacological intervention	Treatment goal
Low HDL cholesterol	Reduce weight Increase physical activity Stop smoking Increase intake of monounsaturated fats	Nicotinic acid[a] • Increases HDL particles (15%–35%) Fibrates • Reduce fasting and postprandial triglyceride levels • Shift small, dense LDL to large, buoyant particles • Increase HDL particles (10%–35%) Statins • Reduce fasting and postprandial triglyceride levels • Reduce LDL particles • Increase HDL particles (5%–15%) • Reduce major coronary vascular events	Increase HDL particles to >40 mg/dL in men, >50 mg/dL in women
Hypertension	Reduce weight Increase physical activity Reduce saturated fat intake Reduce sodium intake Limit alcohol consumption	ACE inhibitors[a] • May slow progression to diabetes • Decrease CVD events • Delay progression of microalbuminuria Angiotensin receptor blockers • May improve dyslipidemia associated with metabolic syndrome • Delay progression of microalbuminuria	Blood pressure <130/80 mm Hg

TABLE 9–5. Treatment interventions and goals for metabolic abnormalities *(continued)*

Metabolic abnormality	Diet and physical activity interventions	Pharmacological intervention	Treatment goal
Hyperglycemia	Reduce weight Increase physical activity Reduce intake of total carbohydrates	Metformin[a] • Slows progression to diabetes in individuals with insulin resistance (less effective compared with lifestyle changes) Thiazolidinediones • Slow progression to diabetes in individuals with insulin resistance	Fasting glucose <110 mg/dL

Note. ACE=angiotensin-converting enzyme; BMI=body mass index; CVD=cardiovascular disease; HDL=high-density lipoprotein; LDL=low-density lipoprotein.

[a]Suggested first-line therapy.

[b]For patients with BMI ≥30 kg/m².

Source. Adapted from Bermudes RA: "Metabolic Syndrome: Five Risk Factors Guide Therapy." *Current Psychiatry* 4:73–88, 2005. Copyright 2005, Dowden Health Media. Used with permission.

KEY CLINICAL CONCEPTS

- A thorough metabolic risk assessment and regular monitoring of metabolic risk constitute the new standard of care for all psychiatric patients, even those without prescriptions of atypical antipsychotics.
- Metabolic risk can be quantified such that further monitoring, interventions, and psychiatric treatments can then be individually determined.
- When metabolic risks are identified, dietary changes, exercise, smoking cessation, and other lifestyle changes should not be discounted for the severely mentally ill.
- Switching medications, especially within the atypical antipsychotic class, may reverse medication-induced metabolic changes.
- Medical management of hypertension, dyslipidemia, and obesity should begin in collaboration with a primary care physician if lifestyle and medication changes do not reverse metabolic problems.
- Even modest improvements in metabolic parameters can result in significant reductions in T2DM and CVD in those with mental illness.

References

Addington J, el-Guebaly N, Addington D, et al: Readiness to stop smoking in schizophrenia. Can J Psychol 42:49–52, 1997

Addington J, el-Guebaly N, Campbell W, et al: Smoking cessation treatment for patients with schizophrenia. Am J Psychiatry 155:974–976, 1998

Addington J, el-Guebaly N, Duckak V, et al: Using measures of readiness to change in individuals with schizophrenia. Am J Drug Alcohol Abuse 25:151–161, 1999

American Diabetes Association: Risk Test, Text Version. Available online at http://www.diabetes.org/risk-test/text-version.jsp. Accessed November 1, 2005

American Diabetes Association, American Psychiatric Association, American Association of Clinical Endocrinologists, North American Association for the Study of Obesity: Consensus development conference on antipsychotic drugs and diabetes. J Clin Psychiatry 65:267–272, 2004

Bamia C, Trichopoulou A, Lenas D, et al: Tobacco smoking in relation to body fat mass and distribution in a general population sample. Int J Obes Relat Metab Disord 28:1091–1096, 2004

Barrett-Connor E, Khaw KT: Cigarette smoking and increased central adiposity. Ann Intern Med 111:783–787, 1989

Basson BR, Kinon BJ, Taylor CC, et al: Factors influencing acute weight change in patients with schizophrenia treated with olanzapine, haloperidol, or risperidone. J Clin Psychiatry 62:231–238, 2001

Bermudes RA: Metabolic syndrome: five risk factors guide therapy, easy-to-use clinical values tell when to intervene. Current Psychiatry 4:73–88, 2005

Bonow RO, Smaha LA, Smith SC Jr, et al: World Heart Day 2002—the international burden of cardiovascular disease: responding to the emerging global epidemic. Circulation 106:1602–1605, 2002

Briffa D, Meehan T: Weight changes during clozapine treatment. Aust N Z J Psychiatry 32: 718–721, 1998

Califano JA: The wrong way to stay slim. N Engl J Med 33:1214–1216, 1995

Casey DE, Carson WH, Saha AR, et al: Switching patients to aripiprazole from other antipsychotic agents: a multicenter randomized study. Psychopharmacology (Berl) 166:391–399, 2003

Centorrino F, Fogarty KV, Cimbolli P, et al: Aripiprazole: initial clinical experience with 142 hospitalized psychiatric patients. J Psychiatr Pract 11:241–247, 2005

Chengappa KN, Kambhampati RK, Perkins K, et al: Bupropion sustained release as a smoking cessation treatment in remitted depressed patients maintained on treatment with selective serotonin reuptake inhibitor antidepressants. J Clin Psychiatry 62:503–508, 2001

Chou KR, Chen R, Lee JF, et al: The effectiveness of nicotine-patch therapy for smoking cessation in patients with schizophrenia. Int J Nurs Stud 41:321–330, 2004

A clinical practice guideline for treating tobacco use and dependence. A U.S. Public Health Service report. The Tobacco Use and Dependence Clinical Practice Guideline Panel, Staff, and Consortium Representatives. JAMA 283:3244–3254, 2000

Cohen SA, Fitzgerald BJ, Khan SR, et al: The effect of a switch to ziprasidone in an adult population with autistic disorder: chart review and naturalistic, open-label treatment. J Clin Psychiatry 65:110–113, 2004

Conoy D, Wareham N, Luben R et al: Cigarette smoking and fat distribution in 21,828 British men and women: a population-based study. Obes Res 13:1466–1475, 2005

Craig WY, Palomaki GE, Haddow JE: Cigarette smoking and serum lipid and lipoprotein concentrations: an analysis of published data. BMJ 298:784–788, 1989

Dansinger ML, Gleason JA, Griffth JL, et al: Comparison of the Atkins, Ornish, Weight Watchers, and Zone diets for weight loss and heart disease risk reduction. JAMA 293:43–43, 2005

Dobbelsteyn CJ, Joffres MR, MacLean DR, et al: A comparative evaluation of waist circumference, waist-to-hip ratio and body mass index as indicators of cardiovascular risk factors: the Canadian Heart Health Surveys. Int J Obes Relat Metab Disord 25:652–661, 2001

Eliasson B, Attvall S, Taskinen MR et al: Smoking cessation improves insulin sensitivity in health middle-aged men. Eur J Clin Invest 27:450–456, 1997

Eliasson B, Hjalmarson A, Kruse E, et al: Effect of smoking reduction and cessation on cardiovascular risk factors. Nicotine Tob Res 3:249–255, 2001

Evins AE, Mays VK, Rigotti NA, et al: A pilot trial of bupropion added to cognitive behavioral therapy for smoking cessation in schizophrenia. Nicotine Tob Res 3:397–403, 2001

Evins AE, Cather C, Rigotti NA, et al: Two-year follow-up of a smoking cessation trial in patients with schizophrenia: increased rates of smoking cessation and reduction. J Clin Psychiatry 65:307–311, 2004

Expert Group: Schizophrenia and Diabetes 2003 Expert Consensus Meeting, Dublin, 3–4 October 2003: consensus summary. Br J Psychiatry Suppl 47:S112–S114, 2004

Expert Panel on Detection, Evaluation, and Treatment of High Blood Cholesterol in Adults: Executive Summary of the Third Report of the National Cholesterol Education Program (NCEP) Expert Panel on Detection, Evaluation, and Treatment of High Blood Cholesterol in Adults (Adult Treatment Panel III). JAMA 285:2486–2497, 2001

Fagard RH: Exercise characteristics and blood pressure response to dynamic physical training. Med Sci Sports Exerc 33(suppl):S484–S492, 2001

Fawcett J, Barkin RL: Review of the results from clinical studies on the efficacy, safety and tolerability of mirtazapine for the treatment of patients with major depression. J Affect Disord 51:267–285, 1998

Fisfalen ME, Hsiung RC: Glucose dysregulation and mirtazapine-induced weight gain. Am J Psychiatry 160:797, 2003

Flegal KM, Trojano RP, Pamuk ER, et al: The influence of smoking cessation on the prevalence of overweight in the United States. N Engl J Med 333:1165–1170, 1995

Ford ES: Risks for all-cause mortality, cardiovascular disease, and diabetes associated with the metabolic syndrome: a summary of the evidence. Diabetes Care 28:1769–1778, 2005

George TP, Sernyak MJ, Ziedonis DM, et al: Effects of clozapine on smoking in chronic schizophrenic outpatients. J Clin Psychiatry 56:344–346, 1995

George TP, Ziedonis DM, Feingold A, et al: Nicotine transdermal patch and atypical antipsychotic medications for smoking cessation in schizophrenia. Am J Psychiatry 157:1835–1842, 2000

George TP, Vessicchio JC, Termine A, et al: A placebo-controlled study of bupropion for smoking cessation in schizophrenia. Biol Psychiatry 52:53–61, 2002

George TP, Vessichhio JC, Termine A: Nicotine and tobacco use in schizophrenia, in Medical Illness and Schizophrenia. Edited by Meyer JM, Nasrallah HA. Washington, DC, American Psychiatric Publishing, 2003, pp 81–98

Grundy SM, Cleeman JI, Merz CN, et al: Implications of recent clinical trials for the National Cholesterol Education Program Adult Treatment Panel III Guideline. Circulation 110:227–239, 2004

Harvey PD, Bowie CR: Ziprasidone: efficacy, tolerability, and emerging data on wide-ranging effectiveness. Expert Opin Pharmacother 6:337–346, 2005

Herman WH, Smith PJ, Thompson TJ, et al: A new and simple questionnaire to identify people at increased risk for undiagnosed diabetes. Diabetes Care 18:382–387, 1995

Himelhoch S, Daumit G: To whom do psychiatrists offer smoking cessation counseling? Am J Psychiatry 160:2228–2230, 2003

Hummer M, Kemmler G, Kurz M, et al: Weight gain induced by clozapine. Eur Neuropsychopharmacol 5:437–440, 1995

Isojaryi JL, Laatikainen TJ, Knip M, et al: Obesity and endocrine disorders in women taking valproate for epilepsy. Ann Neurol 39:579–584, 1996

Jones B, Basson BR, Walker DJ, et al: Weight change and atypical antipsychotic treatment in patients with schizophrenia. J Clin Psychiatry 62(suppl):41–44, 2001

Katzmarzyk PT, Leon AS, Wilmore JH, et al: Targeting the metabolic syndrome with exercise: evidence from the HERITAGE Family Study. Med Sci Sports Exerc 35:1703–1709, 2003

Kilbourne AM, Cornelius JR, Han X, et al: Burden of general medical conditions among individuals with bipolar disorder. Bipolar Disord 6:368–373, 2004

Kinon BJ, Basson BR, Gilmore JA, et al: Long-term olanzapine treatment: weight change and weight-related health factors in schizophrenia. J Clin Psychiatry 62:92–100, 2001

Lambert TJ, Chapman LH, Consensus Working Group: diabetes, psychotic disorders, and antipsychotic therapy: a consensus statement. Med J Aust 181:544–548, 2004

Lamberti JS, Bellnier T, Schwarzkopf SB: Weight gain among schizophrenic patients treated with clozapine. Am J Psychiatry 149:689–690, 1992

Lane HY, Chang YC, Cheng YC, et al: Effects of patient demographics, risperidone dosage, and clinical outcome on body weight in acutely exacerbated schizophrenia. J Clin Psychiatry 64:316–320, 2003

Lasser K, Boyd JW, Woolhandler S, et al: Smoking and mental illness: a population-based prevalence study. JAMA 284:2606–2610, 2000

Leadbetter R, Shutty M, Pavalonis D, et al: Clozapine-induced weight gain: prevalence and clinical relevance. Am J Psychiatry 149:68–72, 1992

Leon AS, Sanchez O: Meta-analysis of the effects of aerobic exercise training on blood lipids. Circulation 104(suppl):414–415, 2001

Lieberman JA, Stroup TS, McEvoy JP, et al: Effectiveness of antipsychotic drugs in patients with chronic schizophrenia. N Engl J Med 353:1209–1223, 2005

Liese AD, Hense HW, Brenner H, et al: Assessing the impact of classical risk factors on myocardial infarction by rate advancement periods. Am J Epidemiol 152:884–888, 2000

Lissner L, Bengtsson C, Lapidus L, et al: Smoking initiation and cessation in relation to body fat distribution based on data from a study of Swedish women. Am J Public Health 82:273–275, 1992

Littrell KH, Hilligoss NM, Kirshner CD, et al: The effects of an educational intervention on antipsychotic-induced weight gain. J Nurs Scholarsh 35:237–241, 2003

Livingstone C, Rampes H: Lithium: a review of its metabolic adverse effects. J Psychopharmacol 2005 Sep 20 (Epub ahead of print)

Maeda K, Noguchi Y, Fukui T: The effects of cessation from cigarette smoking on the lipid and lipoprotein profiles: a meta-analysis. Prev Med 37:283–290, 2003

Manson JE, Ajani UA, Liu S, et al: A prospective study of cigarette smoking and the incidence of diabetes mellitus among U.S. male physicians. Am J Med 109:538–542, 2000

Marder SR, Essock SM, Miller AL, et al: Physical health monitoring of patients with schizophrenia. Am J Psychiatry 161:1334–1349, 2004

McEvoy J, Freudenreich O, McGee M, et al: Clozapine decreases smoking in patients with chronic schizophrenia. Biol Psychiatry 37:550–552, 1995

McFall M, Saxon AJ, Thompson CE, et al: Improving the rates of quitting smoking for veterans with posttraumatic stress disorder. Am J Psychiatry 162:1311–1319, 2005

Meltzer HY, Perry E, Jayathilake K: Clozapine-induced weight gain predicts improvement in psychopathology. Schizophr Res 59:19–27, 2003

Menza M, Vreeland B, Minsky S, et al: Managing atypical antipsychotic-associated weight gain: 12-month data on a multimodal weight control program. J Clin Psychiatry 65:471–477, 2004

Nakanishi N, Nakamura K, Matsuo Y, et al: Cigarette smoking and risk for impaired fasting glucose and type 2 diabetes in middle-aged Japanese men. Ann Intern Med 133:183–191, 2000

National Institutes of Health: Clinical guidelines on the identification, evaluation, and treatment of overweight and obesity in adults: the evidence report. Obes Res 6(suppl):51S–209S, 1998

Newcomer JW, Nasrallah HA, Loebel AD: The atypical antipsychotic therapy and metabolic issues national survey: practice patterns and knowledge of psychiatrists. J Clin Psychopharmacol 24(suppl):S1–S6, 2004

Pouliot MC, Despres JP, Lemieux S, et al: Waist circumference and abdominal sagittal diameter: best simple anthropometric indexes of abdominal visceral adipose tissue accumulation and related cardiovascular risk in men and women. Am J Cardiol 73:460–468, 1994

Sairenchi T, Iso H, Nishimura A, et al: Cigarette smoking and risk of type 2 diabetes mellitus among middle-aged and elderly Japanese men and women. Am J Epidemiol 160:158–162, 2004

Shimokata H, Muller DC, Andres R: Studies in the distribution of body fat, III: effects of cigarette smoking. JAMA 261:1169–1173, 1989

Straker D, Correll CU, Kramer-Ginsberg E, et al: Cost-effective screening for the metabolic syndrome in patients treated with second-generation antipsychotic medications. Am J Psychiatry 162:1217–1221, 2005

Stroup TS, Lieberman JA, McEvoy JP, at al: Effectiveness of olanzapine, quetiapine, risperidone, and ziprasidone in patients with chronic schizophrenia following discontinuation of a previous atypical antipsychotic. Am J Psychiatry 163:611–622, 2006

Thompson PD, Crouse SF, Goodpaster B, et al: The acute versus the chronic response to exercise. Med Sci Sports Exerc 33(suppl):S438–S445, 2001

Umbricht DS, Pollack S, Kane JM: Clozapine and weight gain. J Clin Psychiatry 55(suppl):157–160, 1994

U.S. Preventive Services Task Force: Screening for lipid disorders in adults. Rockville, MD, Agency for Healthcare Research and Quality, 2001. Available online at http://www.ahrq.gov/clinic/uspstf/uspschol.htm. Accessed October 11, 2005

Villablanca AC, McDonald JM, Rutledge JC: Smoking and cardiovascular disease. Clin Chest Med 21:159–172, 2000

Wetterling T, Mussigbrodt HE: Weight gain: side effect of atypical neuroleptics? J Clin Psychopharmacol 19:316–321, 1999

Williamson DF, Madans J, Anda RF et al: Smoking cessation and severity of weight gain in a national cohort. N Engl J Med 324:739–745, 1991

Wong ND, Pio J, Franklin SS, et al: Preventing coronary events by optimal control of blood pressure and lipids in patients with the metabolic syndrome. Am J Cardiol 91:1421–1426, 2003

Ziedonis DM, George TP: Schizophrenia and nicotine use: report of a pilot smoking cessation program and review of neurobiological and clinical issues. Schizophr Bull 23:247–254, 1997

INDEX

Page numbers printed in **boldface** *type refer to tables or figures.*

303

Heredity. *See also* Genetics
  in severe mental illness and diabetes
    mellitus, 121
High-density lipoprotein (HDL)
    cholesterol, 58
  coronary heart disease and, **288**
Histamine, in medication-associated
    weight gain, 172–173
HIV infection, 210
Homocysteine levels, as cardiac risk factor,
    148
Hormones, in medication-associated
    weight gain, 173
HPA. *See* Hypothalamic-pituitary-adrenal
    stress hormone axis
3-Hydroxy-3-methyl-glutaryl coenzyme A,
    for management of dyslipidemia, 45
Hypercholesterolemia, **273**
Hypercortisolemia, 203
Hyperglycemia
  pathophysiology, 7–8
  risk of type 2 diabetes and. *See* Glucose
    metabolism, effects of atypical
    antipsychotics
  treatment interventions and goals, **297**
Hyperlipidemia. *See* Serum lipids, effects
    of antipsychotics
Hyperprolactinemia, in medication-
    associated weight gain, 173
Hypertension
  as cardiac risk factor, 145–146
  as complication of obesity, **60**
  metabolic syndrome and, 37, **38**, 39
    management, 44–45
  treatment interventions and goals,
    296
Hypertriglyceridemia, 245–246, **273**
  treatment interventions and goals,
    295
Hypoglycemia, as side effect of insulin, 17
Hypothalamic-pituitary-adrenal (HPA)
    stress hormone axis
  glucose regulation and, 132
  impact of mental illness and
    cardiovascular disease, 148–149

Impaired glucose tolerance.
    See Prediabetes
Incretin mimetics and incretin enhancers,
    for treatment of diabetes, 20
Insulin
  hepatic resistance, 8
  impaired secretion, 7–8
  resistance, 8–9, 250. *See also* Serum
    lipids, effects of antipsychotics
    definition, **2**
  sensitivity, 8, 225
  side effects, 17
  for treatment of diabetes, 17–18, **18**
  for treatment of metabolic syndrome,
    44
  weight gain and, 18
Insulin-dependent diabetes. *See* Type 1
    diabetes
Insulinopenia, 10–11
Interferon, in medication-associated
    weight gain, 174
Interleukins, in medication-associated
    weight gain, 174
Internal adipose tissue, definition, **57**

Joint National Committee on Prevention,
    Detection, Evaluation, and
    Treatment of High Blood Pressure,
    37, **38**, 44–45, 49
Juvenile-onset diabetes. *See* Type 1
    diabetes

Ketosis-prone diabetes, 11
Kuopio Ischemic Heart Disease Risk
    Factor Study, 33

LDL. *See* Low-density lipoprotein
    cholesterol
Leptin, in medication-associated weight
    gain, 172, 175
Lifestyle modification programs, 278
  for management of metabolic
    syndrome, 42–44, 47–48
  to prevent cardiac risk factors,
    146–147